PRACTISING SOCIAL WORK
IN A COMPLEX WORLD

... EDITION

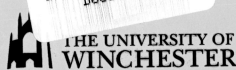

Co-edited titles by Robert Adams, Lena Dominelli and Malcolm Payne:

Social Work: Themes, Issues and Critical Debates, 3rd edn
Critical Practice in Social Work, 2nd edn
Reshaping Social Work Series (series editors)

Other titles by Robert Adams

Protests by Pupils; Empowerment, Schooling and the State
Prison Riots in Britain and the USA, 2nd edn*
Skilled Work with People
The Personal Social Services: Clients, Consumers or Citizens?
*Quality Social Work**
*The Abuses of Punishment**
*Social Policy for Social Work**
*Foundations of Health and Social Care**
Empowerment, Participation and Social Work, 4th edn*

Other titles by Lena Dominelli

Beyond Racial Divides: Ethnicities in Social Work (co-author)
*Feminist Social Work Theory and Practice**
Social Work: Theory and Practice for a Changing Profession
Women and Community Action
Revitalising Communities in a Globalising World
*Anti-Racist Social Work**
Introducing Social Work
*Anti-Oppressive Social Work Theory and Practice**
Revitalising Communities in a Globalising World

Other titles by Malcolm Payne

*Social Care Practice in Context**
Globalization and International Social Work: Postmodern Change and Challenge
    (co-author)
What is Professional Social Work?, 2nd edn
Modern Social Work Theory, 3rd edn*
*The Origins of Social Work: Continuity and Change**
Anti-bureaucratic Social Work
*Teamwork in Multiprofessional Care**
*Social Work and Community Care**
Linkages: Effective Networking in Social Care

* Also published by Palgrave Macmillan

EDITED BY ROBERT ADAMS
LENA DOMINELLI AND
MALCOLM PAYNE

PRACTISING SOCIAL WORK IN a COMPLEX WORLD

SECOND EDITION

palgrave
macmillan

First edition 2005, entitled *Social Work Futures: Crossing Boundaries,
Transforming Practice*
Reprinted twice
Second edition 2009

Published by
PALGRAVE MACMILLAN

Palgrave Macmillan in the UK is an imprint of Macmillan Publishers Limited,
registered in England, company number 785998, of Houndmills, Basingstoke,
Hampshire RG21 6XS.

Palgrave Macmillan in the US is a division of St Martin's Press LLC,
175 Fifth Avenue, New York, NY 10010.

Palgrave Macmillan is the global academic imprint of the above companies
and has companies and representatives throughout the world.

Palgrave® and Macmillan® are registered trademarks in the United States,
the United Kingdom, Europe and other countries.

ISBN-13: 978–0–230–21864–2
ISBN-10: 0–230–21864–4

This book is printed on paper suitable for recycling and made from fully
managed and sustained forest sources. Logging, pulping and manufacturing
processes are expected to conform to the environmental regulations of the
country of origin.

A catalogue record for this book is available from the British Library.

A catalog record for this book is available from the Library of Congress.

10 9 8 7 6 5 4 3 2 1
18 17 16 15 14 13 12 11 10 09

Printed in China

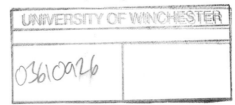

Contents

List of figures and tables

Notes on the contributors

Robert Adams worked in the penal system for several years before running a community-based social work project for Barnardo's. He has been an external examiner on qualifying social work programmes in the UK since the mid-1980s. He has written on and researched extensively in youth and criminal justice, social work, the personal social services, protest and empowerment. He has edited more than 80 books and written more than a dozen books. He was Professor of Human Services Development at the University of Lincoln and has been Professor of Social Work at the University of Teesside for more than a decade.

Sarah Banks is Professor in the School of Applied Social Sciences, Durham University, and co-editor of the journal, *Ethics and Social Welfare*. She has researched and published extensively in the field of professional ethics, particularly in relation to social, community and youth work.

Di Barnes is Research Fellow in the Centre for Applied Social and Community Studies at the University of Durham. Her recent research has focused on mental health policy and service evaluation and Di has a particular interest in advocacy.

Greta Bradley is Senior Lecturer in Social Work at the University of York, where she researches and teaches community care law and practice. Her current work is on sustainable social work with particular reference to supervision.

Viviene Cree is Professor and Head of Social Work at the University of Edinburgh. She has spent 16 years working in community work and social work, and another 16 years as an academic and researcher. Recent publications include *Becoming a Social Worker, Social Work: Voices from the Inside* (with Ann Davis) and *Social Work: Making a Difference* (with Steve Myers). She is co-editor of the international journal *Social Work Education* and joint series editor of the BASW/Policy Press series, 'Social Work in Practice', launched in 2008.

Lena Dominelli is Professor of Applied Social Sciences and Head of Social and Community and Youth Work at the University of Durham. She is an academician in the Academy of the Learned Societies for Social Sciences. From 1996 to 2004, she served as President of the International Association of Schools of Social Work. She is widely published, with a number of important sole-authored books to her name, particularly in the areas of feminism, anti-racism, globalisation and social policy.

Nick Frost is Professor of Social Work (children, childhood and families), Faculty of Health, Leeds Metropolitan University. This post is a partnership with Leeds Children's and Young Person's Social Care. He is co-author of *Developing Multi-professional Team-*

work for Integrated Children's Services and most recently of *Understanding Children's Social Care* (with Nigel Parton).

Helen Gorman has been a social worker, educator and researcher in health and social welfare. She has written publications on older people, community care, care management, social care law and continuing professional development. Her PhD research focused on skills development and adult learning. She has been a research supervisor for a number of years, and currently tutors students on MA and doctoral programmes for the Centre for Labour Market Studies at the University of Leicester.

Angela Grier is Senior Lecturer in the School of Social Sciences, Leeds Metropolitan University, where she teaches youth and community workers, social workers and students on a joint criminology degree, and is part of the team developing a new BA in criminology. Previously, she was a probation officer for nine years and a worker with Irish travelling families. She has co-authored several journal articles on aspects of criminal justice.

Debra Hayes is Senior Lecturer in the Department of Applied Community Studies at Manchester Metropolitan University. She has worked for the Greater Manchester Probation Service. Since her time at Manchester Metropolitan University, her research and writing has focused on immigration and asylum issues, and in particular their relationship to the delivery of welfare and the role of social work.

Stephen Hicks is Reader in Health and Social Care in the School of Community, Health Sciences and Social Care at the University of Salford. He is a founder member of the Northern Support Group for lesbian and gay foster carers and adopters, and is co-editor of *Lesbian and Gay Fostering and Adoption: Extraordinary Yet Ordinary*.

Beth Humphries is a social work academic and researcher. She has practised, taught and written about the profession for many years, and has worked in a number of universities in the UK. She has a particular interest in social research and its relationship to social justice. Her specialist research area is the implications for social work of increasingly draconian internal controls on immigrants and asylum seekers. Beth is currently Visiting Professor at Manchester Metropolitan University.

Glenys Jones is a social worker who has taught at the universities of Bangor, North Wales and Lancaster. She has extensive research experience focusing on policy and practice in the care of old people. She moved into local authority social service management, where the main focus of her work was service development and change. She was Director of Social Services in two north-east authorities. She was also Chair of the Association of Directors of Social Services older people's committee, and in this capacity worked in national forums on the change and development agendas leading to the White Paper *Our Health, Our Care, Our Say*.

Carol Lewis has many years' experience of teaching on qualifying programmes, as well as teaching research methods and supervising doctoral students as a Senior Lecturer in Social Work at Bournemouth University. Before this she spent many years in local authority children and families work, as practitioner and manager. She has contributed to the research strategy for social work developed by JUC SWEC (Joint Universities Council Social Work Education Committee). Her research interests include qualitative and emancipatory methods and also practitioner and service user engagement in research activities. She is an external examiner for two MA programmes in social work.

Mark Lymbery is Associate Professor of Social Work at the University of Nottingham. He has a long-standing interest in the development of interprofessional social work, with a particular emphasis on the needs of older people. He is the author of *Social Work with Older People*, the joint author of *Social Work: An Introduction to Contemporary Practice* and the joint editor of *Social Work: A Companion to Learning*.

Jill Manthorpe is Professor of Social Work at King's College, London and Director of the Social Care Workforce Research Unit. She has a background in teaching on social work and other professional training programmes. Her current research spans social work education, the development of individual budgets and adult safeguarding. Recent books include texts on psychosocial interventions in dementia care, older workers in Europe and depression in later life.

Fiona Measham has conducted research in the field of drugs and alcohol, gender, licensed leisure, historical and cultural criminology for 15 years, and has been a criminology lecturer at Lancaster University since 2000. She is co-author (and the lead researcher) of *Illegal Leisure* and *Dancing on Drugs*, based on two large-scale studies of young people's alcohol and drug use. Recent research includes a study on 'binge' drinking and bounded consumption, a historical analysis of the attempted criminalisation of English barmaids and ongoing research on the criminology of transgression and regulation of leisure.

Andy Millward was, until his retirement in November 2006, the Head of Business for Older People with Nottingham City Council's Adult Services, Housing and Health Department. One of his main professional and managerial interests over a long period has been in the field of collaborative working and partnership between social care and secondary and primary care.

Audrey Mullender is Principal of Ruskin College, Oxford and an elected academician of the Academy of Social Sciences. She is a past editor of the *British Journal of Social Work* and has herself published over a million words in the social work field, including 19 books. She has jointly authored studies of children's perspectives on living with domestic violence, women's voices in domestic violence services, groups for domestic violence perpetrators and mapping family support services in domestic violence across the UK.

Terence O'Sullivan is Senior Lecturer in Social Work at the University of Lincoln and author of *Decision Making in Social Work*.

Joan Orme is Professor of Social Work at the University of Glasgow. She has researched workload measurement from the perspective of trade unions and management and is firmly committed to the need to ensure that workload issues are considered as part of effective practice for the protection of service users and workers.

Ian Paylor is Senior Lecturer in Applied Social Science at Lancaster University. His teaching and research interests are in the field of substance use, youth justice and the 'art' of evaluation.

Malcolm Payne is Policy and Development Adviser at St Christopher's Hospice, London, having been Director of Psychosocial and Spiritual Care there for more than five years. He is Honorary Professor, Kingston University/St George's University of London, and was formerly Visiting Professor, Opole University, Poland and Professor at Manchester Metropolitan University. Recent publications include papers and research on aspects of palliative care, including *Creative Arts in Palliative Care* (edited with N. Hartley). He is author of *What is Professional Social Work?*, *Social Work Practice in Context* and *Modern Social Work Theory* (3rd edn).

Julia Phillipson is an independent social care consultant based in Wales. She undertakes a wide variety of project work including policy and practice development particularly in relation to social work education. Julia has always been involved with practice teaching and remains intrigued by the possibilities of supervision that she provides, assesses and teaches about.

Jackie Powell is Professor of Social Work Studies at the University of Southampton. She is a professionally qualified social worker who previously worked in several social and healthcare settings as practitioner and then 'contract researcher'. She has a longstanding commitment to facilitating older people's involvement in the research process and is active in the implementation of various capacity-building activities to promote research within both the academic and practice workplace.

Liz Sayce is Chief Executive of RADAR (Royal Association for Disability and Rehabilitation). Previously she was Director of Policy and Communications at the Disability Rights Commission and she also worked as Policy Director of Mind. She has published widely on mental health and disability rights.

Terry Thomas is Professor of Criminal Justice Studies in the School of Social Sciences, Leeds Metropolitan University. He was a former social services department social worker and team leader and is the author of *The Police and Social Workers*, *Privacy and Social Services* and *Sex Crime: Sex Offending and Society* and a co-author of *Policing Europe*.

Susan Wallace is the Education Programmes Manager in the Criminal Justice Social Work Development Centre for Scotland, located within Social Work at the University of Edinburgh. She is a qualified social worker and practice teacher. Her interests include assessment, report writing, risk and human rights.

List of abbreviations

ACMD   Advisory Council on the Misuse of Drugs
ASBO   antisocial behaviour order
ASSD   adult social services department
BASW   British Association of Social Work
CQC   Care Quality Commission
CSCI   Commission for Social Care Inspection
DCSF   Department for Children, Schools and Families
DDA   Disability Discrimination Act
DfES   Department for Education and Skills
DH   Department of Health
DTO   detention and training order
DTTO   drug treatment and testing order
DRC   Disability Rights Commission
DWP   Department for Work and Pensions
EBP   evidence-based practice
EHRC   Equality and Human Rights Commission
ESRC   Economic and Social Research Council
GP   general practitioner
GSCC   General Social Care Council
HRA   Human Rights Act
ISSP   intensive supervision and surveillance programme
IFSW   International Federation of Social Workers

JUC SWEC   Joint Universities Council Social Work Education Committee
LA   local authority
LGBT   lesbian, gay, bisexual and transgender
NAT   National Treatment Agency
NHSCCA NHS and Community Care Act
NICE   National Institute for Health and Clinical Excellence
PCT   primary care trust
PSR   pre-sentence report
QALY   quality adjusted life year
RAE   research assessment exercise
RCT   randomised controlled trial
SCIE   Social Care Institute for Excellence
SMC   Scottish Medicines Consortium
UN   United Nations
WHO   World Health Organization
YJB   Youth Justice Board for England and Wales
YOI   young offender institution
YOT   youth offending team

Introduction

What is this book about?

This book provides material for the later stages of the professional qualifying degree programme for social workers as well as for practitioners returning to study. Its theme throughout is the achievement of integrative practice. In pursuing this, it focuses on three aspects you will need to tackle in practice:

- Complexities in practice (Part 1)
- Management, leadership and change (Part 2)
- Research in practice (Part 3).

How does this book fit into our trilogy of social work books?

Practising Social Work in a Complex World, the third book of our trilogy (published in its first edition under the title *Social Work Futures*) takes forward the major tasks facing you in the later stages of your professional study programme – namely, integrating your understanding of themes, issues and debates in contemporary social work (examined in Book 1, Adams et al., 2009a) and the capacity to practise social work critically (dealt with in Book 2, Adams et al., 2009b) with more complex professional skills. What are these major tasks facing you now? They entail dealing with complex situations wisely and confidently in partnership with service users, their families, carers and communities (Part 1 of this book), and with other agencies and colleagues in other professions, and coming to grips with leadership and management roles adopted by others and by ourselves (Part 2 of this book) and developing the skills of researching (Part 3 of this book).

This is a summary of what we cover in the three books in the trilogy:

Book 1: *Social Work: Themes, Issues and Critical Debates*
This introduces the distinctive character of social work as a focus of practice and debate. It looks at social work processes, locates social work in its different contexts and begins to explore some of the lasting debates that arise about practice in different settings.

Book 2: *Critical Practice in Social Work*

This moves from exploring what practice entails in terms of professional values and methods to developing actual expertise in practice, as a critical practitioner.

Book 3: *Practising Social Work in a Complex World*

This tackles the more advanced tasks associated with integrative practice, which correspond with the challenges you will face in the later stages of your social work qualifying degree. Some of the assessment tasks will require you to integrate various aspects of what you are learning and practising – theories with practice being a commonly stated one. This book is designed to help you with this task.

Readers of previous editions of the three books in this series will find that the topics covered in each volume have changed to reflect feedback and our own judgement about the order in which particular topics should be introduced when readers use the books in sequence.

Every effort has been made to trace all the copyright holders but if any have been inadvertently overlooked the publishers will be pleased to make the necessary arrangements at the first opportunity.

Developing integrative practice

1

The further development of social work practice entails the practitioner coming to grips with four major aspects. We devote this introductory chapter to considering these:
- *The theme of integrative practice, which runs through this book*
- *How you tackle the complexities that arise as your practice develops*
- *How you engage with management and leadership tasks and roles in practice*
- *How you can develop research in your social work practice.*

Chapter overview

What does 'integrative' mean to us?

We begin by examining the word 'integrative', which, we suggest, will preoccupy you increasingly as you move to the later stages of your professional qualifying programme in social work. 'Integrated studies', 'integrated case studies', 'integrated practice' and 'integrated practice studies' are common features of the final stages of these programmes. However, it is wrong to write of practice as 'integrated' as though it is already finished. We prefer to use the term 'integrative' to indicate that the process of integrating is ongoing and possibly never completed. As long as we are still reflecting critically on our knowledge, understanding and practice, we are still working on its material, bringing our thoughts, emotions and experience together, connecting them with our actions in our practice. This is an integrative activity. So, as we near qualification, our social work becomes integrative for four reasons:

- An important aim of social work is integration, solidarity and connectedness within the societies where it operates
- An important social work role is to integrate, through coordination, collaboration, partnership and planning, a range of care services with the lives of the human beings it helps

- Social work aims to help clients, service users and carers achieve personal integrity in their social, family and community identity, to feel whole, valued, consistent and socially connected
- Social work values integrity in its workforce, that social workers deliver what they promise and are open and transparent in their dealings with the people they help, who are often much less powerful in society and in social care services than social worker are themselves.

These may seem ambitious aims, but they are obvious if we think about the opposites. We would not think much of a social work that aimed for a disjointed, aggressive society, disorganised services and social isolation and alienation among the people it helped and dishonesty and opacity in its workforce.

Being integrative in our practice involves 'imaginising'. This is not just being imaginative, although that helps; it is a word used in the organisational change literature, referring to creating a different image of what we are doing and what we understand. We can do this in a number of different ways:

- Bringing together ideas from practice and the literature and seeing where they fit and do not fit. If they do not fit, what needs to change? In might be some aspects of our practice or the literature, or perhaps we need to rethink our understanding of our practice or the literature. If they do fit, this might confirm our practice, or stimulate us to think how we can build on what seems to be agreed, or question the certainty that seems to be emerging. Are there uncertainties and complexities that we have not yet thought through?
- Bringing different aspects of our lives and our practice together in a person. We embody social work for the people we work with, service users, their families and carers and our colleagues in other professions. Our practice demonstrates what social work is to them. We seek to be genuine and act with integrity; therefore different and perhaps conflicting aspects of ourselves have to be incorporated into the professional person we present to clients and colleagues. For example, we recognised (Adams et al., 2009a) how the international definition of social work (IFSW, 2000) incorporated three elements of social work that are sometimes in tension or lead us in different directions towards social order, social transformation and therapeutic help for individuals and groups.
- We suggested above that integrative social work is by its nature incomplete; therefore we are always in the process of forging a new practice, and a new embodiment of ourselves. We are incomplete throughout our lives, so also are our clients and their families, so as a matter of principle, there is always opportunity for more satisfying and successful lives, however we or our clients define it.
- We have proposed throughout these books (Adams et al., 2009a, 2009b, 2009c) that solidarity, social cohesion and social resilience are an important objective of all social work practice. We seek to help someone, or a group or community in the hope that they will be able to contribute better to an improved society.

- There are barriers to solidarity, social cohesion and social resilience, and one of our aims is to help people overcome those barriers. These may be difficult relationships, poverty and social conflict, or the debilitating effects of social and economic inequalities.

- The values of social work, set out in its international definition (IFSW, 2000) and discussed elsewhere by us (Adams et al., 2009a, Ch. 1), include social justice, there-fore an awareness of and an attempt to respond to the social consequences of inequalities and oppression are a necessary part of our thinking as we help people.

- Individual and social empowerment is one of the ways in which we try to deal with the barriers to solidarity, social cohesion and resilience and promote social justice. Empowerment aims to give people the opportunities to understand and do some-thing about the social sources of the forces that affect their lives. This is important for people with little power or influence on the events shaping their lives, as the experience of being effective in solving one particular problem is a platform for increasing their confidence and feelings of self-worth and building the strengths and skills to achieve other objectives in their lives.

- All this contributes to bringing about a better society; they are small steps, they may be small-scale changes, but each individual achievement makes things better for the people involved in it and can strengthen them to take further steps.

How does research contribute to practice?

We adopt a particular focus on researching practice in Part 1 of this book. Throughout these books (Adams et al., 2009a, 2009b, 2009c), in various ways, authors have discussed the importance and the difficulties of the evidence base that social work relies on. We have suggested that critical reflection and critical commentary are part of research, because these techniques stimulate better practice by looking at it in new ways as we practise. If we can find new ways of practising, we can contribute to social improvement more effectively.

Therefore, it is important that we develop a sympathetic attitude to research in our own practice and contribute to other people doing the same. The development of research in practice can only be a collective activity, not an individual one. If we carry out a research study, for a dissertation or because we want to audit our practice, we will rely on others to test out our thinking and/or methods. Research activity depends on us and our colleagues being 'research minded' – the starting point of every piece of prac-tice is thinking about the most effective way of achieving our aims and those of our clients and their family (Adams et al., 2009a, Ch. 19). Partnership with social work and multiprofessional colleagues helps to develop the knowledge, and the skills in carrying out research will help us to become 'research capable'. These expressions, 'research minded' and 'research capable', tend to be used by managers outside practice. In Part 1 of this book, we examine how research knowledge and expertise equip the practitioner to ask questions about what counts as knowledge, critically reviewing the existing evidence base from previous research and developing a more informed practice. We also go through the different stages involved in researching practice.

If you see research as a project that leads to a report or a publication, it is tempting to say that you are too busy to do research, because it is not part of your core responsibilities. However, research is an essential component of your work as a critical practitioner, for the following reasons:

- You are researching all the time, finding out about people's lives and writing assessments, reports for courts and other professionals and reviewing your practice and the outcomes of your work in particular cases.
- As a practitioner, you are engaging constantly with service users' social experiences, so you are finding out about trends and changes in society and you need to think about how these changes should affect your practice.
- Research can help you to get outside the way everybody is thinking at the moment, the dominant paradigm, and offer a different way of viewing it; this may well benefit the people you are working with, users, carers and your colleagues.

It enables the critical practitioner to reflect heretically. Heresy may sound shocking, but it literally means considering a range of interpretations and approaches, some of which may not agree with taken-for-granted beliefs and standards. This is in recognition that some aspects of social work are contested and involve engaging with controversial opinions.

This approach to researching builds on what we have examined in *Critical Practice in Social Work* (Adams et al., 2009b). Your critical engagement with practice is made more creative and valuable because experiential evidence is valid and useful in different ways from accumulated evidence from research studies. The implications of the details of research findings for one particular service user and family must be disentangled from the wider implications for all people; nevertheless, achievement for one person contributes a knowledge and skill bank to help others.

A new practice comes from bringing different elements of knowledge and skill together, understanding their interaction in new ways. This is a chain reaction; one improvement leads to further developments.

EXaMPLE

Continuity – a continuing stream

The social worker is practising beyond merely caring and helping. The social worker is saying what needs to be said. But sometimes it will be rejected. It challenges.

It may involve challenging individual attitudes and patterns of relationships. It may involve challenging a social reality that is oppressive, for example racism in the neighbourhood or sexism or sexual exploitation in the family.

It will often be uncomfortable, even painful, at the time. In retrospect, it may be judged valuable.

Its 'utility' becomes apparent with hindsight.

What do we mean by complexity?

Part 2 tackles a number of different aspects of complexity in practice. While we recognise that complexity is not unique to social work, it is apparent that social workers deal with many of the more complex and intractable problems of people's lives. Chapter 2 deals with how the practitioner grapples with complexity. Complexity comes from the problems faced by clients, the people involved with them and the multiprofessional team working together with clients, their families and carers. It can suggest a number of meanings:

- The reforming of complex families after separation or divorce creates multiple families and multiple clients, carers and family members. There may also be several different agencies fielding several different professionals with differing legal and administrative responsibilities and financial systems to work by. An example is where an older person is receiving community care funding for a care package at home, has children from more than one family to be involved in decision-making, a GP, a district nurse and an Age Concern advocate.
- There are multiple problems, for example a mentally ill person may also have learning disabilities or misuse drugs.
- It is not only the quantity of problems that may contribute to the complexity; it may be that their interaction raises additional difficulties. For example, the complexity may come from the number of different professions involved because they have different models of care. A healthcare professional may see an individual whose illness should be the priority, while a social worker may see a family that needs to be held together. The law and ethics mean that only the doctor's patient can decide on their treatment, while family cohesion may mean that several family members should be involved in the discussion.
- The complexity is inherent in the difficulty of the problems. Many of the issues that social workers face are intractable. A mother with a mental illness may love her family and be loved by her children, but they may still be at risk from her instability.

Social work methods that derive from evidence-based research often produce a practice that seeks to simplify and focus practitioners' aims: a problem must be selected from the many and worked through to completion, then a further issue taken up. This adds to further complexity of the interaction of the research and situation that the practitioner faces. The imperatives of the service may make this a luxury.

◇◇◇◇ CaSE EXaMPLE ◇◇◇◇◇◇◇◇◇◇◇◇◇◇◇◇◇◇◇◇◇◇◇◇◇◇◇◇◇◇◇◇◇◇◇

Salman (76) is caring for Karima (74), his wife of 45 years, who is increasingly affected by dementia. The adult social services department (ASSD) offered the couple the opportunity to receive direct payments for the carers who come three times daily to provide physical care and meals for Karima. The couple could work with a local organisation for older people from minority ethnic groups, which would manage the budget for them and employ the carers, whom Salman would select. This would give them greater flexibility and control of Karima's care, and enable them to use the care to meet a wider range of needs. While it increases their freedom, it also puts more pressure and responsibility on the couple, and Salman is not sure he wants to accept this; he prefers having things organised for him. He would also rather that leading members in his minority community, who run the organisation, did not know about his private affairs. The ASSD makes this sugges-tion because the service would connect better with their faith and ethnic background and because government policy wants to shift provision towards more self-direction of services, partly because research has shown that, in general, service users prefer this and it also reduces the ASSD's workload. However, when this idea is put to Karima, she refuses, because she likes the (white) local woman who has been the main carer provided by the ASSD.

In this apparently simple situation of implementing a government policy designed to benefit the lives of service users, we can see many ambiguities in feelings, and in the reasons why decisions have been made and actions taken. In general, ethnically appro-priate service providers and service users usually welcome greater self-direction, but particular circumstances may lead to more complex and ambiguous reactions. The interests of service users, carers and agencies may conflict, rather than be mutually supportive. There is also a distinction between support and empowerment; not every-one feels that empowerment is supportive, just as not all support is empowering.

Complexity thinking

We may respond to these aspects of complexity by trying to reduce it, and this is often the route that policy and research takes, in order to reduce the number of variables. However, we reject this course; social work is the complexity profession, it seeks to take account of and respond to the complexities and ambiguities that people face in real life, and therefore we emphasise complexity thinking as the most appropriate course of action for a social worker to take.

Our practice develops complexity continually as we revisit and reflect critically on basic ideas we encountered earlier in our practice. This is an important and often under-estimated process, like rereading a beloved book or repeatedly listening to a significant piece of music. Revisiting ideas through reflection, critical thinking and doing enables us to re-evaluate them in the light of our developing practice and reading about practice, as our understanding of those ideas becomes deeper and more refined. It also allows us to test and change ideas about the situation that faces us throughout every moment of our practice.

Central to this book is the thought that practice means more than the work we do with service users, more than 'doing'. As we saw (Adams et al., 2009b), theories and values are embedded in all that we do and practice also entails reflection, reflexivity and being critical in and through action. These elements put what we do in wider context during our education but also continuously as we practise later in our careers. All this involves a complex combination of practical skills, knowledge, values, thoughts, feelings and actions.

'Practice' is a word that can mean doing, or rehearsing, as in the practice a musician or actor does before a performance. We argue that the social work practitioner engages in practice much as a musician performs. Each performance is unique. Practice, therefore, is a creative act of choosing in a planned way between myriad possibilities.

Doing is the visible, more obvious part of social work, but it is not irrelevant to or separate from the critical thinking, reflecting and evaluating that accompanies action. Often, practitioners accuse managers and college tutors of taking refuge in planning or theory at one remove from the 'coal face' of interaction with service users and practice situations. Academics equally complain that practitioners and managers follow procedures or assumptions without thinking critically about them. Managers say that practitioners and academics want to criticise everything in a negative way, when they have a duty to deliver a service according to legislation and public policy. We suggest that social work requires a concern for the complexity of the way all these things interact together: users, their needs and wishes; policy and public objectives; reflecting and evaluating; continuity and critique. The mutual criticisms made by different interest groups within social work imply alternatives. Therefore, to practise, manage or develop ideas and policy, we have to engage with those alternatives and find ways of thinking about our aims and how we can achieve them differently.

One way of thinking about alternatives is in 'dichotomies' – either/or decisions. Practitioners are often accused of doing too much or too little, intervening too readily in people's lives, or not intervening enough. They are criticised for making the wrong decision or being indecisive. The difficulties encountered by practitioners in balancing or mediating between these equally undesirable alternatives arise partly from the complexity of the situations with which they work. Practice often feels like choosing between unsatisfactory alternatives – if only there were more resources, or a more imaginative or supportive team. Casting the situation in dichotomous terms means missing the opportunities for helping people to progress their aims for a better quality of life contained within every piece of practice.

Complexity thinking presses us away from dichotomous thinking. It is against the oversimplified way of thinking that says: if we do this, we cannot do that; if we think this, we cannot think that. Instead, complexity thinking is *inclusive* thinking, holding within it the logic that enables us to hold competing claims and contradictions while looking for solutions. We look for alternatives and different sides of the situation and try to grasp them and integrate them into a discourse. Because the meanings that a social group give to events or actions are always constructed in a discourse, social meanings always include complex and competing elements, reflecting competing and shared interests in the situation – they are never one thing or the other. How we react to them and interact with others as they react to them provides opportunities for moving in different directions and opening up new possibilities.

EXAMPLE

A woman may come to see her male partner as abusive. She may then experience a dilemma: should she stay for the financial security that his household affords, or leave for her own safety? But she has children she is concerned about and so it is not just a matter of the violence affecting her, awful though that is. There is a possible risk of violence to the children of the relationship. If we include the children in the picture, other scenarios open up and these are likely to guide our reactions. The dominant discourse presents this as a choice between going or staying. But complexity thinking suggests that there are other alternatives and assists in thinking about more nuanced responses. These might include: going now, with the intention of negotiating a return on better conditions; staying now, but setting up arrangements to go to a safe place if violence returns; and going now with the aim of starting a new life elsewhere. The 'going/staying' discourse is limiting. Complexity thinking extends the gaze of the woman and the practitioner to highlight other opportunities for resolving the dilemma.

Thoughtfulness in practice

Critical reflection is central in practice, and we argue that it is indivisible from doing. One of the more obvious aspects of practice apart from the doing is the quality of thoughtfulness that should be the foundation for all our actions, including decisions. Thoughtfulness is, or should be, the six-sevenths of the iceberg of practice lying below the surface of visible actions.

Thoughtfulness is a quality inherent in all good practice. It invariably accompanies action, reflection, decision-making and evaluation. Thoughtfulness lies behind much care work, close to sensitivity and self-awareness. Is this quality of thoughtfulness inherent in us, or is it a skill we can acquire? It can be both. Some of us may be naturally more thoughtful, but we can all learn thoughtfulness. The everydayness of the word 'thoughtfulness' is not helpful, but, unfortunately, much of social work is like that. The basic ingredients of social work are described by words like 'caring', 'thoughtful', 'reflective', 'critical', 'decisive' – words used in everyday speech. In social work, they have an additional meaning – combining doing with thinking in complex ways.

EXaMPLE

An elderly person in a hospital bed is ready, according to the doctor, for discharge. She cannot go home: the social worker must find a bed in a nursing home quickly or the SSD may be charged the cost of her remaining in the hospital bed under the Community Care (Delayed Discharges) Act 2003. The social worker can explain this to her, discuss her preferences and the views of her family, and set about finding a bed that meets her wishes. This is 'doing'. But to be seen as 'thoughtful' involves talking through the strong feelings of loss and change that will be taking place for the woman and her family, including the possibility of never seeing a loved family home again, or having to sell it to pay nursing home costs. This is 'thoughtful', because the people involved will see it as sensitive. Although this does not deal with the structural constraints that other professional and policy objectives place before the practitioner, we argue that it is transformational because it allows the woman and her family the best possible chance of making the transfer with a sense of satisfaction and forward movement.

So being thoughtful is also doing, and a more complex doing than the actions required by social and agency policy. It is also transferable to other families who may come to appreciate the skill of social workers, and value the public services provided.

All this sounds complicated because complexity thinking includes different aspects of the situation, it means that we interact with complex realities instead of an oversimplified model of the situation. A further example will explain what is happening in reflexive critical reflection.

CaSE EXaMPLE

Ed, a young man being looked after by the local authority, is fascinated by fast cars and commits several offences of taking cars without the consent of the owners. His residential social worker spends time with him talking over the situations in which he steals cars: usually when he is with a group of friends, has been drinking and needs the car to get home. They discuss ways in which some of the factors can be removed: arranging transport in advance, drinking locally, drinking less, finding a different group of friends. Then, Ed takes a car and crashes it, under the influence of alcohol. The social worker meets him after he returns from A&E, and at the beginning of the interview feels himself getting angry. Ed is sullen and unresponsive, until the worker explodes when expressing concern about the risk that Ed might have been killed, and will now get into trouble. Ed shouts back that the worker is only concerned that there will be trouble for him because he did not keep Ed under control.

There are many things to reflect critically on in this situation. This incident has a history: both Ed and the worker are revisiting the past in the present angry incident, and changing the meaning of the past by what they are doing now. The worker finds he is emphasising their rational attempts at behavioural planning. Reflecting on his anger, he realises that it is not only about the failure of his attempt at treatment, but fear of Ed being injured or dying. At first the worker experiences shame at being angry, but reflection tells him that demonstrating his fear may get a more positive reaction from Ed. So when Ed emphasises the treatment aspect of the past, the worker's response is not first to reinforce the treatment (this is what behavioural models of practice would propose), but to emphasise his fear for Ed's safety. But reflection tells him that mixed in with his emotional reaction, the incident might reinforce the treatment, by emphasising to Ed the relationship between them. Therapy relies on relationships to work, as well as well-worked-out, rational treatment plans.

In the reflexiveness of this incident, complexity thinking identifies the discourse that is going on in the reflection. Discourses are one step away from the immediate thinking and reacting: they express the overall pattern of what is going on. It is about the personal interacting with the rational and professional. We see the worker first reacting with anger (the experience), reflecting on the experience and working out some complexities within it. He is standing outside the experience to reflect on it while it is going on – 'in-action', as Schön would say. But as soon as he does this, he gains understanding about the connection of the experience with the reflection: reflexively, one way of thinking changes the interpretation of the experience, so that it is not only about treatment but also about personal concern. The reflection on the experience changes the action. Instead of hiding his anger, the worker sees it not only as a reaction to the failure of the treatment but also as a demonstration of concern. This then allows him to reinterpret his action to incorporate both his insights: he sees how it can enhance his relationship and how this will enhance the treatment. By experiencing inside himself and reflecting also outside himself, he brings together many different aspects of the incident. In the future, this may cause him to reflect – 'on-action', as Schön would say – that he needs to judge personal reactions not only in terms of being non-professional, but also in terms of the value of demonstrating personal involvement.

Intervention implies crossing boundaries into people's private domains where they have different rights and oppressions. It may involve partnership work with people, users and their carers, multiprofessional colleagues and administrative and ancillary colleagues within social care agencies. Partnership working is essential to achieving the fundamental objective of social work: to increase the resilience of individuals, groups and communities in dealing with problems in their lives through solidarity and equality in society.

How do social workers engage with management and leadership?

Social workers are likely to directly encounter management and leadership issues in a great variety of circumstances, both directly and indirectly:

- Directly, newly qualified social workers are likely quite quickly to become involved in some tasks that require them to exercise leadership and management skills. Management and practice are not clearly separated functions in the organisation providing social work services for children, families and adults, and practice requires people to manage their own work and take on leadership and management roles within a group of colleagues working on particular cases.
- Indirectly, all social workers practise in organisations and teams where day-to-day work involves them coming into contact with management and leadership activities.
- Most organisations in which social workers practice have undergone rapid changes over the past generation.
- Organisations providing services have proliferated, as their provision has been distributed to many providing organisations and groups in the independent sector, both voluntary and private, and practitioners are involved in shared management tasks in many of these organisations; this also helps them to have influence on behalf of the people with whom they work.
- Managements of social work organisations have taken on more managerialist roles. 'Managerialism' is the term used to refer to views and policies of management as a controlling activity with a view to meeting organisational rather than professional goals.

Nevertheless, management focusing on the strategic and the organisational structures, processes, operations and culture remains fairly constant throughout the different settings where social work is practised. In such settings, leadership roles for staff may entail not only strategic activities but those concerned with bringing about change at different levels inside the organisation, and in the activities the organisation shares in work with others. Such joint working is a familiar area of practice for social workers.

The concern of management with strategic change gives social workers an opportunity, since much of their practice concerns bringing about change in individual, family and other group settings. Much of their practice also takes place in conjunction with others. As we have already noted, practitioners should be encouraged to develop practice that incorporates research. Bringing together these three tasks, therefore, is a primary responsibility of social workers:

- Good management
- Good research
- Good practice.

The notion of integrative practice applies at the interface with individual service users. The role of the practitioner may be to enable people to bring about change in their lives. This may be painful at the time. For example, in human relationships, it may be difficult at the time for people to take decisions, but afterwards they may look back and reach a balanced view. Both social workers and their agencies need to work at being equipped to help people with this and other painful experiences, afterwards integrating them into strategic thinking for the future. Therefore, the evidence of difficulties in local communities or the stress of excessive demands on social workers mean both an individual response from practitioners in the way they manage their work, but also an agency response in the way in which it manages its resources.

Conclusion

In this chapter, we have argued that social work needs to be integrative, to work constantly on achieving an integrated experience of the help provided to service users, to see service users as whole people within the context of a whole social environment. Integrative practice means thinking about how the social pressures of inequality and poverty and the social resilience of families and communities may be brought together. In practice and in management, this requires complexity thinking, because practitioners have to handle, that is, integrate, many complexities into their thinking and their doing. We also suggested that this means integrating thinking and doing, which in turn means that social work research and social work agencies have to provide the support and resources that enable complexity to be handled integratively.

Part 1

UNCERTAINTY AND COMPLEXITY IN PRACTICE

In Chapter 1, we began to engage with one of the core challenges of social work – the complexity of people's lives – and introduced the notion of social work as an integrative activity. Social work is concerned with helping and empowering people to manage the interface between their problems and vulnerabilities as individuals and their relationships with other people, groups and the community. There are many uncertainties in people's lives and these conditions can also affect commissioning and providing organisations and the practitioner.

This first part of the book considers the implications for practice of working with different aspects of complexity in conditions of uncertainty. Chapter 2 offers a general framework and discusses its application across the entire field of social work. We consider then how this impacts on key areas. Chapter 3 focuses on the problem of domestic violence as an aspect of anti-oppressive practice with deep-seated implications for all family members. Chapter 4 looks at work with children and families in relation to the themes of risk and protection. Chapter 5 examines some major issues arising in work with young offenders. Sexuality is explored in Chapter 6, and work with older people in Chapter 7. Chapter 8 covers work with disabled people and people with mental health problems, and Chapter 9 explores social work with asylum seekers. The part ends with Chapter 10, which examines work with people engaged in illicit drug use.

Encountering complexity and uncertainty

2

This chapter is about what it takes to move through the process of gaining expertise. As we learn through study and experience, we develop the capacity to work with more difficult and demanding cases. The complexities and uncertainties of these will challenge us to extend and work across boundaries, with an enhanced awareness of the connectedness of our practice and how we contextualise it. We should be able to practise reflexively, thereby maintaining our professional and personal development side by side.

Chapter overview

Starting points

This chapter considers the different components of your developing expertise as a critical practitioner, building on what we have written in the previous chapter and the first two books in this trilogy (Adams et al., 2009a, 2009b). Table 2.1 outlines the relevant topics we have considered earlier.

Table 2.1 Relevant topics considered elsewhere in this trilogy (Adams et al., 2009a, 2009b, 2009c)

Social Work: Themes, Issues and Critical Debates	
Chapter 1	The nature of social work The specialness of the 'social' in social work How social work differs from social care
Critical Practice in Social Work	
Chapter 7	Reflective practice Theories and approaches
Chapter 20	Developing critically reflective practice Perspectives on becoming critically reflective Expertise

Practising Social Work in a Complex World	
Chapter 1	Integrative practice
	Complexity thinking

Practice becomes more advanced as the level of uncertainty and complexity increases. We have referred to these words earlier but I want to delve further into their meaning now, because this is relevant to social work at a more advanced level, both pre- and post-qualification.

Understanding what we mean by uncertainty

There are three main types of uncertainty:

1   *Ontological uncertainty:* 'Ontology' refers to our beliefs and our being. It is relevant to consider that the qualifying social work course challenges not just our ignorance and requires us to learn 'things' and 'how to' knowledge, that is, skills, but also challenges our conception of who we are and what we believe in, that is, our values. So ontological uncertainty can present us with fundamental challenges, because it touches doubts, gaps in our understanding, incomplete tasks, debates on which we haven't a fixed view, and unresolved emotions. You are likely to feel uncertainty when you begin a new practice learning opportunity while on your qualifying course. As your qualifying programme moves towards its conclusion, there is no doubt that you will be placed in situations of greater uncertainty, in the sense that there are fewer guidelines on what to do. You will be undertaking a final placement and, eventually, moving into your first post as a qualified practitioner. Both situations present challenges. Most obviously, there is a need to come to grips with the culture of the organisation, its ways of working, procedures and personalities in the office.

2   *Epistemological uncertainty:* 'Epistemology' means the study of the nature of knowledge, the basis and assumptions for knowledge, and the validity and extent of knowledge. At first sight, this is self-contradictory. Surely knowledge, by definition, is what we know. However, constructionist, critical and postmodern perspectives on the social sciences (see a brief discussion of these in Adams et al., 2009b, Ch. 20) present the reality that what we take for granted as knowledge is, *according to social constructionism*, socially constructed, *from a critical perspective* contested and *from a postmodern perspective* multiple knowledges rather than one knowledge as 'the essential truth'. So epistemological uncertainty refers to situations where the situation faced by the practitioner is ambiguous, or even capable of more than two interpretations. This arises particularly in social work where the cases are complex, the problems they show up are unpredictable and the range of possible outcomes is not clear.

3   *Procedural uncertainty:* This is a feature of work in organisations faced by many practitioners, where a new setting is novel and strange to them. It is also the case that

staff in organisations providing services may face a multitude of practice hurdles, which arise because of the diversity and novelty of some of the cases.

Responding to uncertainties

We can see immediately different possible ways in which the agency, or the newcomer practitioner, may try to 'solve' the problems of uncertainty outlined above.

CaSE EXaMPLE

Reducing ontological uncertainty

Richard is in the final stages of his qualifying social work programme. He is in a practice learning setting in a project diverting young offenders from custody. Because of his background in the penal system, he wants to see the 'welfare' element of delving into the experiences and perceptions of the young people reduced and a short cut taken to facing them with the simple choice between restitution or restorative justice in the community and custodial punishment.

Richard has some learning to do. He is uncomfortable with his ontological uncertainty, but the way to resolve it isn't to cling to his 'obvious' prior assumptions and adopt a reductionist approach. He needs to seek out the ambiguities and multiple realities and meanings in the situations and perceptions of the young people with whom he is working. The realities of their lives may be untidy and full of inexplicable aspects. A tension exists between the inherent uncertainties involved in practice and the strategies adopted by organisations in managing them. One of the main strategies is to try to reduce uncertainties by 'playing safe', that is, by managing risks. Another is by creating various prescriptive formulae such as procedures, which practitioners have to follow in order to fulfil their responsibilities.

CaSE EXaMPLE

Reducing epistemological uncertainty

Varna is undertaking her final practice learning in a children and families team specialising in teenage pregnancy. She is frustrated by her team colleague with a background in school-based work, who wants to provide for all teenagers, regardless of circumstances, a sex education programme developed in an isolated rural community, irrespective of the different beliefs and cultures in this urban, mixed Asian, African-Caribbean and white community.

CaSE EXaMPLE

Reducing procedural uncertainty

Tara undertakes her final practice learning in a very busy team trying to cope with an influx of work arising from the arrival in the town of several thousand migrant workers and asylum seekers. Her team colleague Jim has convinced the team leader to instruct all team members to use the forms he has devised to be used in work with all cases, regardless of circumstances. His argument is that these will achieve three things:

1 they will identify aspects of risk in each case
2 they will be more efficient
3 they will be cost-effective.

Tara is resistant. Her argument is that the starting point in each case should be to use social work skills to find out four things:

1 the person's perception of their situation
2 their feelings about it
3 their views about what they want help with
4 what they expect and hope for as the outcome.

Clearly, the team colleague has a point and Tara has a serious point as well. We can highlight it by simplifying somewhat the real world into two main types of procedures:

- *Open procedures*: These are based on sequences of actions that amount merely to checklists and are relatively innocuous. They may be useful as reminders to the practitioner and as guides to ensure that the stages of the necessary interventions are carried out.
- *Closed procedures*: These are based on prior assumptions about the nature of the person's problems and their eligibility. They tend to restrict the territory of the practitioner and can weaken or undermine critical practice.

Tara is challenging the working culture of the team. She will be in a difficult position if the team leader insists she follows the procedures, in the face of her own judgement.

Understanding what we mean by complexity

Complexity arises through the accumulations of different kinds of factors that contribute to people's problems and vulnerability. These factors may be analysed according to their nature and characteristics. These characteristics include:

- *Intensity* – how 'dense' they are, how strong their effect is on the person's life.
- *Extensity* – their scale, how much of the person's life they affect, for example rela-

tionships with other people. Together these constitute the relationship between the amount and range (heterogeneity) of problems and the length of time (Ciuccarelli et al., 2008).

- *Connectedness* – with which other factors they link.
- *Intersectionality* – how the different factors interact to create and contribute, for example, to exclusion, discrimination and disempowerment. 'Intersectionality' refers to the capacity to engage with the ways in which complexity is constructed, notably objective constituents such as 'race', class and gender and sociocultural aspects such as divisions and hierarchies of power, which contribute to categories such as inclusion, exclusion, domination, subordination, enablement and vulnerability. Egeland and Gressgard (2007) point out that the concept of intersectionality requires that these categories are not simply added up (additive), but are constructed in mutually constructive and interactive ways. In other words, people's problems are likely to have consequences for them that do not just increase in seriousness arithmetically but geometrically. Thus, individuals and families experiencing stresses and problems on multiple dimensions are disproportionately vulnerable and likely to require unusually high levels of support and other services.
- *Contextuality* – what their relationship is to the different contexts of the person's life, for example housing, employment, health and the community.

How complexity contributes to more advanced practice

We have described aspects of complexity in Chapter 1. This is a significant aspect of the cases that require greater social work expertise, either late in the qualifying programme or post-qualification. Complexity is an integral feature of much social work and as practice develops, it becomes manifest in the ways summarised in Table 2.2.

Table 2.2 Components of complexity

Nature of the problem	Diversity Range Depth
Different roles required	Listener Counsellor Therapist Advocate Welfare rights adviser
Different grades of staff involved	Practitioner Coordinator Manager Mixed roles
Interprofessional arrangements	Specialist practitioner consulting Other practitioners Multidisciplinary team Multiprofessional team

Working in partnership with people	People who use services Carers Neighbourhood and community members Other individual professionals Other professional teams
Extending understanding and skills	Drawing on different 'knowledge' disciplines Drawing on different 'how to' knowledge, that is, practice skills
Boundary work	Extending boundaries of existing practice Crossing boundaries, that is, making connections Contextualising practice in relation to boundaries

The problems many people experience are not like illnesses that can be cured. We cannot 'solve' the situation of an abused or bereaved person, any more than we can make decisions which, in a conflict-torn family or other group, will satisfy everybody. Sometimes, service users, their carers, family and friends are in conflict and one person's solution is another person's nightmare.

Social work offers a distinct and, on occasions, unique view. By definition, social workers occupy boundary positions between people and diverse views of their situations and different choices about what they should do next.

The raw material of social work is people's everyday lives, from which none of us can detach ourselves. Practitioners unavoidably share the life course with people receiving services, including many of the problems involved in growing up and growing older. Of course, divisions and inequalities in society privilege some of us and protect us from poverty, discrimination and harm. Also, we can maintain boundaries between us, the worker, the professional, and us as the private person. From time to time, though, our thoughts and feelings are bound to 'leak' back and forth across these boundaries. We need to acknowledge the impact of this on our practice, as life events such as illness and bereavement affect us in our work with other people.

The complex difficulties of people's lives create the need to seek understanding from the different disciplines – areas of knowledge such as social policy, law, sociology, psychology, anthropology and 'how to' knowledge of practice skills – on which social workers draw in their practice. The most obvious is in settings where multiprofessional and multidisciplinary teams are involved. Social workers are not unique in this. Other practitioners in the health and social services, such as occupational therapists, health visitors, community physicians and nurses, in their work with social workers share many common perspectives on work with people. In such circumstances, boundaries between organisations, professions and disciplines may be crossed, or even shift.

Government policies emphasise the need for joined-up thinking. Organisational approaches such as systems perspectives have been adopted as one way forward. Others include lateral thinking, creative thinking, or what Morgan (1986) calls 'imaginisation', critical reflection and the contextualising of practice. There have been attempts to control, punish, eject and, more positively, train practitioners out of problems.

Understanding boundaries

In social work with children and families, social workers intervene in situations where families are divided by force of circumstances, such as exclusion or armed conflict leading to emigration of refugees or asylum seekers. More locally, when partners separate, for example, complex situations may arise involving contact between children and adults, especially where there is disagreement, violence or abuse between family members. Social work is intimately involved at these pressure points in people's lives. In the process, global, ethnic, cultural and religious boundaries all may be encountered.

In work with adults, social workers contribute to decisions involving health and social care practitioners about the care that people receive from a range of services, ranging across boundaries between residential, day and community care services.

Social workers do not have a monopoly over ideas about boundaries – they are embedded in all human affairs. Biologists, psychologists and sociologists rely on the notion of boundaries to distinguish between individuals, groups and communities, as well as to refer to commonalities and interactions. Boundaries do not always divide. They may clarify differences and encourage communication and joint activity. This is important, not least because social workers can exploit it to enable people to change their lives.

When we consider boundaries and the idea of separating one area of activity from another, we are also implicitly acknowledging the importance of connectedness and the idea of practitioners making connections across boundaries.

The image of 'boundary' is a rich one. In one's practice, it can exist physically or metaphorically, providing a support, a barrier or a bridge between disciplines, professions, organisations or domains of knowledge and skill. It can change through time; the learning practitioner practises within limits, or boundaries, whereas post-qualification, the boundaries shift or are crossed without restriction.

We may grumble about a boundary such as a fence denying us access to something we want. We may applaud a boundary we perceive as serving a useful function: distinguishing our territory, or serving as protection from threats to our health or safety. In part, our differing view may depend on which side of the boundary we are, how we construct its meaning and whether we are privileged or excluded by it. Some boundaries, such as legal and organisational limits, may seem clear-cut and less ambiguous in their meaning, but it is probably safe to assume that no boundary or limit will be agreeable to everybody. It is realistic to remain ambivalent towards most boundaries. This is more uncomfortable, since it means that we recognise their strengths as well as their weaknesses. It is a critical view, appreciating the complexity of the situation.

We sometimes view boundaries as a symbol of safety and personal or group security; at other times they may be an irritation, as we seek to cross them or tear them down. We most obviously encounter the notion of boundaries when working in organisations.

The fact that organisations have boundaries, yet at the same are interconnected, is an incontestable reality in situations where services have to be organised and delivered. Social work services are delivered through increasingly complex arrangements involving a growing diversity of providing organisations and agencies working together. Where do the ambiguities arise? Quite simply, working together – whether liaison, cooperation, coordination or collaboration – is not just complicated but problematic as well. Organisations and ways of organising can be both liberating and oppressive.

The implications for people – managers, practitioners, service users, carers and members of the general public – are complex and take some teasing out.

Sometimes, our boundary crossing affects not only our tasks, but our sense of who we are: our definition of ourselves as worker or service user becomes blurred, fragmented or contradicted by circumstances. Our experience as practitioners may contrast with what we feel when we become users of those same services. If we become a carer for a relative or spouse, in addition to our role as a practitioner in health and social care, we may have to manage tensions between our identity as practitioner and our identity as service user or carer.

In order to illustrate the interplay between boundary crossing, the complexity of situations and associated practice tensions and dilemmas, we shall use a case example.

CASE EXAMPLE

Kis, a man aged 65, has been married for more than 30 years to Kati, aged 59. Kis has suffered anxiety and depression and for many years has had a drink problem. Kati finds it increasingly difficult to cope with Kis, but is unwilling to consider alternatives that would give her respite. She leaves the house only for short periods, for essential shopping. Kati and Kis were refugees from Eastern Europe and, although having lived in England for many years, have a limited command of English. This makes Kati less confident when dealing with health and social services agencies.

The couple come to the notice of social services when Kis has a fall and Kati goes to the local social services department to ask if she can borrow a wheelchair. The duty officer recognises the complexity of the situation. She invites Kati to talk to a female social worker, Mari, from a similar ethnic background. Mari is able to appreciate the extent of Kati's problems because Mari's mother, who has suffered from dementia for several years, has just been admitted to a nursing home. Mari is faced privately with the decision about whether to sign the consent form for her mother to have a potentially life-saving, but also risky and life-threatening, operation. Shortly afterwards, Mari and a community nurse from the community-based, multidisciplinary mental healthcare of older people team visit Kati and Kis at home. Their needs are assessed, with their full participation. As a result, respite care is organised for Kis, who is admitted to a hospital ward, linked with a day centre.

This summarised case example illustrates the complexities of situations that may face social workers. It is instructive to try to identify as many types of boundaries as possible, recognising that different people will perceive them differently and a comprehensive list is probably unattainable. However, the list in Table 2.3 makes a start.

Table 2.3 Types of boundaries

Global and ethnic boundaries	The multidisciplinary team takes responsibility for allocating a multi-lingual social worker to work with Kis and Kati, as a way of crossing ethnic boundaries between agency service providers, service users and carers
Boundaries of language	Mari, the social worker, is aware of the language boundaries preventing Kis and Kati having full enough access to other people, services, groups and communities. She takes responsibility for facilitating communication across these boundaries
Boundaries of culture and religion	Mari, who is from a Muslim background, is aware of religious and cultural differences between her and Kis and Kati, who are Christians
Community, group and family boundaries	In the multiethnic, multifaith locality in which Kis and Kati live, they are aware of different kinds of boundaries between them and other families, groups and communities
Individual boundaries	It is not uncommon for some practitioners, like Mari, to be juggling multiple roles, across the boundaries between their personal and professional lives, between their responsibilities as workers and their personal circumstances as carers or, less commonly, service users
Organisational boundaries	Mari, as the social worker, has to engage with a range of organisations outside her own employing agency, including the local hospital, primary healthcare team, residential home and day centre, quite apart from visiting different practitioners in their work settings in the NHS trust. Any decisions taken by social workers in multiprofessional or multidisciplinary teams to involve Kis and Kati in particular ways in the assessment, planning, implementation and review of the work done with them will affect the work of other practitioners with them, such as community nurses and occupational therapists
Professional boundaries	Mari's collaboration with different professionals such as occupational therapists and community nurses necessitates interaction back and forth across boundaries between differing professional values, approaches, methods and skills
Disciplinary boundaries	A clinical psychologist working with the community care team has a very different perspective on the family to that of the social worker. Mari works with the psychologist, although the disciplines informing their practice are different. The disciplinary boundaries between the psychologist and the social worker are maintained, but they collaborate across them

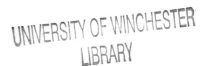

Self-critical practice: the need for self-critical reflection

There is a need for Mari to maintain a self-critical approach to her own work. This involves her using reflexivity, as she identifies her own emotions and harnesses them in her struggle to achieve self-criticality. She needs to develop self-criticality as a way of examining her practice critically and not simply evaluating what has happened, as though this is independent of her and other practitioners. All the practitioners involved could ask many questions. Three key questions encourage this process of critical reflection:

1   What have I learnt from this piece of work?
2   In what ways could the situation have worked out better for Kati and Kis?
3   In what ways could I have practised differently so as to achieve these better outcomes?

Delving further into the ambiguities of boundaries

The concept of boundary is value laden, ambiguous and multifaceted. According to Walsh (2000: 107), in his study of nursing practice, boundaries are 'lines of demarcation that help us make sense of the world by separating entities such as territory, occupations or objects from one another'. This statement clarifies one aspect of boundaries, their function as organisational and professional lines of division.

Consequently, one group of managers and practitioners may regard professional and organisational boundaries as needing to be crossed to improve the coordination and integration of services. On the positive side, Walsh notes that interprofessional boundaries help people receiving services to distinguish between different practitioners and enable professionals to know what roles the different practitioners are performing. However, Walsh (2000: 107) reminds us that professional boundaries may become positions to defend, in which case they become negative and harmful to people receiving services, as different professions spend time in conflict with each other rather than fighting ill health and disease. Morgan (1986: 170) describes how individuals, groups and departments in another setting may regard it as necessary to work defensively to maintain boundaries around their practice. In this way, they may hope to avoid the threats they perceive to their autonomy, maintain their independence and defend their existing ways of working.

Staff in group care settings work as multidisciplinary teams. They work in partnership with individuals, their carers, families, social workers, health and education services. The roles of the workers span key worker, supporter, carer in one-to-one work with service users and carers, involvement in teamwork, groupwork and advocacy and in work with other professionals and agencies. This is a powerful illustration of the ability of some formerly residentially based organisations to reframe their work by recasting boundaries between the institution and associated community networks. It is all too easy for organisations to function as though the organisationally based group is at the 'core' of practice and external groups are at the 'periphery'. This may be part of the reason why vulnerable individuals and groups continue to be marginalised and excluded. Continual vigilance is needed to prevent this happening.

Shifts in policies and practices concerning disabled people need to be appreciated in their wider social and political context. Brigham (2000: 27–42) discusses how, in the late nineteenth and early twentieth centuries, people with learning disabilities came to be regarded as a threat. Women were targeted by policies directed at controlling their sexuality, restricting their fecundity and curbing their alleged immorality. In the process, boundaries between public and private domains, social classes, 'races', men and women and normality and abnormality have been redrawn. These changes have taken place in the context of changing attitudes to the public and private spheres of society and the production and consumption of goods (Hirschman, 1998: 13–17). Boundaries exist between public and private, inclusion and exclusion, selfishness and selflessness, individualism and the collective, the personal and the social, possessions and shared ownership, trespassing and migration.

While boundary crossing may be associated with positive or negative ideas, often social policy has made it difficult for refugees, asylum seekers, travellers and others dispossessed and seeking new opportunities to migrate.

In all these areas, the question is how far it is possible for social workers to assert and advocate on behalf of excluded individuals and groups, when social work's boundaries are being configured and reconfigured. In other words, social work is part of the wider context of health, welfare and other services and issues concerning how practitioners respond are linked with legal, policy, organisational and managerial decisions about how responsibilities are assigned to different professional groups.

Tackling practice tensions and complexities

We consider now the issues raised by the case of Kis and Kati. There are four main tensions:

1   The work needs to be done by the social worker and other members of the team, with the full involvement of Kis the service user and Kati his carer. Nevertheless, the more the social worker involves them, the more this creates expectations that other members of the multidisciplinary team will need to match.

2   There is a need to balance risks against quality of life. There is a risk that if Kis continues to live at home, he will be less inconvenienced but will suffer a quicker deterioration in his health. On the narrow criterion of reducing risks, he would be safer in a residential setting. On the other hand, if he stays at home, perhaps his quality of life will be sustained for longer. There is no 'answer' to this. It depends on one's vantage point.

3   From Kati's point of view, she experiences relief that Kis is in hospital, but also mourns his absence. The uncertainties are inherent in the complexities of everyday life that many people encounter, and from which Mari as a social worker cannot be

exempt. Mari has to manage the tensions between her work as a practitioner and her identity as a carer.

4   There is a tension between Mari's aim as a carer to enable her mother to remain as independent as possible and the priority to manage her situation so as to minimise risk. Practice is not about assessing a case and finding the technical means to 'solve' problem situations. There may be no 'solution'. Whichever decision is made, there may be gains and losses for the different people involved.

Tackling complexities

The complexities are made more manifest because there are no easy or straightforward ways to a solution for any of the three main people involved. Kati is in a double-bind. She wants to continue to care for Kis at home but she wants him to be treated successfully and his condition to improve. Kis is in a dilemma. He wants relief from his long-term depression and finds his drink problem debilitating, but does not want to go through the stressful and painful process of treatment. Mari faces a dilemma. Should she sign the form giving permission for her mother to have the operation and run the risk of her dying during the operation, or do nothing in the knowledge that without the operation her mother will die within a short time?

Moving practice forward

What ways forward exist that will offer prospects of tackling, or at least managing, the kinds of practice tensions and dilemmas faced by Kis, Kati and Mari? On one hand, it seems uncontroversial that social workers should establish clear boundaries around their practice. On the other hand, there are many circumstances in which social workers should practise more effectively with others, across professional and organisational boundaries. Surely boundaries are clear, whether as markers around organisational territories, activities, roles or meanings, or as ways of demarcating and defending best practice. The closer we examine these ideas, the easier it is to dispel illusions of simplicity and certainty around the ideas of boundaries and boundary crossing. We need to explore how these difficulties are manifested in social work and how practitioners may be better equipped to tackle them. The goal is to help us to deconstruct the idea of boundary crossing and enable a more constructive engagement with the meaning of boundaries in our practice.

Contemporary policies aspire towards seamless services, so as to meet people's complex psychological, medical, emotional and social needs in a coordinated way. This implies that a range of health and social services managers, professionals and practitioners work together. Cable (2002: 2–3) points out how policy in the UK since the mid-1980s has converged with publications by the World Health Organization. In 1973, a WHO committee asserted that benefits, in terms of increased job satisfaction as well as more effective, holistic care, would result from greater interprofessional integration of healthcare services (WHO, 1973). In 1979, the WHO supported the need for an emphasis on the distinct organisation of primary, secondary and tertiary health and social care services (WHO, 1979) and a decade later argued for improved interdisciplinary teamwork in the interests of the holistic care of people (WHO, 1988).

Health and social care policy in the UK since the late 1980s, based on the Griffiths Report (DHSS, 1988) and enacted in the National Health Service and Community Care Act 1990, reflected this consistent emphasis on improving coordination between, and integration of, health and social care services. Cable (2002: 5) argues that these aspirations have not led to 'the development of clear and coordinated policy in relation to either global directives or local need'. He refers to a catalogue of potential conflicts:

- care versus cure
- central control versus local control
- bureaucracies versus collegiate structures
- managerial versus professional dominance
- public versus private funding of services
- the integration versus the separation of particular health and social care services, professions and practices.

In order to tackle these intractable problems, it is vital that all employees and volunteers in all participating organisations take responsibility for their work, across organisational boundaries. It is also vital that the agencies set up a partnership agreement in which all participants are accountable for the service. This involves sharing tasks and taking responsibility for managing and delivering the service.

Let us revisit the case of Kis and Kati for a view about how Mari the social worker may use the ideas of boundary crossing in developing positive practice.

◇◇◇ CASE EXAMPLE (cont'd) ◇◇◇◇◇◇◇◇◇◇◇◇◇◇◇◇◇◇◇◇◇◇◇◇◇◇◇

The situation improves. The social worker contributes to a multidisciplinary community care assessment of Kis's circumstances. Kis's anxiety and depression begin to ease. The team agree to a discharge plan following a discharge care plan approach meeting, attended by Mari, ward staff including the ward manager and psychiatrist and nurses, as well as staff from the day hospital, following guidelines for discharge planning and aftercare. As part of this, it is recommended that Kis spends alternate nights at home. Three weeks later, he is discharged from the ward. The social worker sets up an arrangement with the GP, community nurse and pharmacist in the local primary care unit that Kis's medication will be monitored to ensure that he continues to take it. The social worker also contacts a local voluntary organisation offering visitors to older people with drink problems. A volunteer begins to visit Kis and Kati regularly, to act as a bridge between them and the services they need and empower them to deal with their difficulties.

This example shows how Mari, the social worker, works effectively within and across the following kinds of boundaries:

- aiming to provide a seamless service, to enable carers and people using services to cope better, achieve change and improve their life chances
- providing continuity of services as service users and carers move between hospital, community and continuing care day and residential settings
- providing multidisciplinary assessments, reassessments and reviews
- working with individuals, families, groups and communities.

Let us reflect on some wider lessons raised by this boundary crossing case, under three main headings of identifying potential boundary crossers, networking and developing skills.

Identifying people with potential as boundary crossers

Sometimes boundaries are crossed, sometimes they are blurred, shift or disappear. There are unavoidable contradictions and dilemmas for practitioners. In order to tackle these, social workers need to draw on critical perspectives on geographical, conceptual, value-based, organisational, disciplinary and professional boundaries between different areas.

It is necessary to identify reticulists, both agency staff and volunteers, with the ability to facilitate interagency working. (Reticulists are people with responsibilities and skills in bridging organisational and professional boundaries.) In some circumstances, working across boundaries is essential to achieving the particular goals that are desirable for people receiving services. Evidence suggests that it is difficult to impose boundary crossing from above on the organisation or team (Lart, 1997).

Rule-following may be customary, accompanied by the beliefs and assumptions that support this (Morgan, 1986: 128–30). Significant change in established ways of practising and thinking is necessary. Any change is likely to require unlearning and relearning. Lart (1997) evaluated the Wessex Project, which introduced planned discharge for prisoners with mental health needs, using the care programme approach where appropriate. The project began in a context where no other agency saw this area of work as their particular responsibility. Lart examined the vital sharing of tasks and responsibilities in the multi-agency team, and the key role played by reticulists, in situations where crossing professional boundaries is essential to the continuance of day-to-day practice.

Networking

The failure of welfare policies to meet the needs and wants of the people who should receive services is, in part, a failure of organisation and service delivery. Schön (1971) developed the analysis that transformations are needed in the model of government responses to these failures. Schön (1971) argues that it is fine for policy makers to govern change from the centre, but power needs exercising by people at the 'periphery', where services are actually delivered, to ensure that they meet needs. The complexity and variety of local needs contradict the requirement for uniformity at the centre, where general policy is formulated and administered. Even regionally and locally, formal bureaucracies managing services, to the extent that they replicate this 'centre-periphery' model, impose restrictions and control, rather than abolishing need, acknowledging diversity and ensuring justice. Schön (1971: 189) states: 'The need is for differentiated, responsive, continually changing but connected reaction.' His argument is for mechanisms encouraging systems at the local periphery to transform themselves and connect with each other. This depends on two contributions: from leaders and through networks. If informal networks are strong, they support a nuclei of leadership and local arrangements hold together without any necessary central direction or support for the transformations (Schön, 1971: 189–90). While formal networks exist to serve the management of an organisation – purchasing, processing, advertising and delivering – Schön is writing of informal networks here. These, he states, are

> the informal or 'underground' networks connecting persons, groups and organisations. These are used to circumvent, supplement or replace the operations of formal organisational systems. (Schön, 1971: 191)

Such networks are often ad hoc, remedying shortcomings between the large providers of services and local problems that people perceive as requiring services. These networks may have a short life or, if poor conditions persist, may acquire permanency. Schön (1971: 192) instances poor, black communities where informal networks of so-called 'nannies' look after young and sick people. He coins the term 'shadow network', to refer to the informal arrangement 'filling the gap between fragmented services and a more highly aggregated functional system' (Schön, 1971: 195).

Other writers have emphasised the key contribution of workers, not all senior line managers or even employed staff, as crossers of boundaries and networkers. Sarason and Lorentz (1998), in their study of the informal mobilisation of support for schools in the US, identify people with a flair for boundary crossing as the key to more effective coordination. They argue that these people may not be staff occupying senior positions. They may not be employed by the organisation, but may work in the community, occupying key positions in networks and maintaining significant relationships. Sarason and Lorentz discuss the need for recognition of the essential, although usually informal, contribution of the coordinator. They view coordination and drawing people together as taking place not in formal organisations and meetings, but in the neighbourhood, communities and informal networks. Much of their book is taken up with examining the five elements they regard as essential if this is to be successful:

1 Regarding, and drawing on, people as resources
2 Recognising obstacles to redefining resources
3 Accepting the unique contribution of networks and networking to making the most of resources
4 Building on the particular character and role of coordination through networks

5   Identifying how resource exchange energises and reinforces collegiality and a sense of community (Sarason and Lorentz, 1998).

Developing skills

We can recognise many social work qualities and skills in the four aspects of the role of the coordinator identified by Sarason and Lorentz (1998: 95):

1   Developing a real, authentic knowledge of the territory, through 'curiosity' rather than through knowledge passively obtained
2   Scanning with fluidity, that is, seeking commonalities and easily and speedily recognising them, and imaginativeness
3   Perceiving assets and building on strengths
4   Using power and influence as well as selflessness.

We can go further than this in identifying the kinds of skills that social workers need, in order to use and work within, as well as transcend, boundaries in their practice. According to Sarason and Lorentz (1998: 115), coordinators possess a constructive way of thinking, that is, the ability to avoid focusing on people's deficits and see opportunities for connecting between people and organisations that to others may seem entirely separate. This enables them to contribute effectively to a range of partnerships in their work with others. In order to flourish, these partnerships need to:

- Be flexible and able to make use of new and unexpected opportunities
- Be open-ended, so they produce benefits now and in the longer term
- Go beyond simple mechanistic arrangements where services are provided in exchange for information from the service user, and become true collaboration where the participants create genuine 'added value'
- Be dependent not solely on line management in the organisation but also supported by local networks and interpersonal relationships.

All these research findings should encourage us not just to replicate existing practice but to develop a transformational practice. We can show how this could work by inventing an agency and speculating first on a worst-case scenario and then on a best-case scenario where practitioners are motivated and are given the scope and power to tackle problems creatively.

CaSE EXaMPLE

Transforming practice

Prime Serve is a fictitious not-for-profit organisation contracted to provide community care for adults in Midshire. Among other activities, Prime Serve employs staff to coordinate a large number of volunteers working with multi-disciplinary staff in different local agencies.

Several problems have arisen among agencies in partnership with Prime Serve. A number of meetings have been held to examine these. All these meetings have agreed that improvements are necessary, but so far little progress has been achieved. The reasons for this are not clear to the staff involved. An already long list of possible reasons has been added to at each meeting.

In the worst-case scenario, procedures may dominate. Care managers in the local authority are clear about the problems. A senior manager produces an organisation chart to demonstrate that the problems lie 'out there', are not his responsibility and he cannot be held accountable for them. The organisation chart view of the situation prevails. The job descriptions of staff state that they carry out the procedures prescribed and do not go beyond these. They are taken as forbidding staff to cross boundaries, or only cross those authorised by management. Boundary crossing in other areas, such as networking, is perceived as a threat.

Now let us consider the transformational, best-case scenario. In this, a consultant or practitioner colleague advises the agencies on how to surmount the difficulties that have arisen. The consultant discusses the issues with staff in the agencies and the volunteers working for Prime Serve. The consultant suggests a series of informal dialogues and informal and formal meetings between the people working for local agencies and Prime Serve, to examine how to improve collaborative working. Staff are empowered to use their initiative to go beyond the boundaries of their job descriptions, the role of their employing organisation, to seek and tackle problems they identify, recruit local workers and through them promote networks to maintain improvements in services. Reframing what practitioners are coordinating is not considered 'out there', and is brought within the scope of the practitioner. This may involve disengaging with embedded perceptions and practices and being willing to embrace new practice. This is an intrinsically anti-oppressive, equality-driven, non-stigmatising, person-valuing process. It involves non-directed, flexible, imaginative interaction, such as networking, which fosters interdependence. It necessitates that managers and practitioners grasp how boundary crossing works, formally and informally, at different levels and in different sectors.

Conclusion

Critical practice develops by engaging with uncertainty and complexity, as encountered in each particular case. Through this engagement, we encounter the notion of boundaries. It is common to write of boundaries as though they are mainly organisational and managerial, but there are many different kinds. In particular, social work straddles boundaries between geographical, religious, ethnic and cultural, value and disciplinary divides. In many ways, social workers occupy unique positions in complex situations, where other practitioners work within a designated professional territory and social workers draw on a variety of disciplines and have the capacity to work across many different kinds of boundaries.

Whether social workers positively regard boundary crossing and the associated challenges posed depends on the extent to which they are committed to developing beyond procedurally bound practice and seek to change practice significantly. Boundary crossing may be more creative, but is more demanding. It requires more commitment to work with all parties towards outcomes that aspire to empower service users and carers, but en route may be more stressful and resource consuming.

Practitioners setting out to meet the diversity and full extent of people's needs can use notions of boundary crossing to engage in work that is more capable of being transformational. The rest of the chapters in Part 1 of this book illustrate the major practice challenges of social work that engage with the complexities of achieving this.

For further discussion of criticality, see Adams et al., 2009b, Chapter 1, and for becoming critical, see Adams et al., 2009b, Chapter 21.

Banks, S. (2001) *Ethics and Values in Social Work*, 2nd edn, Basingstoke, Palgrave – now Palgrave Macmillan. Good source of discussion on practice involving ethical dilemmas.

Payne, M. (2000) *Teamwork in Multiprofessional Care*, Basingstoke, Palgrave – now Palgrave Macmillan. Rich on aspects of boundaries and boundary crossing.

Sullivan, H. and Skelcher, C. (2002) *Working Across Boundaries: Collaboration in Public Services*, Basingstoke, Palgrave – now Palgrave Macmillan. Source of much material on aspects of joint working.

Persistent oppressions: the example of domestic violence

3

This chapter critically examines social work responses to domestic violence, acknowledging in the process its somewhat problematic and consequently neglected situation. It discusses important questions that should be raised from the distinct but related viewpoints of women, children and men.

Chapter overview

Social work has been slow in accepting domestic violence as within its legitimate sphere of interest. At one time, the typical response was to reject domestic violence as 'not a statutory responsibility'. The shift in attitude came when a link was established between the abuse of women and the safety and wellbeing of children (Mullender et al., 2002). This made the issue 'core business' for social services departments, but has tended to result in a narrow focus on domestic violence as a child protection concern, rather than a recognition that social work skills have a great deal to offer to all the parties involved. These encompass emotional support and practical assistance for abused women, direct work with children who are recovering from living with domestic violence and tackling violent men's behaviour.

This chapter will explore these domains of practice from a critical perspective, raising the following issues:

Regarding women:
■ Why do women feel unable to tell their stories to social workers?
■ What could social work offer women that would actually help them to be safe and improve their quality of life?

Regarding children:
■ Why is practice not child centred?
■ Could models of direct work with children be more widely adopted that focus on safety planning and recovery from distress and upheaval?

Regarding men:
- 'What works' with men?
- Is there room for social work skills in preprogrammed cognitive behavioural intervention?

This chapter will conclude by highlighting how the skills of social groupwork could be particularly helpful in challenging the behaviour of violent men and helping women and children to move forward with their lives. In respect of all three areas of intervention – with women, children and men – what will be revealed is that social work holds many of the answers to domestic violence, particularly through the use of groupwork. First, however, to explain the title of the chapter, we will turn to a brief consideration of the persistence of domestic violence over time and across cultural and socioeconomic groupings.

The persistence of domestic violence

Domestic violence will be understood here as typically combining physical, sexual and emotional abuse and intimidation and, characteristically, as the misuse of power and the exercise of control by one partner over the other in an intimate relationship (see www.womensaid.org.uk). It is predominantly perpetrated by men against women (across all ethnic and socioeconomic groupings), sometimes the other way round, and also occurs in same-sex couples, who may find it even more difficult to obtain help owing to homophobic attitudes and heterosexist assumptions. Disabled women may be particularly vulnerable to abuse, for example when their abuser is also their carer. Domestic violence also forms one aspect of elder abuse.

Although there has never been a national prevalence study of domestic violence in the UK, a well-conducted and generalisable local survey found that 1 in 3 women in a random household survey in north London admitted to having experienced, at some point in their lives, violence in an intimate relationship worse than being grabbed, pushed or shaken, with similar rates across all social and ethnic groupings (Mooney, 2000). These figures indicate that domestic violence is endemic right across society. Turning to incidence, when women are asked about events in the 12-month period prior to interview, figures are remarkably consistent, with 12 per cent in the Mooney study having been victims during that period and 13 per cent in the British Crime Survey reporting at least one incident of violence in the past year (Walby and Allen, 2004). More than half of all incidents of rape and serious sexual assault are perpetrated by a current or former male partner (Walby and Allen, 2004, based on the confidential self-report in the British Crime Survey) and, in 2001, of the 125 victims of domestic killings in England and Wales, more than 4 out of 5 (82 per cent) were women. Even where women are not killed, their health (BMA, 2007) and mental health (Humphreys and Thiara, 2003) often suffer significantly.

The proportions of disabled women who have experienced abuse may be higher still (Hague et al., 2008). In the home, if her partner is also her carer, the woman's dependency may trap her in the abuse, as may the daunting prospect of reconstructing a complex care package elsewhere. Her disability may also be used against her if her abuser restricts her mobility, her outings or her access to medication.

The predominant pattern across society is one of men's violence towards women (Hague and Malos, 2005). Although women can certainly be violent towards men, it is important to recognise that this is often in self-defence and that women are far more likely to be frightened, injured and badly hurt than men, with attempted strangulation and forced sex almost entirely male-on-female phenomena (Walby and Allen, 2004). There is also abuse in some same-sex relationships, between lesbians and between gay men, and obtaining help may be more difficult because of negative attitudes in the wider society (www.broken-rainbow.org.uk).

Abusers trade on the fact that men were traditionally not only expected but required to keep women in order in the household, with the issue still emerging from being a butt of humour into construction as a potentially resolvable social problem. The turning point in the UK came around 1990, when police policy shifted to regarding a domestic assault as a crime like any other, and men as responsible for their own abusive behaviour (see Morley and Mullender, 1994, for a historical summary). More recently, the Protection from Harassment Act 1997 has allowed intervention in situations where more subtle methods are used to sustain intimidation but, overall, it remains difficult to secure effective legal remedy against domestic violence (Hester, 2005).

The failure to offer women effective help

Women are the experts in their own issue (Hague et al., 2003). They report that, even though domestic violence is now on the sociopolitical agenda as never before, assistance remains patchy and often accompanied by judgemental and woman-blaming attitudes (Mullender and Hague, 2000). Too little has changed since women in the classic studies (for example Dobash et al., 1985) spoke of trying one agency after another and encountering constant obstacles and delays. Homophobia and inaccessible services (Hague et al., 2008) make the situation worse for lesbian and disabled women, while institutional racism has also been identified in domestic violence responses from statutory agencies (Mama, 1996; Rai and Thiara, 1997). Women who do not have British nationality may have been lied to by their abuser about their citizenship and residence rights. Officials dealing with immigration, asylum and refugee status do have an element of discretion, which they can operate in cases of real danger, but may tend to demand proof that abused women are not always in a position to provide. The lack of services for abused women with no recourse to public funds because they are subject to immigration controls remains an important campaigning issue (www.womensaid.org.uk, see Domestic Violence A-Z, BAMER issues).

Yet women turn to professionals only when the violence has become frequent and severe and they have exhausted all the resources of self, family and friends. Encountering a lack of effective help may then escalate the danger, especially as many professionals continue to believe that, if the woman leaves, she will be safe, ignoring the dangers of post-separation violence for women and children (Humphreys and Stanley, 2006).

Refuges are the only agencies that women consistently believe can offer them safety and which they entrust with the full details of their experiences (Hague et al., 2001). Women's organisations specialise in offering survivors of violence respect, with emergency, outreach and advocacy projects all playing a key role. Consequently, women evaluate such services positively (Mullender and Hague, 2000). In all other contexts, they fear disbelief, revulsion, blame and, often, possible consequences in terms of child protection intervention (Humphreys and Stanley, 2006).

Rediscovering social work skills: a way forward?

Because the problem of domestic violence thrives in isolation and intimidation, behind closed doors, groups are one of the most powerful ways of challenging its impact. They help women to see that violence is not their fault because it is widespread, show children who have lived in violent homes that they are not the only ones this has ever happened to, and create a context in which workers and other group members can challenge the perpetrators to confront their own behaviour and its impact. These dynamics for change cannot be recreated through individual work. While recognising that feminist counselling and other interventions can also be helpful, groupwork is considered here as a particularly useful approach.

The remainder of this chapter will explore what groups can achieve with women, children and men in relation to domestic violence and will argue for a reclaiming of groupwork skills as a key element in the struggle to combat men's abuse of women as a persistent oppression.

Groups for abused women

Groupwork offered by women to women has always been the foundation of a feminist approach to domestic violence services. Such groups aim at a process of healing and growth. They focus on helping women to understand that the abuse is not their fault and that the abuser must take responsibility for his own behaviour. They support women in naming the abuse and in rebuilding self-esteem and an independent life. Groups may use participative exercises, discussion topics, role-playing and women's own stories and poems to highlight not only the causes and effects of men's controlling tactics and women's enforced submission, but also women's survival strategies and energy for change. The original women's group manual from the world-famous Duluth programme in the US (Pence, 1987) emphasised internalised oppression and cultural expectations, in relation to class, age and ethnicity, as reasons for staying in a bad relationship. It combined individual validation – 'I am a lovable person, I deserve to be treated well' – with the need for social change – 'What can we do that will make a difference?' There are numerous personal accounts of living with abuse and leaving it (www.womensaid.org.uk

would be a good source). Many of these could be adapted for use in groups to explode the myths about why women stay with abusive men (Hague and Malos, 2005) or return to violent relationships, and how they survive, in most cases eventually separating.

Although groupwork with women would be hard to find in most statutory social work and probation settings, social workers do have the necessary tradition (Cohen and Mullender, 2003) and could rapidly revive the skills. There would be opportunities all over local authority settings for social services staff to facilitate supportive discussion wherever women gather together. Groups for women whose children have been identified as having childcare needs, for example, will always include women who are being or have been abused, and could be an ideal context for meeting women's as well as children's needs. In the community, too, any mother and toddler drop-in session, women and health course, or women's class in a minority ethnic community centre could be used to offer support and advice on living with or leaving abusive relationships and affirm women's experiences and plans.

An independent evaluation of support groups for women survivors of domestic violence in the US found that group members experienced substantial improvements in social and emotional functioning and also a reduction in violence (Tutty et al., 1993). These findings support the wisdom of rediscovering traditional social work skills in groupwork where domestic violence is concerned.

The failure to help children – and a way forward

A recognition that living with domestic violence often has an adverse impact on children's behavioural and emotional adjustment (see Mullender and Humphreys, 2000 for a summary) has frequently led to a narrow child protection response. Practice examples of this approach at its worst have included blanket registration on the grounds of emotional abuse (guaranteed to prevent women from mentioning their own abuse to social services), the sending of a routine letter warning of the impact domestic violence could be having on the children (taking no precautions to prevent the arrival of the letter from further exacerbating the man's violence) and numerous individual instances of statutory intervention used to protect children while taking no action to help the woman (Humphreys, 2000).

Although these interventions are intended to be child centred, they do not meet children's needs, either to feel safe or to recover from their experiences. A patchier but far more positive development, drawing on work in Canada and the US, is that of offering groups for children who have lived with domestic violence (Humphreys et al., 2000).

Children's groups

Groups are an ideal way of working with children who have lived through domestic violence (Mullender, 2004). They bring children together so that they know they are not alone in what they have experienced, as the atmosphere of secrecy at home has previously led them to believe. Coming together helps children to talk more freely about feelings they have been keeping bottled up inside, to understand that the violence is not their fault and to learn new ways of keeping safe.

The Community Group Treatment Program for Child Witnesses of Woman Abuse in London, Ontario (Loosley et al., 2006) offers groups for 4–16-year-olds, divided into age bands of two to three years in each group and available to all agencies in the city to make referrals. A rolling programme of groups, drawing together workers from a range of agencies, operates to a set of core principles. These focus on listening to children, helping them to understand that violence is not their fault and that it is unacceptable, developing safety plans with children and helping them to rebuild their self-esteem and capacity to have fun.

Groups are closed, that is, the same children attend throughout, and set their own ground rules, with 'confidentiality' and 'no violence' to the fore. Most are mixed sex and they normally run weekly for 10 weeks, following a programme of topics approached through a range of age-related activities. Facilitators can be one, two or three women (the youngest children need three workers), or a woman and a man. Group sessions may be varied as needed. A teenage group may focus on the subject of dating violence, for example, dealing with personal safety and forms of help available. It is part of the group worker's skill to vary content and activities as the life of the group and the needs of members determine. Younger children tend to respond to more activity and less talking, with a faster pace. A topic can be introduced during a snack, for example, rather than expecting five–six-year-olds to sit still and listen. One issue that remains to the fore is how best to involve mothers. In the London, Ontario programme, work with women happens alongside, to help them understand and support their children, with joint sessions at the beginning and end.

Effective outcomes have been demonstrated from children's groups (Sudermann et al., 2000). They can challenge children's assumptions of responsibility for the violence and teach them to seek help safely and about non-violent conflict resolution. Groups are fun and can help to rebuild self-esteem. Thus, once again, the evidence from research shows that groupwork has much to offer where there has been domestic violence.

Working with perpetrators

Groupwork with the perpetrators of domestic violence also remains in short supply in the UK, although it is spreading – undertaken most often by the probation service or in the voluntary sector and typically based on cognitive behavioural techniques. It can certainly form one part of an active response to domestic violence, requiring abusive men to take responsibility for their own behaviour and attitudes, although completion rates are low and evaluation to date equivocal (Mullender and Burton, 2000). Men's programmes need long-term monitoring, with feedback from partners to ensure that men are not simply using more subtle abuse tactics or claiming to have changed in order to preserve their relationships.

In order to be successful (Mullender and Burton, 2000), groups need to be based on a clear recognition of domestic violence as an endemic crime. Anger management, for example, is not an appropriate response because men who abuse women are not out of control – they choose the time, place and victim. Issues of women's safety need to be prioritised, with a direct channel for the group workers to hear instantly if the woman is revictimised. Accountability to women more generally is also an issue in men's work, including not competing for resources with services for women and children. There remains a debate as to whether some forms of groups for domestic violence perpetrators – for example those which divert from sentencing, or are not linked to the criminal justice system – may themselves minimise or decriminalise domestic violence in comparison with other violent crime. There are good practice principles and minimum standards for programmes in the UK (respect accreditation standard at www.respect. uk.net/respect_docs/Respect%20Accreditation%20Standard.pdf) that can help to avoid many of these dangers.

Groupwork process: the key to change

Recent research has suggested that it may well be groupwork process that obtains the best results and not a simple instructional format. The evidence comes from a four-site, longitudinal study comparing different groupwork models (Gondolf, 2002, 2004), which indicated that altering gender attitudes may be the crucial element. The men were more likely to show attitude change if they had learned to avoid violence through discussion or respect for women and their point of view. This cannot be achieved in a group simply by practising behavioural techniques such as 'time out' when the man begins to feel angry.

These findings are supported by Dobash et al. (2000), in a study of two programmes in Scotland, where discussions in the group were also said by the men to have had most effect on them, along with specific aspects of the content. Dobash et al. (2000: ix) comment:

> Group work it seems is very important in providing a context in which violence can be discussed with others who have had similar experiences and with group leaders who focus clearly on the offending behaviour and provide new ways of seeing and understanding violence.

The skill lies in challenging directly and facilitating meaningful discussion, so as to draw men into confronting one another's denial, minimisation and projection (blaming others). The ability to do this cannot be learned from a manual; it requires adequate training and professional experience both in the group worker and in their supervisor or consultant, as well as adequate resourcing.

Social work traditionally possessed and nurtured immense skill in groupwork as an intervention for change (Cohen and Mullender, 2003; Doel, 2005; Preston-Shoot, 2007). Our work is about more than assessment; we can also help people to move on in their lives.

Conclusion

We arrive, then, at a series of paradoxes:

- Why, when domestic violence is so high up the agenda, do women continue to feel unsafe and not believed?
- Why, when social work is obsessed with child protection, does it give children so little effective help?
- Why, when research has shown that attitudinal change towards women makes perpetrators less dangerous, do a rather rigid, mechanistic, cognitive behaviouralism and talk of 'anger management' persist in practice?

The greatest paradox of all is why the UK is allowing a precious national resource, in the form of the traditional social work skills of 'people change', to wither away in deference to managerialism. In fact, as this chapter has demonstrated, skilled and carefully evaluated groups have a great deal to offer in helping survivors to recover and in challenging perpetrators, yet they are little used nowadays. When the need is so pressing, as it clearly is in relation to domestic violence, this failure to harness the appropriate tools for evidence-based practice looks like wilful neglect.

For further discussion of anti-oppressive practice, see Adams et al., 2009a, Chapter 5, and for feminist perspectives, see Adams et al., 2009b, Chapter 18.

www.womensaid.org.uk Official website of the Women's Aid Federation of England, includes links to numerous articles on all aspects of domestic violence.

www.ncdv.org.uk
www.endabuse.org
www.broken-rainbow.org.uk
www.respect.uk.net
www.womensaid.org.uk

Cohen, M. and Mullender, A. (eds) (2003) *Gender and Groupwork*, London, Routledge. Outline of groupwork theory and practice from a gendered perspective, spanning the UK and US. Includes coverage of groupwork with domestic violence perpetrators and children who have lived with domestic violence.

Doel, M. (2005) *Using Groupwork*, London, Routledge. Good, basic textbook on groupwork. Seeks to promote greater awareness of group processes and application of groupwork methods in social welfare settings.

Hague, G. and Malos, E. (2005) *Domestic Violence: Action for Change*, 3rd edn, Cheltenham, New Clarion Press. Useful handbook on domestic violence, giving a comprehensive summary of knowledge about domestic violence and appropriate responses to it.

Preston-Shoot, M. (2007) *Effective Groupwork*, 2nd edn, Basingstoke, Palgrave Macmillan. Draws on theory and research to discuss the planning, running and management of groups in the contemporary welfare context.

VIVIENE E. CREE and SUSAN WALLACE

4 Risk and protection

Chapter overview

This chapter considers the meanings of risk and protection and examines the relevant legislation, values, rights and responsibilities. It discusses the reality that while 'risk assessment' and 'risk management' are important, they do not offer a simple solution to the uncertainty and unpredictability of people's lives, which can only be safeguarded through critical, ethical, professional practice.

Understanding risk and protection

We are living in a 'risk society' (Beck, 1992). Wherever we look, we are faced with the dangerousness of life in the early twenty-first century. But there is a paradox here. Just as we are confronted by risks at every corner, so we have come to expect that we should be protected from risk as never before. Within the field of social services, there is an increased expectation that risk should be controlled so that vulnerable children and adults are protected. When social work or health agencies fail in this endeavour, the public outcry is characterised by hurt and anger. The underlying message is clear: 'We trusted you, and you let us down.'

This chapter will begin by considering the meanings of risk and protection, before going on to explore a series of broad considerations that are fundamental to risk and protection, including legislation, values, rights and responsibilities. Drawing on evidence from literature and our own work experience in children and families and criminal justice social work, we will discuss the two key concepts of 'risk assessment' and 'risk management'. We will argue that although these concepts are undoubtedly central to what social workers do (and have always done), we should not be lulled into a false sense of security – into thinking that somehow we have 'covered' the risk or guaranteed protection. In offering suggestions for good practice in social work, we are acutely aware that there is no 'quick fix' solution to the uncertainty and unpredictability of life. Our achievement, at best, must be that we behave in a professional, ethical manner, working alongside service users and other professionals to share the responsibilities and challenges that real life brings.

A quick search of any sociological database tells the same story: risk is 'big business' (Adams, 1995). From chemical accidents to low birth weight infants, nuclear terrorism, environmental protection, flood risk, HIV prevention, data protection, consumer risks and child protection, research studies implicitly (and sometimes explicitly) take it for granted that the world is more unsafe than it was in the past, and that something must be done about it.

One of the most influential writers on risk is Ulrich Beck (1992, 1999). He argues that there has been a major shift in the way we view risk. In 'traditional' or 'pre-modern' societies, disasters such as famine, disease and flood were viewed as acts of God, or accidents of fate; there was little that anyone could do to either prevent catastrophes or protect themselves from future adversity. Industrialisation brought with it a new, 'modern' outlook, which presumed that human beings could and should seek to control such misadventure. But, Beck (1992) argues, industrial society did not remove risk; instead, it created new and more damaging risks. While 'modern' industrial society brought wealth and 'goods', it also created 'bads', or threats, including environmental problems such as pollution, and social problems such as unemployment and family breakdown. These were not simply 'negative side effects of seemingly accountable and calculable action' but rather they are 'trends which are eroding the system and delegitimating the bases of rationality' (Beck, 1999: 33). Risks, he argues, have become more difficult to calculate and control; they are global and at the same time local, or 'glocal' (1999: 142). 'Risk society' therefore equals 'world risk society', in which human experience is characterised by unintended consequences and greater knowledge does not ease this state of affairs; instead, more and better knowledge often leads to more uncertainty (1999: 6). 'Expert' and lay voices now compete with one other as the outcomes of modernity are challenged on all fronts, in a process Beck calls 'reflexive modernisation'.

While highly convincing, it seems likely that Beck's thesis may have contributed to a rather pessimistic view of risk and protection. Beck fails to acknowledge the contradictions, ambivalence and complexities that are an inevitable part of the individual's response to risk. Not only this, Tulloch and Lupton (2003) suggest that he does not pay sufficient attention to the roles played by class, gender and 'race' in constructing different risk knowledges and experiences. In their comparative study of attitudes to risk in Britain and Australia, Tulloch and Lupton found that early 'modernist ideas' about the control of risk still dominated people's ideas, as did some pre-modern notions about 'fate'. Although many risks were indeed categorised as 'uncontrollable' by individuals, this was not because they were incalculable or global. Instead, fate or the actions of others were seen as beyond the individual's control (2003: 37). What is more, Tulloch and Lupton point out that risk is not necessarily negative. People choose to take risks all the time, for personal gain, excitement or self-actualisation, or 'simply as part of the human project'. A life without risk may be perceived as 'too tightly bound and restricted, as not offering enough challenges' (2003: 37). Risk-taking is therefore part of the process through which human beings create themselves as individuals; it is a 'practice of the self' (Foucault, 1988).

Risk, protection and the law

Legislation shapes and determines what social workers do, so this is our starting point in considering risk and protection. It will not be surprising, given the discussion already, to learn that there is no explicit legal definition of risk in either English or Scottish law, although it will often be pertinent to both civil and criminal matters in all aspects of social work. There have been significant developments in this direction, however. In Scotland, under the provisions of the Management of Offenders etc (Scotland) Act 2005, new duties were placed on local authorities, the police and the Scottish prison service to establish joint protocols for assessing and managing people who had been convicted of sexual offences and those who had been convicted of serious violent offences. This led to the establishment of multi-agency public protection arrangements, known as MAPPA, through which all registered sexual offenders are now administered (Scottish Executive, 2006). Similar developments were introduced in England and Wales in 2001.

Given the absence of a precise, legal definition of risk, the onus is on the social worker or probation officer to familiarise themselves with the applicable primary legislation and procedures in children and families social work, community care and criminal justice social work. Social workers must also be aware of secondary, procedural legislation as it applies to specific work activities. For example, the Criminal Procedure (Scotland) Act 1995, section 210A(1) requires that the author of a social enquiry report (known as a pre-sentence report in England and Wales) produces a risk assessment of any potential harm a violent and/or sex offender may cause, so that the judge can make a decision about whether to impose an extended sentence. In such a situation, the social worker must know the type of case that could legally result in an extended sentence being imposed, the type of offences that fall into this category (and those that do not) and the type of court procedure being used.

Social workers must also be knowledgeable about key governmental policy directives, and these often emerge as an outcome of a high-profile case where protection has failed. The inquiry into the death of Victoria Climbié (Butler-Sloss, 2003) was one of these watershed moments. This inquiry and a Department of Health report published the same year were instrumental in the changes that appeared in the Children Act 2004 and the programmes instituted through *Every Child Matters* (DfES, 2004). The emphasis (and indeed the language) shifted from the notion of 'protection' to the much wider concept of 'safeguarding': a duty was placed on local authorities to work with all relevant agencies (health, education, social work, police and voluntary agencies) to promote the wellbeing of children and young people. Statutory local safeguarding children boards were set up from April 2006, replacing the former (non-statutory) area child protection committees, and strategy plans for children and young people were published. Scotland has seen a similar set of changes, with the publication of a key policy report

It's Everyone's Job to Make Sure I'm Alright (Scottish Executive, 2002) and the development of integrated children's services plans (Scottish Executive, 2004).

Policy initiatives in relation to risk and protection have not only been the province of social work with children and families. The care of 'vulnerable adults' has experienced a great deal of public attention in recent years (Stanley et al., 1999), and over the past decade, steps have been taken throughout the UK by way of legislation, government policy and practice guidance for health and caring agencies to bring practice in line with measures designed to protect children. In England and Wales, as part of the implementation of the Care Standards Act 2000, the government introduced the protection of vulnerable adults scheme (POVA). This recognised the need to ensure that those deemed unsuitable are prevented from working with vulnerable adults (DH, 2004). POVA effectively acts as a workforce ban on professionals who have harmed vulnerable adults in their care and prevents known abusers from entering the workforce. POVA compliments other initiatives (Social Services Inspectorate Wales, 1999; DH, 2000a), which lay out multi-agency codes of practice aimed at detecting, preventing and tackling the abuse of vulnerable adults. Local councils were given the lead responsibility for ensuring the above guidance is observed in practice, and in 2005, *Safeguarding Adults* was published, setting out a national framework of good practice standards in order to ensure consistent good quality practice with vulnerable adults throughout all local authorities (ADSS, 2005).

Developments in adult protection were again accelerated by a highly publicised failure to protect, this time in Scotland, and another inquiry report (SWSI/MWC, 2004). In March 2002, a woman with learning disabilities was admitted to Borders General Hospital in Scotland having suffered extreme levels of physical and sexual abuse within her household over an extended period. In September 2002, three men were imprisoned for this abuse. This woman had been in receipt of social work services from Scottish Borders Council and its predecessor authorities and from NHS Borders since her early childhood. Her case highlighted the importance of protection not just for children, but for all those who are vulnerable, and led to the passing of new legislation (the Adult Support and Protection (Scotland) Act 2007) and the development of new training requirements in risk and protection for all those working with vulnerable adults. Other chapters in this trilogy (Adams et al. 2009b, Chs 22, 23, 24, 27 and 28) provide more detailed analysis of specific policies in relation to the care of children and adults. However, it is enough to state here that a good knowledge of policy and procedures is critically important for all social workers, because a failure to follow procedural guidelines has been recognised as a contributory factor to 'things going wrong' (Butler-Sloss, 2003).

Adherence to the relevant legislation, policy and procedure thus provides three corners of a working framework that should anchor good practice in relation to assessing and managing risk and protection. The fourth corner must be attention to rights.

LEGISLATION	POLICY
PROCEDURE	RIGHTS

Risk, protection and rights

In considering the issues of protection and risk, it must be recognised that those we consider to be 'at risk' and those whom we believe may present a risk equally have rights; social workers have duties to observe the rights of others and advise them about their rights (Wallace, 2000). Just as Article 19 of the UN Convention on the Rights of the Child (1989) assures a child the right to protection from abuse and neglect, so the Human Rights Act 1998, which came into force in October 2000, guarantees all citizens certain absolute and qualified rights, which all public bodies in the UK (including social services, social work and probation departments) must adhere to when dealing with the public (Walden and Mountfield, 1999).

The Human Rights Act guarantees basic civil, political, social and economic rights. Some are absolute, for example 'Article 3: freedom from torture'. Others are subject to some limitations and qualifications, and in such cases, the Act seeks to balance the rights of the individual against other public interests (Harris et al., 2005). For example, 'Article 8: the right to respect for private and family life' has a proviso that interference by a public body is permissible, if it is in the interests of preventing a crime or protecting the rights and freedoms of others. However, before a public body can overrule an individual's rights in such a situation, five issues must be considered: proportionality, legality, accountability, necessity/compulsion, subsidiarity (see Walden and Mountfield, 1999 for a fuller discussion on these principles). Any infringement by a public body or an employee of another's rights must therefore be justified and transparent.

Given the uncertainties and grey areas that abound in assessing potential risk and questions of protection, social workers must develop a good working knowledge of the European Convention on Human Rights 1950 and the Human Rights Act 1998 and ensure that protocols and practice are compatible with the Convention. This should include making the recipients of social work services aware of their rights in a meaningful fashion, not only in terms of a narrow reading of the Act, but also that they reach a deeper understanding of what they can expect as a recipient of a social work service and what recourse they may have if they are not happy with the service they are receiving (Wallace, 2000). A rights-based framework should ensure sharper, more open and transparent decision-making with clear lines of accountability. The concept of the 'defensible decision' is especially useful here: if you were to hand over your case notes to another professional, would they act in the same manner as you had, because you had taken the correct steps and acted ethically in the process (Kemshall, 2002a)?

Risk, protection and responsibilities

Alongside rights, inevitably come responsibilities. There are commonly two sets of responsibilities to be considered: the responsibilities of the client, service user or offender and their contacts, and the responsibilities of the social worker or probation officer. When a tragedy occurs and a child or vulnerable adult is hurt or dies, thoughts turn very quickly to blame: to whom can responsibility be attributed? Who is to blame? Sir

Louis Blom-Cooper (1993: 20), who has chaired many inquiries into abuse, including homicides, states that the purpose of inquiries is

> to examine the truth ... what happened ... how did it happen, and who if anyone was responsible, culpably or otherwise, for it having happened?

But what is 'the truth'? Whose 'truth' are we to believe? In an examination of the role of the public inquiry in welfare scandals, Butler and Drakeford (2003: 219) argue that the inquiry is itself 'a player in the contested terrain, contributing its own voice to the construction of the original events'. Furthermore, the 'truth' that inquiries seek to uncover

> is influenced by the institutional framework within which the seeking-after is constructed ... If scandals are constructed, then, they are manufactured with a purpose. (Butler and Drakeford, 2003: 221).

The purpose, Butler and Drakeford assert, is to manage the immediate consequences of the scandal and, in so doing, leave the wider institutional order intact. Public attention is thus diverted from organisations onto individuals, and larger questions of historical and structural significance are avoided.

In thinking about the ways in which inquiries focus on the actions of individuals, Peay (1996: 11) tellingly asks: 'subject to this level of analysis, which of us would be likely to be found completely without fault?' The following case example, which describes a real scenario from practice, demonstrates that responsibility cannot be held by a social worker alone, or even by a team of professionals. Parents, relatives, neighbours, friends, health, education and social care professionals and society as a whole must share some responsibility for keeping children safe.

CASE EXAMPLE

Viviene's experience

A health visitor referred a 28-year-old white, single mother to the voluntary sector children and families agency where I worked. Joan was isolated and depressed following the break-up of her marriage, and wanted information about welfare benefit entitlements, as well as an opportunity to talk with a social worker about the marital breakdown. The health visitor also made a referral to the local children's centre for part-time provision to enable Joan's children Lisa (aged 2 years) and Robert (aged 4 years) to enjoy some quality time away from Joan.

As our relationship developed, Joan gradually told me the story of her life; the violence in her marriage and her father's sexual abuse of her when she was a child – abuse that had continued, sporadically, into her adult life. She was eager to try to understand what had happened to her and, with my support, she began to write her story down, and write poems that she shared with me. I introduced her to a local incest survivors group, and she began to grow in confidence as she heard the stories of others. One day, her son Robert began to draw scary pictures at the children's centre, and speak about a 'night monster with a prickly chin' that sometimes came to his bedroom and climbed into his bed. On questioning, he told the daycare worker that the night monster was Pappa (his name for his grandfather). A case conference was called, and Joan had to confront the reality that her father may have abused her son and perhaps also her daughter.

It emerged that while Joan had been making such strides in her own life, her father Peter had continued to play an important role with the family, supporting Joan financially and helping her with everything from decorating to babysitting. It should be stated that, aside from Robert's story (which he retracted a few days later), there was no evidence at this time that either Robert or Lisa had been sexually abused. The case conference recommended that voluntary measures of care should remain in place, and that all those working with the family should continue to monitor the children carefully. Joan assured the case conference that she would never again leave the children alone with her father, and that she would restrict his contact to occasional visits.

The postscript to this case is that six months later the police were called at 1 am to Joan's house. The 10-year-old son of a neighbour had been sleeping in Joan's house (this boy was unknown to the agency) and had telephoned the police to report that he had been attacked by Peter and had defended himself with a knife. Peter was subsequently taken to the police station for questioning and all the sheets in the house were removed for forensic examination. I was called out to the house and arranged for the children to be placed temporarily in foster care; Joan was nowhere to be seen and had been out all night at a party. Following a children's hearing, the children returned home under a statutory supervision order; meanwhile, there was insufficient evidence to pursue any complaint against Peter. I continued to work with Joan alongside a local authority social worker until I left the agency the following year. No further action was taken against Peter.

This case highlights a persistent reality in social work practice: that even when we have done everything possible to protect those with whom we are working, we cannot, with any certainty, know what is going on in a family when we are not present. Two options had been available in this situation, and neither had been in any way palatable: Viviene could seek to remove the children for their own 'protection' from a mother whom they loved and who loved them; or the children could be left at home, albeit with supervision, where sexual abuse may occur. Because of the lack of 'hard' evidence of abuse, only the second option could ever be realised, and the children continued to live at home with as much support and monitoring as was possible. But this could not remove all risk of harm from the children.

Risk, protection and values

As this case demonstrates, the whole process of dealing with risk and protection is fraught with moral and ethical dilemmas for social workers, primarily as a result of the uncertainty of outcomes. There are no 'right' or 'wrong' answers in most cases; assessing risk is never an exact science, and if the wrong decision is reached, this can have grave and profound implications. In any assessment of risk, there are four possible outcomes:

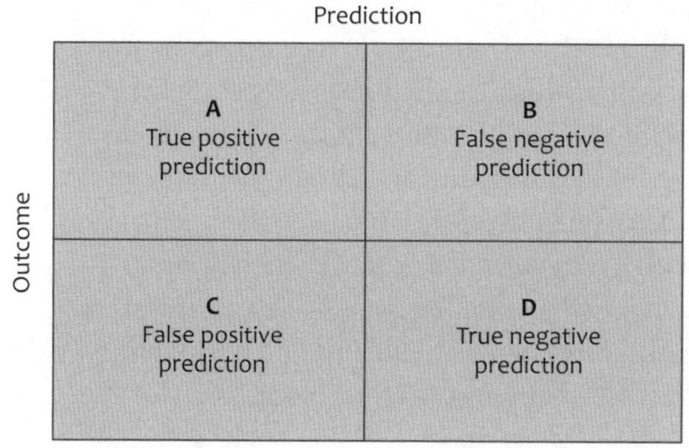

Prediction

A True positive prediction	**B** False negative prediction
C False positive prediction	**D** True negative prediction

(Outcome — vertical axis label on left)

Source: Kemshall, 2002b: 14

- ■ In box A, it is predicted that harm will occur and it does
- ■ In box B, it is predicted that there will be no harm but it does occur
- ■ In box C, it is predicted that there will be harm but it does not occur
- ■ In box D, it is predicted that there will be no harm and it does not occur.

From this representation, the two outcomes that clearly present most difficulties for social workers, service users and the public at large are B and C. In the case of B, vulnerable adults and children may be harmed or killed, and their agencies may be brought into disrepute; while C raises significant ethical dilemmas for practitioners and those concerned with civil liberties (Kemshall, 2002b: 14). MacDonald and MacDonald (1999) assert that we frequently overemphasise low-risk, extreme outcomes (for example child death), and argue that what is needed is a revisiting of the moral assertions made about risk. MacDonald and MacDonald (1999: 43) assert that 'our untutored, intuitive perceptions of risk are likely to be systematically misleading, so that we must use a more stringent, scientific approach in the future'. This is self-evidently a worthwhile goal. But the reality is that all of us must make decisions under conditions of 'manufactured uncertainty', where not only is the knowledge base incomplete, but more and better knowledge often means more uncertainty' (Beck, 1999: 6). Furthermore, 'to be free to act well, is to be free to act badly' – autonomy brings risk, inevitably (Caddick and Watson, 1999: 66).

◇◇◇◇ **CASE EXAMPLE** ◇◇

Susan's experience

Matthew was a 24-year-old white man subject to a supervised release order, having spent 18 months in custody for a series of car crimes. Three special conditions were attached to Matthew's release order:

- he should reside at an address approved by his supervising social worker
- he should seek employment
- he should undergo drug counselling.

I had not met Matthew until shortly before he was due to be released from prison. He had a long history of involvement with the social work department as a child due to a rather chaotic home life, which resulted in him being taken into care. As an adult, he was also well known to the criminal justice system and had served a number of prison sentences. Stealing cars and driving without a licence were his main type of crimes. Departmental records indicated that mental health personnel had seen Matthew on a number of occasions. He had never been diagnosed as suffering from a recognised mental illness; however, concerns had consistently been expressed regarding his mental wellbeing. He impressed as a very troubled soul with a history of self-harm and suicide attempts.

Matthew moved into supported accommodation after his release from prison. As the weeks went by, I became increasingly concerned about Matthew. He acknowledged that he was drinking a lot and using drugs, and he appeared incredibly distressed. I arranged for Matthew to be assessed by a psychiatrist but subsequent events took over. Matthew walked into a police station one evening in November stating that he did not want to carry on and wanted to die. He was taken to A&E where he was seen by the duty psychiatrist, who reported that because Matthew did not suffer from a recognised mental illness, he could not be admitted to hospital for assessment/treatment. The psychiatrist was clearly of the opinion that he needed help, but the system was not able to avail him of this.

A few days later, Matthew's solicitor contacted me. Matthew had been arrested the previous evening for stealing a car. He was due to appear in court later that morning. While in custody, Matthew had bitten his arm very badly and his solicitor was concerned about his state of mind. I shared my own concerns with him. The solicitor decided not to oppose any moves that Matthew should be remanded in custody. This was an unusual action, but we both felt that given his fragile state of mind and inability to access an admission to a psychiatric hospital, prison may well provide a secure and safe environment for him to be monitored.

Matthew was remanded into custody. Discussions immediately began with prison social work and health services. A case conference was convened and the decision was taken that Matthew should be placed under suicide watch and he should undergo assessment and receive support. A week passed, Matthew appeared to be stable and had not caused himself any further injury. On Christmas Eve, Matthew asked to see a nurse. He explained that he was feeling much better and was desperate to be moved into one of the regular remand wings in the prison. He was very persuasive and the duty nurse agreed to his move, although this contravened the established protocol, which stated that such a decision should only be taken by a reconvened case conference. A few hours later, Matthew was found dead in his cell.

This case again highlights profound issues about risk and protection. It demonstrates that, in spite of the willingness of social work and health professionals to work together, Matthew 'fell between two stools', in this case, between the mental health and criminal justice systems. Susan was forced to accept that the only way Matthew could be protected from himself was in prison, but even this was not sufficient to prevent the eventual outcome. The case also shows that where procedures and protocols exist, they should be rigorously followed; the decision to take Matthew off suicide observation should not have been taken by one person, and the nurse's actions left him open to accusations of blame. But does this make him responsible for Matthew's death? Who has the right to interfere with an individual's choice to determine whether to take their own life? These are ethical and moral questions that go far beyond a common-sense reading of risk and protection.

Risk assessment

All social work practice, implicitly or explicitly, involves an assessment of risk. But risk measurement is no easy task, and what might work well in one setting may not readily transfer to another:

> Risk assessment is a process of analysis, not a specific kind of research and not a result, and it must be viewed as a process that is subject to much uncertainty. (Bailar and Bailer, 1999: 285)

Although writing about risk relating to chemical hazards, these sentiments equally apply to risk assessment in social work. The one certainty in social work that does exist is that there are *no* certainties, at best probabilities. In thinking about risk assessment, we need to be clear what the risk is, who presents the risk and to whom. Parsloe (1999: 11) usefully separates out three different kinds of risk:

- Risk to service users from other people, usually their own relatives
- Risk to users themselves from their own behaviour
- Risk to known or unknown others from service users.

Two methods are currently used in assessing risk in social work: actuarial and clinical methods.

Actuarial method in risk assessment

The actuarial (or statistical) method has its roots in the insurance industry; it involves statistical calculations of probability, in which an individual's likely behaviour is predicted on the basis of the known behaviour of others in similar circumstances. This method is relatively easy for social workers to use, since it presents them with a fixed set of questions to ask and a simple way of calculating the level of risk – they simply add up the number of 'high-risk' responses.

There are, however, major methodological limitations in transferring information about the behaviour of a group to an individual risk assessment. For example, in the field of criminal justice social work, where actuarial tools have been employed for several years, many of the risk assessment tools currently in use have been developed using male prison populations. These do not readily apply to other groups such as female offenders, or specific types of offender (Kemshall, 1997; Silver and Miller, 2002). This point is further elaborated by Hart et al. (2007). In an exploration of the use of risk tools in the prediction of violence within the mental health field, they caution that it is of vital importance for practitioners to familiarise themselves with the limitations of tools. This becomes particularly relevant in situations where lengthy periods of incapacitation may be determined on the strength of a 'risk score'. There is also a recognised problem with cultural transferability, when tools developed in one sociocultural jurisdiction are employed in another culture. Many of the risk assessment tools being employed in the UK today have their origins in US and Canadian populations. Smith and Vanstone (2002) indicate that this can lead to deep-rooted problems, which may require much more than merely tipping the cap to 'cultural sensitivity' when using imported materials. Moreover, Silver and Miller (2002) note how easy it becomes for those conducting risk assessments to depersonalise the subject of their assessment so that they come to see the person merely as a collection of 'risk variables'.

Clinical method in risk assessment

Clinical assessment is the traditional and more familiar method used in social work practice, and employs diagnostic assessment techniques relating to personality factors and situational factors relevant to the risky behaviour and the interaction between the two (Prins, 1999). It is highly dependent on the interaction between the social worker and client or service user; interviewing and direct observation are the key components used to collect information on social, personal and environmental factors associated with the problematic behaviour. Its main usefulness has been in terms of making sense of an individual's risky behaviour, by shedding light on the attitudes, motivations and precipitating factors that led to the risky behaviour and assessing their likely responses to 'treatment' (Prins, 1988; Kemshall, 1997).

The clinical method has serious limitations as a predictive tool. Clinical assessment is a highly subjective process, which is affected by the individual background, values and beliefs of the assessor (Kemshall, 1997). In this uncertain world of risk assessment and prediction, the most promising and productive practice would seem to be to draw on a combination of actuarial and clinical assessment methods (Kemshall, 1997). By combining clinical assessment – with all its potential for eliciting 'rich' information relating to an individual – with actuarial information – developed from broader populations with higher predictive accuracy – risk assessments are likely to be stronger, more focused and more useful than simply using one method.

But this does not go far enough. Social work values promote the worth of the individual and the uniqueness of human beings in their social and cultural contexts. By channelling all our energies into the assessment of risk, we may lose sight of social work's traditional values, especially when the service user is regarded by society as 'dangerous', or when their behaviour is seen as abhorrent, as in the case of sexual offenders (Harris et al., 2005). Risk assessment methods illustrate a wider process in social work in which tasks are becoming increasingly routinised and performed in often highly prescriptive ways. McBeath and Webb (2002) assert that accountability, quality control and risk management dominate social work today, with an accompanying emphasis on duties and regulations. This has led to the development of defensive forms of social work, which, they argue, are uncongenial to the development of human qualities likely to promote engagement in discussion of what counts as good practice in social work.

This is a good place to start in terms of a rethink about risk assessment. If the assessment of risk is, as we have stated, at the heart of social work practice, it provides an opportunity to work with service users in an empowering rather than oppressive way. Regardless of whether the service user is a willing recipient of care, for example an older woman who has had a fall at home, or an 'involuntary client', such as a young parent under investigation for neglecting their child, those whom we are assessing should feel part of the process of assessing risk (Trotter, 1999). This means at the outset that attention must be paid to the relationship between the worker and the service user. This is not about encouraging service users to see us as their 'friends'. Instead, it is about being clear with service users what our role is, what our responsibilities and obligations are, what the service user can expect from us and the organisation and what may happen in the future. Only then will service users be able to make informed decisions about the risks they are prepared to take (and not take) and the protection they may require.

Risk management

Risk assessment is not and should not be an end in itself, but is best considered as part of a wider risk management strategy. There have been occasions in the past when the process of registration, for example at a child protection case conference or a sex offender registration conference, has been treated as an end in itself; it has become an administrative procedure, rather than the opportunity to address the future management of risk as part of an ongoing process (Kemshall and Maguire, 2001). This has had disastrous consequences (Butler-Sloss, 2003).

Risk management, like risk assessment, brings its own dangers. An investigation of risk management in the world of business draws interesting parallels with risk management in social work. Traditionally, risk management in business was concerned with assessing how and why a company experienced losses, with a view to minimising those losses. However, heightened sensitivity to risk exposure has led to a huge elevation in the importance of risk management. Instead of being a useful tool, it starts to become 'an unnecessary self-regulation', and companies become far too cautious (Hunt, 2003: 93). This is undoubtedly a real possibility in social work, as workers become afraid to show creativity and initiative, and become procedure driven and overly concerned with self-protection.

Davis (1996) points out that risk management is often interpreted simply as a risk minimisation strategy. In terms of mental health, this means locating risk 'in a deficient and potentially dangerous minority of individuals who need to be identified, registered and managed by medication and surveillance' (1996: 113). In doing so, real issues for the majority of service users are often ignored, and little attention is paid to the ways in which 'social, economic, cultural and interpersonal environments influence vulnerability as well as a potential for violent, harmful and self-neglectful behaviour' (1996: 114). Davis thus shifts attention from the 'dangerous' individual to the wider context, including the relationship between the service user and the agency, the locations where practice takes place, the different agencies involved and the organisational structure. Mental health service users must be empowered to take risks to be whole human beings. In order for this to happen, workers must be adequately supported and supervised in their own organisations.

But there is another important point here. Social workers are never alone in carrying the management of risk (although it may feel like this at times) and it is vital that there is a clear sharing of tasks and responsibilities between all those in an individual's social network. This is likely to include formal supports, through social work, health professionals, teachers and the police, and informal supports, through relatives, family friends, local community groups and so on. Most children, Beckett (2003) indicates, look to their parents for protection first and then to neighbours, friends and other family members. This means that social workers must be prepared to work in partnership at all levels and appropriately share information and responsibility, in such a way that service users know what is happening and why.

Checklist for good practice

We have considered some of the general themes underpinning risk and protection in social work. These raise a number of fundamental questions for practice:

- ■ What is the risk? Is it positive or negative, and for whom?
- ■ What is the relevant legislation?

- What procedures and policy frameworks apply to the situation?
- Whose rights and whose responsibilities need to be safeguarded?
- What values issues need to be considered?
- What methods of assessment should be used and why?
- How can decision-making and tasks be shared between agencies?
- What support systems are in place for you as a worker?
- What are the lines of accountability? How can these be shared?
- How will the work be monitored and reviewed?

Conclusion

In reviewing this chapter, a number of themes emerge. First, we have argued that risk and protection are a huge preoccupation in social work, as they are in society as a whole. Massive sums of money have been earned by North American companies that have tapped into this preoccupation with risk, seeing a gap in the market to produce risk assessment tools that have eagerly been snapped up in the UK. Our questions remain: how far have these actually met the needs of the situation? And more provocatively, are these tools in fact a 'smoke screen' to convince ourselves and others that we are doing something positive in a situation over which we may have little control?

But this seems overly pessimistic. Our second thesis is that although risk is everywhere, it is not necessarily negative. Social work should be about much more than minimising risk; it should be about maximising welfare (Munro, 2002). This means that in some situations, we will be encouraging people to take risks – to continue to live at home in spite of physical or mental frailty, join a self-help group, go to school, apply for a college course. In this way, social work is a balancing act in which we encourage service users to take risks and learn by their mistakes. Each new abuse scandal becomes another 'nail in the coffin' for preventive practice. This must be resisted at management and organisational level (Spratt, 2001) if social work's core values and skills are to be upheld.

Third, we have argued that while 'risk' and 'protection' may be social constructions, perceived differently by different people at different times, this does not make them imaginary. On the contrary, as our two case examples demonstrate, risk can have serious consequences for individuals and their families. Social workers must therefore work from the basis of a sound understanding of legislation, policy, procedure and rights. They must be prepared to examine their practice from a moral and ethical perspective and work from the basis of theories that aim to challenge, not support, oppression, in other words, they must act with integrity (Cree, 2000: 209). Lastly, they must seek to work in real partnership with service users, other professionals and members of society to ensure that the risks which are taken have positive outcomes and that protection allows vulnerable children and adults to live creative, full and, if at all possible, 'safe' lives.

For further discussion of risk and decision-making, see Chapter 16, and for family-based social work, see Adams et al., 2009b, Chapter 25.

www.victoria-climbie-inquiry.org.uk Victoria Climbié report.

www.adss.org.uk/publications/guidance/safeguarding.pdf Safeguarding Adults framework.

Beck, U. (1992) *Risk Society: Towards a New Modernity*, London, Sage. A critical analysis of societal risks created by uncertainties arising from social developments.

DH (Department of Health) (1995) *Child Protection: Messages from Research*, London, HMSO. Useful reflections on child protection research, even though somewhat dated.

Parsloe, P. (ed.) (1999) *Risk Assessment in Social Care and Social Work*, London, Jessica Kingsley. A useful collection, showing the range of meanings attributed to 'risk' and the unevenness of research coverage.

Prins, H. (1999) *Will They Do It Again? Risk Assessment and Management in Criminal Justice and Psychiatry*, London, Routledge. A thoughtful study of risks presented by 'dangerous' people with criminal and/or psychiatric propensities.

Scottish Executive (2007) *Effective Approaches to Risk Assessment in Social Work: An International Literature Review*, Edinburgh, Scottish Executive. A useful international review of the literature.

Tulloch, J. and Lupton, D. (2003) *Risk and Everyday Life*, London, Sage. An examination of how people think about, experience and respond to risk in everyday life.

Webb, S. (2006) *Social Work in a Risk Society: Social and Political Perspectives*, Basingstoke, Palgrave Macmillan. A very thoughtful yet accessible discussion of the ideas, concepts, policies, modes of organisation and practices associated with risk in social work.

Troubled and in trouble: young people, truancy and offending

5

This chapter examines work with young people who offend, in the context of changing policy since the late twentieth century, from 'welfare' and 'minimalism' to today's more directed and authoritarian 'interventionism'. It focuses on the 'popular punitiveness' currently directed at young people, the identification of truancy and interventions to deal with it, antisocial behaviour, young people who commit sexual offences and the persistent young offender.

Chapter overview

Social workers work with young people who have behaviour problems, are truanting from school, and are engaged in criminality and other antisocial behaviour; this work now takes place in local authority children's services and multi-agency youth offending teams (YOTs), alongside police officers and other practitioners. Social work is carried out in these teams and within the extensive legal frameworks and national standards that now circumscribe social work with young people who offend.

This work with young people takes place against a political backdrop that is often hostile to young people:

> One of the biggest challenges we face is how to deal with young offenders who believe that their age makes them untouchable, who flout the law, laugh at the police and leave court on bail, free to offend again. The public are sick and tired of their behaviour and expect the criminal justice system to be able to keep them off the streets. (Home Secretary David Blunkett, quoted in Home Office, 2002a)

and is supported by an equally virulent media that seems to see all young people as drug-using members of gangs who truant from school and drink underage, who wear hooded clothes and carry guns and knives as a fashion accessory (see, for example, Townsend, 2006). At their worst, young people are seen as a feral race apart, with no fear of the police or criminal justice system (Butt, 2005).

In this chapter we seek to explore the changing nature of work over the past 30 years with young people who offend, from a position of 'welfare' and 'minimalism' to today's more directed and authoritarian 'interventionism', said now to be even 'criminalising' many of our young people (see, for example, *Independent*, 20 June 2005). The ex-head of the Youth Justice Board went so far as to call it the 'gratuitous criminalising' of children (*Safer Society*, 2007). Four areas of work are singled out for particular attention as examples of the 'popular punitiveness' currently directed at young people: the identification of and the interventions to deal with truancy, antisocial behaviour, young people who commit sexual offences and the persistent young offender.

'Popular punitiveness' is a phrase coined to describe the way in which politicians, using the umbrella of the rhetoric of 'law and order', have been 'tapping into, and using for their own purposes, what they believe to be the public's generally punitive stance' (Bottoms, 1995: 40). Garland (2001: 13) has elaborated on the idea:

> A few decades ago public opinion functioned as an occasional brake on policy initiatives: now it operates as a privileged source. The importance of research and criminological knowledge is downgraded and in its place is a new deference to the voice of 'experience', of 'common sense', of what 'everyone knows'.

From 'welfare' to 'minimalism' to 'interventionism'

The history of youth justice policy between the 1960s and the early 1990s has been divided into two phases: 'welfare' and 'minimalism' (Pitts, 2003).

The welfare era reached a peak in the late 1960s and early 1970s. The social sciences, through social work, appeared to offer a means to resolve social problems and therefore associated behaviour such as youth offending. When questions were asked about whether these new approaches actually worked (Martinson, 1974), the optimism of welfare was deflated and followed by an era of minimalism; the 1980s saw crime as almost a 'routine activity' for young people who were best left alone wherever possible to 'grow out of it' and practitioners were best occupied in trying to divert them away from the criminal justice system. When New Labour came into power in 1997, a new era of 'interventionist' youth justice came into being.

The Crime and Disorder Act 1998 defined, for the first time, the 'principal aim' of the youth justice system, which was 'to prevent offending by children and young persons' (s. 37). Critics were quick to point out that this definition said nothing about any 'welfare' component of the work to be carried out, even though section 44 of the Children and Young Persons Act 1933 still required courts to 'have regard to the welfare of any child or young person' brought before them.

A new national body – the Youth Justice Board (YJB) of England and Wales – was to have oversight of the youth justice system; most activities would remain localised but the YJB would promote good practice, issue national standards, and provide funding. It would also commission research, which was back on the agenda for practitioners in terms of their practice being evidence based to ensure that it was evaluated and actually did 'work'.

The Crime and Disorder Act 1998 restructured youth justice services at the local level by creating youth offending teams (YOTs). Social workers were to be relocated from social services department into the multi-agency YOT to work alongside seconded probation officers, police officers, education workers and (sometimes) healthcare professionals. The presence of social workers in YOTs presumably meant that 'welfare' was still seen as important but it would have to take its place alongside other practitioners from different backgrounds and cultures, possibly with different aims and objectives (Souhami, 2007).

◇◇◇◇ CASE EXAMPLE ◇◇◇◇◇◇◇◇◇◇◇◇◇◇◇◇◇◇◇◇◇◇◇◇◇◇◇◇◇◇◇◇◇◇◇◇◇◇◇

Alan is 15 and lives with his mother and brother in a rural area. A few months ago, following an argument with his mother's 'boyfriend', he 'stole' her car and drove it around a supermarket car park at 2 am in the morning. Nearby residents called the police who arrested him. No one was hurt but £500 worth of damage had been caused to the car's bodywork. A reprimand was considered insufficient and prosecution followed.

The social worker in the YOT wrote a pre-sentence report (PSR) for the youth court and proposed an action plan order (APO) as the best way forward. Alan was assessed as being very remorseful and unlikely to reoffend; the APO (lasting three months) was considered to be sufficient intervention to bring home to him the risk to himself and others. Alan had no previous convictions, attended school regularly, where he was described as 'industrious', and had no apparent social 'deficit' that needed meeting.

However, the youth court imposed a two-year supervision order. Alan met his supervisor (the author of the PSR) twice a week – as required by national standards. The supervision was seen as somewhat perfunctory and with no real aim. Plans were in hand to apply for a revocation of the supervision order after 12 months.

The social work role appears almost non-existent in this case example. The court ignored the options outlined in the PSR and work on improving credibility in the courts might be needed now; the resulting imposition of top-down national standards was clearly inappropriate and denied any professional discretion to the social worker.

Social work with children and young people in danger of offending or actually offending takes place within local authority children's services and the multi-agency YOTs. The age of criminal responsibility – set at 10 years – provides a socially constructed line that has divided the work of these two agencies when offending takes place.

The Crime and Disorder Act 1998 left the age of criminal responsibility unaltered, but did make children more responsible for their actions by removing the so-called 'doli incapax' doctrine (the doctrine that there was a rebuttable presumption that a child aged between 10 and 14 years could not form the necessary criminal intent; see Bandalli, 1998 for more on this). Paradoxically, it also made parents more responsible for their children's behaviour by introducing parenting orders designed to teach better parenting skills (Goldson and Jamieson, 2002).

It is only possible here to give a flavour of the Crime and Disorder Act and its initial moves towards greater interventionism; we consider the Act's antisocial behaviour order (ASBO) in more detail below. Some of the Act's provisions did give space for more social work input within them, for example drug treatment and testing orders and parenting orders. In the following sections, we consider the interventionism introduced into four particular aspects of young people's behaviour: truancy, antisocial behaviour, the young sexual offender and the persistent young offender.

Young people who engage in antisocial behaviour

One new direction taken by the New Labour government was that towards combating antisocial behaviour. What exactly antisocial behaviour was and how it differs from criminality has always been a matter of debate. It has variously been described as 'subcriminal', 'low-level disorder' and 'public nuisance', but others have pointed out that this can also mean behaviour that is non-criminal; on the other hand, if it includes criminal behaviour, why call it just antisocial?

The developing idea of antisocial behaviour appears not to have started with the public, the police or social workers but with housing officials. Elizabeth Burney (1999) has carefully documented the early history of antisocial behaviour from the mid-1990s. Beset with problems and complaints landing on their desks, housing officials lobbied for new laws to tackle this seemingly growing behaviour that included noise, abuse, graffiti and inconsiderate behaviour.

From these origins, antisocial behaviour was always going to be focused on working-class areas and local authority housing estates. When it cropped up in town centres in the guise of 'binge drinking' and associated disorderly behaviour, it fell outside immediate policy concerns. Later initiatives such as drinking banning orders and alcohol disorder zones (Violent Crime Reduction Act 2006) tried to remedy this situation.

The American academic Michael Tonry (2004: 57) has pointed out that the British public did not really know what antisocial behaviour was until the government drew their attention to it:

> By making anti-social behaviour into a major social policy problem and giving it sustained high-visibility attention, Labour has made a small problem larger, thereby making people more aware of it and less satisfied with their lives and their government.

The implication was that now the government had to keep doing 'something' to contain the problem they had revealed.

The tackling of antisocial behaviour initially left social workers in a quandary. The new approaches left little space for understanding and welfare and even suggested the 'failure' of social worker and social work values (Jerrom, 2003). The Blair government was now ready to 'abandon long established taboos on judgementalism and on discussions of personal behaviour' (Deacon, 2002: 105). It was part of the rhetoric of communitarianism that said that if you have 'rights', you also have 'responsibilities'. Ideas were floated that suggested reduced benefits to those who committed antisocial acts (DWP, 2003) or refused to take treatments for drug dependency (HM Government, 2008: 27–32). Unemployed young people claiming incapacity benefit might also face tougher assessments to stop them from forming a long-term habit of not working (Grice, 2007).

The police were given new powers to disperse groups of young people on the streets and curfews could be imposed to prevent young people being out on the streets after a certain time in a certain area. Most high profile was the new antisocial behaviour order – ASBO.

ASBOs were a form of injunction applied for in the civil courts by police or local authorities on people said to be causing 'harassment, alarm or distress' (1998 Act, s. 1). The recipient of the ASBO is given a list of activities they must desist from and sometimes a geographic area they must stay out of. Most ASBOs ended up being on children and young people.

Failure to comply with the conditions of an ASBO meant an appearance in the criminal court where sentences rather than injunctions could be imposed. Some saw this as an unhelpful fast track into custody:

> The primary effect [of ASBOs] has been to bring a whole range of persons, predominantly the young, within the scope of the criminal justice system and, often enough, behind bars without necessarily having committed a recognisable criminal offence. (Council of Europe, 2005, para. 83)

It meant that two young people in a city could be acting in exactly the same way but one – subject to an ASBO – now faced a criminal court and possible custodial sentence, while the other one – not subject to an ASBO – may not necessarily have broken any law at all. No longer 'equal under the law', some young people could start to experience a separate 'jurisprudence of difference'.

One of the most difficult aspects of the ASBO for the social worker was the publicity that could attend the making of a successful application. Social workers, used to a veil of confidentiality falling over their work with young people in the youth courts, now realised that no such veil fell over ASBOs. The courts listening to applications were the magistrates courts, where there were no automatic reporting restrictions and the press duly provided names and addresses and sometimes photographs of young people. On top of that some local authorities decided to produce their own publicity leaflets to distribute door to door in an offender's locality to let the community know who was now subject to an ASBO (see Grier and Thomas, 2003, where examples of leaflets are reproduced).

The official line was that this publicity allowed communities to know something was being done and to help them proactively report anyone breaching the conditions of their ASBO. Others thought it was an unnecessary 'labelling' of young people that would only amplify their behaviour by acting as a 'badge of honour' or cause unknown damage to their development (see House of Commons, 2005, vol. 2: evidence 15 and 28). The Home Office minister responsible for this area of policy said she was unaware of any research looking at the effects of publicity on young people and she had '(no) intention to commission that kind of research' (House of Commons, 2005, vol. 3: evidence 111).

Practitioners did try to ameliorate the negativity of the ASBO and campaign groups became more critical, for example ASBO Concern. The individual support order (ISO) introduced in 2004 was a more positive add-on to ASBOs and allowed for more social work to be provided to young people. Researchers suggested that a more balanced approach to this work was needed, which developed a positive side (Millie et al., 2005).

'Respect', a government campaign launched in January 2006, sought to relaunch the need to be hard on antisocial behaviour to achieve more 'respect' from young people, but appeared to be not much more than a somewhat sloganising 40-page action plan (see www.respect.gov.uk). The Respect agenda was wound up by Gordon Brown, the new prime minister, who took over in July 2007, hinting at a softer line.

Young people who do not go to school

In the 1990s, one of the best known New Labour sound bites had been the need for 'education, education, education'. What was left unsaid was what you did with children and young people – and their sometimes collusive parents – who did not want education and did not want to go to school. Some 272,950 pupils were said to be persistent absentees in 2006/07 (SFR, 2008).

New Labour set out a new authoritarian approach towards non-school attendance and truancy. The education welfare officer or education social worker recognised that some truants had problems at home or were even phobic about schools, while for others truancy may have become just another 'routine activity'.

The Crime and Disorder Act 1998 (s. 16) gave the police new powers to intervene when children were found in public places when they should have been at school. Under the previous law, the police had been powerless because truancy was not a criminal offence. On the other hand, if you believed truancy to be a precursor to youth crime, perhaps 'something should be done' in the name of crime prevention; the parliamentary debate on the Crime and Disorder Bill heard that 5 per cent of offences committed by children were said to occur during school hours (Hansard HC Debates, Standing Committee B, 9 June 1998, col. 778).

In future, truancy would still not be an offence but the police would have powers – in collaboration with education departments – to patrol the streets to pick up truants. This use of police power was not an arrest, and the law was unclear on exactly what degree of force could be used by the police. The new powers did take the police into new areas that were primarily civil rather than criminal. Having removed the child to designated premises or the school in question, the police handed over to the education social worker for follow-up work.

Within schools, concern about levels of bullying have come to the fore and have been identified as a cause of truancy (Bindel, 2006). Bullying has also moved with the times to use technology. Cameras in mobile phones have allowed filming of assaults ('happy slapping') and bullying text messages have been sent between young people. In general, there has been a noticeable air of violence in some schools, with staff not being immune from becoming victims (Neill, 2008).

The only criminal offence connected to non-school attendance is committed not by the child but the parent. Unless parents are exercising their right to educate their child at home, they have a legal duty to register the child with a school and then ensure regular attendance – failure to do either is an offence. Social workers working with families have always been aware of this final sanction but their interventions sought to avoid it. Now the sanctions were to get heavier.

Parents failing to secure the attendance of their children became liable to a fine of £2,500 and/or three months in prison. Much publicity surrounded the imprisonment of an Oxfordshire woman in May 2002 (*Guardian,* 14 May 2002) and the government later proposed new 'fast-track' arrangements to bring parents to court within 12 weeks in cases of truancy. Section 23 of the Anti-social Behaviour Act 2003 went further, with its provisions to introduce on-the-spot fines for parents of truants.

Although all these punitive sanctions would no doubt be discussed between education and social workers before implementation, the rising levels of authoritarianism may question just how much the social worker is being drawn into what is about to befall the family with whom they are working. It would also raise questions about the further 'criminalising' of young people's behaviour by involving police in this new area of work.

Marginally more welfare oriented and supportive are the parenting orders (Crime and Disorder Act 1998, s. 8) and parenting contracts (Anti-social Behaviour Act 2003, s. 19), both available as a court disposal where elements of truancy have been identified. Social workers may be implementing both these initiatives. The parenting contract is not a legal contract but any non-compliance might be used as evidence for further court hearings; it formalises earlier initiatives by social workers and others known as ABCs (acceptable behaviour contracts) and builds on a well-established tradition of using contracts in social work (see, for example, Corden and Preston-Shoot, 1987).

Young people who commit sexual offences

Most of the concern about sexual offenders in recent years has been directed at adult offenders who target children and young people as their victims. It has, however, long been recognised that young people may themselves commit sexual offences. Guidance accompanying the Children Act 1989 advised that 'such adolescent abusers are themselves in need of services' (Home Office et al., 1991, para. 5.24.1–2).

The extent of the problem was explored in an influential report (NCH, 1992), which estimated that a third to a quarter of all sexual offending could be by young people under 21. Since this report, social work services to young sexual offenders have improved and spread across the country (Masson and Hackett, 2003).

At the same time as this acceptance of social work help to young sexual offenders, contradictory policies have sent shots across the bows of a welfare approach. In 1993, the law was changed to make it easier to prosecute young sexual offenders by lowering the age at which it was thought possible to rape, from 14 down to 10. Critics bemoaned the English desire to punish rather than help young offenders:

> the real concern is that the 13 year old boy prosecuted for rape is just another example of the law turning its back on a sympathetic approach to young children by treating them as criminals and putting them through the same justice system as adults. (Rhead, 1994)

Later research revealed the new laws to be little used and not particularly helpful (Soothill, 1997).

When the sex offender 'register' was introduced in 1997, young offenders, convicted or cautioned, had their names included alongside adults; they, or their parents, were required to notify the police every time they changed name or address, with non-compliance leading to a criminal sanction. The only concession given to young people was that the time period for which they had to register would be half of that imposed on adults.

From the outset, the inclusion of young people on the register was challenged as being unhelpful (NSPCC, 1997). Although it was not supposed to be part of the punishment, the idea that juveniles should be on the register for only half the time imposed on adults seemed to come more from the justice sphere of thinking than from any welfare orientation; arguments might even be made that young people should be on the register twice as long as adults if welfare provisions were being made to prevent them becoming adult sexual offenders in the long term (see, for example, Myers, 2001).

When the government reviewed the working of the register in 2001, it looked at a number of welfare options that included taking young people off the register altogether and giving a separate register for young people to a non-police agency (Home Office/ Scottish Executive, 2001: 28–9). These welfare-oriented options were welcomed in many quarters and the majority of respondents to the consultation paper opted for some change along the lines now put forward (the responses are accessible at www.sexualoffencesbill.homeoffice.gov.uk).

The White Paper that followed, however, simply ignored the position of young people who commit sexual offences (Home Office, 2002b), but it did show the new 'authoritarianism'. Section 91 of the Sexual Offences Act 2003 introduced a custodial sentence for young people not complying with registration requirements to strengthen the existing non-custodial sanctions. Why this new sentence was needed was even more of a mystery because compliance was never a problem. For all registrants, of whatever age, compliance was reported to be as high as 97 per cent and 'steadily improving' (Home Office/Scottish Executive, 2001, para. 4) and on top of that, the Home Office (para. 3) had admitted that it did not even know how many of those on the register were under 18 (see also Thomas, 2003).

Young people who persistently commit offences

If, for some young people, criminal activity was seen as fairly normal and even a 'routine activity' that would eventually be left behind, others posed a more serious problem. In the early 1990s, the 'persistent' young offender had been identified as someone responsible for an inordinate amount of crime.

In 1993, the home secretary's announcement of the new secure training orders were premised on the idea that they were needed for 'that comparatively small group of very persistent juvenile offenders whose repeated offending makes them a menace to the community' (Hansard HC Debates, 2 March 1993, col. 139). The 'persistent offender' was also offered up as part of the explanation for why youth crime statistics were actually falling at this time:

> one explanation for the apparent discrepancy between ACPO's [Association of Chief Police Officers] picture of greater juvenile offending and the decline in the number of juvenile offenders is a growth in the number of persistent offenders. (House of Commons, 1993, para. 15)

The idea of a core group of offenders who needed isolating and containing for the benefit of the majority is not a new one. The Victorians had called these offenders 'habitual criminals' that needed identifying. In the 1990s, the press named them 'blip boys', to suggest that they were different from other offenders and caused their own 'blips' in the crime statistics. Later, they would appear as the drug-dependent offenders who committed 'acquisitive crimes' to pay for their drugs or the 'active offenders' responsible for most of the nation's crimes and whose DNA we needed to record:

> it was estimated in early 2000 that the target of all *active offenders* would involve taking samples from 2.3 million to 2.65 million individuals. (Home Office, 2005a, para. 3, emphases added)

More considered research, however, found the 'persistent young offender' somewhat hard to pin down (Hagell and Newburn, 1994) and raised the possibility that this was another form of 'folk devil' emerging from a 'moral panic'. A report from the Centre for Crime and Justice Studies also questioned just how law abiding the supposed law-abiding majority actually was and pointed out how many people were potential and actual offenders when they chose to be (Karstedt and Farrall, 2007).

The youth courts already had the power to remand violent and sexual offenders aged over 15 years and those who had offended when absconding from local authority accommodation; in 1998, the age criteria had come down to 12. The problem was that 'persistent' young offenders did not usually commit violent and sexual crimes, and were not necessarily absconding from anywhere. The response in 2001 was simply to lower the criteria for direct remands to cover 12–16-year-olds 'who commit persistent, *medium low level offences* and who courts believe continue committing offences whilst on bail' (Home Office, 2002c, emphases added; Criminal Justice and Police Act 2001, s. 130); the absconding criterion was repealed.

The UN is among the critics of the UK's high use of custody for children and is:

> particularly concerned that more children between the ages of 12 and 14 are now being deprived of their liberty [and] ... deeply concerned at the high and increasing numbers of children in custody, at earlier ages for lesser offences. (UN, 2002, para. 57)

The argument that custody for young people was damaging and brutalising in itself seemed to have been lost along the way. The Howard League, concerned that young people detained in the prison estate appeared to be outside the remit of the Children Act 1989 and in particular its child protection provisions, sought clarification from the courts. The courts ruled that this 'disapplying' of the Children Act to certain children was simply 'wrong' in law. Local authorities with young offender institutions (YOIs) and secure training centres in their area had to start talking to each other about how child protection provisions in particular could be made manifest in custodial settings (Wise, 2003). This official denial of welfare had been going on for 10 years before it was put right.

One attempt at avoiding the negative aspects of custody has been the adoption of the intensive supervision and surveillance programme (ISSP). The ISSP was specifically aimed at the persistent young offender, to bring structure into often chaotic lives (Home Office, 2001). The ISSP was not originally an order of the court but could be built into other orders. As its name suggests, the ISSP offers rigorous community-based surveillance, with up to 25 hours a week contact with a young person (see Moore et al., 2004 for an early evaluation). The government now wants to make the ISSP a formal order of the court, where it can become 'the main response to serious and persistent offending' (Home Office, 2003, para. 20); provisions were duly included in the Criminal Justice and Immigration Act 2008.

Intensive supervision and surveillance programmes and some remands for young people can now also be accompanied by electronic monitoring and the wearing of an ankle tag. Any misgivings that these might be stigmatising and unhelpful 'Orwellian' additions to the youth justice system appear to have disappeared. Indeed, the Home Office was even happy to adopt Orwell's terminology and, without any trace of irony, proudly reported the new developments as 'a Big Brother-style approach to dealing with persistent offenders' (*Crime Reduction News*, April 2003: 4).

Another idea put forward involved the identification in schools of children as young as five or six as the adult offenders of tomorrow. This identification would be based on such factors as disruption in classrooms and non-school attendance. This idea had been tried in the early 1990s but discontinued because of ethical concerns and the seeming dangers of labelling (see, for example, *Daily Mail*, 15 February 1991). Now it was back on the agenda and deemed politically acceptable. Early intervention was better than costly custody that came too late and had limited results.

In 2006, the government announced that 77 'parenting experts' (clinical psychologists) would be appointed to help families prevent and divert their children's antisocial behaviour; this was to be the family intervention project but the press immediately dubbed them 'supernannies' after the reality TV programme of the same name (Ward and Wintour, 2006). This intervention was to be followed up with 20 pilot schemes involving up to 1,000 young people and their families. Contracts would again be used and if there was 'persistent offending', one way forward was to provide 'an assertive and persistent' approach to help turn young lives around (DCSF, 2008: 11). How these new services fitted with existing social and youth work endeavours was left unsaid.

case example

Robert is 15 years old and comes from an inner-city area of a large conurbation. He is currently the subject of a 12-month detention and training order (DTO) and residing in a local authority secure children's home – he was considered too vulnerable for a custodial setting. Robert has committed offences of criminal damage, assault, sexual assault and burglary; he has 39 previous convictions of a similar nature.

A meeting has been convened to discuss Robert's care for the second half of his DTO, which will be served in the community. Robert was made the subject of a care order seven years ago and has had numerous placements during that time. Before coming into care, Robert was brought up by his grandmother and believed his real mother was his sister; he was physically and sexually abused by various male visitors to the home. Robert has three siblings in care.

The meeting is attended by the YOT's social worker who will be supervising Robert for the six months of his DTO in the community and by the social worker who will be finding him suitable accommodation; placement with his mother is considered unrealistic. Robert's behaviour is considered unpredictable and even 'dangerous'; he is 6 ft 2 ins and weighs 18 stone. The education authority is seeking a school for Robert; he has a statement of special educational needs. A psychiatrist reports being unable to help because Robert has an 'untreatable' personality disorder.

The meeting was inconclusive as no placement or school exists as yet for Robert. A six-month ISSP was considered inappropriate because it would be too demanding for him. The possibility of further secure accommodation under the Children Act s. 25 will be looked into; Robert leaves his present secure accommodation in eight weeks' time when the DTO ends.

This case example illustrates the damage that can accumulate within one child by ineffective social work interventions; the outstanding work now required is overwhelming and leaves the social worker with almost nothing but a 'containing role', while awaiting a new crime or other event to take place. The requirement to 'protect the public' that is now placed upon social workers through national standards and other guidance is both nebulous and unrealistic, especially when accompanied by a lack of resources and a wariness from other agencies and professionals.

Conclusion

Contemporary social work with young people takes place in the shadows of new 'popular punitivism' and authoritarian interventions. Social work and welfare is offered to children and young people up to a point and then punishment falls in on them from the sky; once labelled as offenders, it is hard for us to see them as children first. As Dame Elizabeth Butler-Sloss, president of the Family Division of the High Court has said:

> as a society we are highly protective of children for so long as they remain innocents. Once those children get into trouble, however, society becomes unforgiving. (cited in *Youth Justice Board News*, July 2003: 9)

The police have moved into new areas such as truancy and antisocial behaviour. Social workers in YOTs now share offices with police officers and probation officers and we are told that 'we've got out of the mindset that you're either in welfare or in law enforcement' (Home Office minister Paul Goggins, cited in *Youth Justice Board News*, December 2003: 6). Whether or not social work in YOTs is surviving intact only time will tell, as they balance social work help to children in need at the same time as assessing risks and trying to reduce crime. Some social workers in YOTs feel glued to their computer screens and driven by the process of their activities ('form-filling') rather than being able to engage in 'real' social work.

Other elements of the 'new youth justice' give more optimism to social work. Restorative justice may be able to find space in reparation orders, action plan orders and referral orders. Restorative justice sees offending and antisocial behaviour as a 'wrong' committed on an individual or the community that needs to be put 'right' as a problem-solving exercise (Johnstone, 2002). Reports look promising, suggesting

> against the expectation of many commentators ... Referral Orders seem to come remarkably close to providing the basis for constructive and thoughtful youth justice. (Earle et al., 2003)

The requirement increasingly put on social workers to be evidence based in their work, mindful of research and ready to have work 'evaluated' may be a double-edged blessing. On the one hand, it can constrain creativity and autonomy but, on the other, it might prove useful in combating the excesses of 'popular punitivism'.

Social workers are otherwise in an unenviable position working with young offenders. As the criminal justice agenda gets evermore interventionist in family life, it does so at the expense of more generalised family support. Criminal justice strategies become the preferred way of resolving – or repressing – social problems and social workers could get caught up in the undertow. Although there are now signs of a more positive welfare approach, the level of debate among politicians is still depressingly low, with resort to rhetoric such as the need for 'national service' and yet more police on the beat. When they suggest a more understanding approach, they are ridiculed by other politicians and the press as wanting to 'hug a hoodie' (Thomas, 2007).

For further discussion of youth offending policy and practice, see Adams et al., 2009b, Chapter 26.

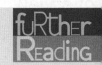

Boxford, S. (2006) *Schools and the Problem of Crime*, Cullompton, Willan Publishing. Useful source of material on school-related crime.

Crawford, A. and Newburn, T. (2003) *Youth Offending and Restorative Justice: Implementing Reform in Youth Justice*, Cullompton, Willan Publishing. Good reference work on contemporary approaches to restorative justice and related initiatives.

Garland, D. (2001) *The Culture of Control: Crime and Social Order in Contemporary Society*, Oxford, Clarendon Press. Stimulating examination of ideas, policies and practices.

Pitts, J. (2001) *The New Politics of Youth Crime: Discipline or Solidarity*, Basingstoke, Palgrave – now Palgrave Macmillan. Interesting critical exploration of the politics of youth crime.

Smith, R. (2007) *Youth Justice: Ideas, Policy, Practice*, 2nd edn, Cullompton, Willan Publishing. Up-to-date treatment of youth justice theories, strategies and practice.

Stephenson, M., Giller, H. and Brown, S. (2007) *Effective Practice in Youth Justice*, Cullompton, Willan Publishing. Critical discussion of the evidence base of youth justice research.

Thompson, N. (2002) *Building the Future: Social Work with Children, Young People and their Families*, Lyme Regis, Russell House. Accessible text dealing with aspects of practice.

STEPHEN HICKS

6 Sexuality

Chapter overview

This chapter examines the ways in which sexuality has been thought about within social work theory, policy and practice from the 1970s through to the present day. It discusses various models, asks which versions have been dominant or sidelined, and proposes an approach based on analysis of the practical and theoretical implications of sexuality as 'discourse'.

Introduction

What challenges face social workers working with lesbians, gay men or bisexual people? How has social work theorised questions of sexuality? Are contemporary ideas really all that helpful? These are the questions that this chapter seeks to address via an examination of the ways in which 'sexuality' has been constructed in social work theory and practice. The chapter will focus mainly on lesbian and gay issues within social work and welfare in the UK, but will inevitably also be concerned with the ways in which sexual 'normality' is produced and maintained.

I have organised the chapter into an overview by decade, looking at the 1970s through to the current day. This is a structural device only and is not meant to suggest a sudden switch or change of ideas. In addition, this is not a progressive narrative, working from the 'dark ages' through to an enlightened present. Actually, I intend to show how some ideas about sexuality have changed very little over the past 30 years or so, and there is a great danger in assuming that our contemporary view is the more liberated. Readers should also remember that this chapter is not an impartial account and I shall try to make my own preferences obvious. I begin with a discussion of 'sexuality as discourse', before moving on to give an overview of each decade. I relate theories to social work practice implications, taking the question of lesbian and gay parenting as my exemplar. The final section reviews the status of social work knowledge in this field and asks what happens 'after sexuality'.

A 'discourse' approach to sexuality and social work

The very term 'sexuality' is itself problematic because it is usually taken to refer to something possessed by a person, as in 'what is your sexuality?' This, of course, relies on a way of thinking that divides bodies, desires and actions into a series of discrete 'types', such as 'the lesbian', 'the gay man', 'the bisexual' or 'the heterosexual'. However, while these terms appear simply to describe the way people are, 'lesbian', 'gay' and so on are actually socially achieved ideas that are part of a wider set of sexual discourses that regulate what can and cannot be known or said. They specify particular ways of thinking about sexuality, but it is important to remember that there have been, and will be, other models. In addition, these terms are not simply different and equivalent, because discourses of sexuality are also linked to questions of legitimacy and power. Thus, heterosexuality is privileged and normalised, while homosexuality is accorded an 'abnormal' and lesser status. It is assumed, therefore, that everyone must have a 'sexuality' (Heath, 1982), which is organised into a series of types, hierarchically related, and in which heterosexuality is promoted as the norm.

I intend to take a discourse approach to sexuality in this chapter (Mills, 1997). The word 'discourse' is used here to refer to groups of statements that are regulated but also have effects. That is, a discourse of sexuality regulates what can and cannot be known, allowing some ways of thinking but attempting to exclude others. It also forms the objects of which it speaks. Cheek (2000: 23) provides a helpful definition of discourse:

> Discourses create discursive frameworks which order reality in a certain way. They both enable and constrain the production of knowledge in that they allow for certain ways of thinking about reality whilst excluding others. In this way they determine who can speak, when, and with what authority, and conversely, who can not.

This approach was first applied to social work knowledge by Philp (1979: 84), who argued that:

> beneath the apparent theoretical freedom in social work there is a form, an underlying constitution to everything that is said. This form creates both the possibility of a certain form of knowledge for social work and also limits social workers to it.

Philp drew on the writings of Foucault, so it is vital to remember here that Foucault's (1981) version of 'discourse' is one concerned with social practice and effect. Discourse is not solely focused on language and representation, it is 'a material practice with definite, public, material conditions of operation' (Kendall and Wickham, 1999: 45). This means that social work discourse makes use of institutional categories (for example the 'approved foster carer'), defines subjects (for example the 'gay man') and produces social effects (for example whether or not a lesbian or gay applicant is approved as a foster carer; but also the notion of 'the gay foster carer'). As O'Brien (1999: 151) notes, social work practice is 'deeply implicated in the construction of power relations in sexuality'.

Taking a discursive approach to sexuality and social work will be new to, and may even frustrate, some readers. This is because I do not present a 'how to work with lesbians and gay men (or indeed heterosexuals or bisexuals)' model for a number of reasons:

- I am critical of models that assume an obvious set of sexual types with their attendant characteristics. This kind of approach tends to suggest that social work merely needs to determine the 'special needs' of lesbians and gay men in order to avoid discrimination. I intend to argue that 'anti-discriminatory practice' (Thompson, 1993) adopts this model, and instead I suggest a more reflexive approach to the very idea of 'sexuality' and social work (Hicks, 2008a).
- People who use the terms 'lesbian' or 'gay' to refer to themselves are so diverse that to specify 'their needs' is to reduce that very complexity to a limited, and dominant, version of those categories, not least in terms of race (Lorde, 1984).
- Like Chambon and Irving (1999: xiv), I think that the role of social work theory is not to present 'how to' guidance, but rather to challenge 'the boundaries of our vision'. Succinctly, instead of asking, 'how do we work with lesbians and gay men?', I ask, 'how does social work produce the very categories "lesbian" and "gay"?'

I ask this because social work is a profession in which sexuality is constituted as an object of inquiry and classification, and expert status is used to define people's sexuality in ways they may not agree with. For example, social work practice is capable of enforcing the view that some people ought not to be sexual (disabled people, older people) or that their sexual behaviour should be curtailed. And this is because social work is an activity that constructs ideas about people and their 'needs' through the operations of discourse. A person's 'needs', their 'sexuality', the very idea that they have needs or have a sexuality are all defined through negotiations between the social worker and the client or service user, a situation that involves the operations of power. As Hall et al. (2006: 21) state, social workers and clients 'deploy morally informed categorisations which are not only established and maintained in interaction, but also derive their nature from available discourse routines'.

The 1970s

Much of social work theory during the 1970s was completely silent on questions of sexuality (for example Pincus and Minahan, 1973), and, where addressed at all, the dominant response was to define homosexuality as a 'pathology', meaning a disease that is studied, debated and defined through professional discourses. Homosexuality was a problem in need of help (in extreme form, a sickness requiring cure), or a danger that threatened the welfare of others, especially children and other vulnerable adults. The features of this discourse of pathology are exemplified by the 1975 National Council for Civil Liberties' survey of local authority social services committees' views on homosexuality. This noted that the authorities saw homosexuality as a form of disability, criminality or illness (Ferris, 1977: 32). Thirteen authorities reported active discrimination to prevent homosexuals working in residential settings, with children or the 'mentally handicapped' (the term that was then used):

> It is one of the more worrying findings of this survey that three authorities specifically mention the fear of sexual involvement with children as a reason for discrimination against homosexuals, while the replies of several others ... seem to imply a lingering belief that homosexuals are likely to be sexually predatory either towards children or more generally. (Ferris, 1977: 19)

There is little recorded evidence of a liberal equality position on sexuality and social work during the 1970s, and this did not gain prominence within social work theory until the 1980s. However, Carpenter's account, as a lesbian in the youth service of the 1970s, does highlight liberal views and the ways that those who held them were threatened by any real challenges to heterosexual superiority. Carpenter (1988: 172) recalls how heterosexual workers implied that she was 'always "pushing lesbianism down their throats"', and notes that lesbians' work to challenge heterosexual privilege was interpreted as a threat, since liberals preferred to see sexuality as a private, individual matter.

In response to models that tolerated homosexuality at best, and pathologised it at worst, radical social movements made very different arguments. Lesbian feminists developed various analyses of what they termed 'heterosexual privilege', in which they argued that heterosexuality, far from being 'natural', was a political institution designed to restrict the sexual behaviour and choices of women and deny the lesbian possibility (Rich, 1980). Similarly, the gay liberation movement questioned the supposed normality of heterosexuality, and argued that tolerance of homosexuality did not represent true liberation. Instead, gay liberationists stated that lesbians and gay men should 'come out of the closets' and openly declare their sexuality (Young, [1972]1992).

These lesbian feminist and gay liberationist ideas strongly influenced the development of radical social work theory in the 1970s, which argued that part of the role of the social worker should be, in fact, to challenge 'heterosexual superiority' (Milligan, 1975: 96). The *Case Con* editorial collective, for example, stated that versions of homosexuality as a sin, sickness or vice were 'ideologies perpetrating the supremacy of heterosexual norms and the oppression of homosexuals' (Charing et al., 1975: 2). Thus, radical social workers rejected the pathology models of homosexuality so prevalent in social work theory of the time, also arguing that expert psychiatric help was actually a contributor to such oppression. Remember, for example, that homosexuality was listed as a classifiable 'mental disorder' by the American Psychiatric Association until 1973. Radical social work also rejected the liberal tolerance model, calling this the 'cultural submission of the minority to the majority' (Milligan, 1975: 100), and made the important point that social work theory and social work practitioners cannot, and should not, be neutral on questions of sexuality. Neutrality was not seen as possible or even desirable, which may come as something of a shock to generations of social work professionals brought up on the idea that they should always be 'non-judgemental' and 'accepting of the person'.

Lesbian custody

case example

Sharon was married to Dave for 10 years and they had two children. Towards the end of their marriage, Dave had an affair and the relationship ended in divorce. Sharon subsequently met and started a new relationship with a woman called Marcia. For some time, she tried to keep this from Dave as she was worried that he would try to take the children away from her. When Dave found out about Sharon's relationship with Marcia, he was angry and instigated legal proceedings to win custody of the children. He argued that lesbianism was unnatural and he didn't want his children living in such a household.

During the 1970s, what was then called lesbian 'custody' of children was a key area in which issues of sexuality were very much to the fore. Social workers, lawyers, psychologists and other professionals were involved in cases in which the 'fitness' of lesbian mothers to care for their children was in dispute, and in which lesbians' children were removed from their care purely on the basis of their sexuality. Expert psychiatric or psychological opinion was used to reinforce the idea that lesbianism was a form of sickness or mental disorder.

Not all lesbians lost custody of their children, but in the cases where they won, it is possible to detect models that display liberal tolerance. For example, courts made distinctions between a lesbian 'preference' and 'practice', requiring those who were awarded custody of their children to be discreet about their sexuality. In one case, a lesbian was directed to live apart from her partner (Hunter and Polikoff, 1976: 698), and courts judged that political activism in relation to gender or sexuality was inappropriate. Radical models of sexuality emerged mainly in feminist commentaries and articles rather than in the court arena itself (Hunter and Polikoff, 1976).

Practice implications for social work

Social work practitioners should think about:

- How they can challenge discrimination based on sexuality within their practice, including work in the field of childcare.
- How they can challenge pathological views of lesbians and gay men.
- The evidence they can draw on to show that sexuality is no determinant of parenting skills (Golombok, 2000), alongside the need to ensure that children are protected from harm.
- Ways to recognise that being lesbian or gay is a political choice made in the face of 'compulsory heterosexuality', and not just a private or irrelevant matter.
- How they might link these ideas to a commitment to an anti-homophobic and pro-feminist social work practice.

■ How social work can be used to challenge anti-lesbian and anti-gay ideas as part of a wider commitment to social change.

The 1980s

In the 1980s, sexuality issues acquired slightly more prominence in social work theory. In the US, for example, major texts dealing with lesbian and gay issues appeared for the first time (Schoenberg et al., 1984; Hidalgo et al., 1985). However, it is important to be clear that pathologising models of sexuality did not disappear. In addition, much standard social work theory was still completely silent on questions of sexuality (for example Howe, 1987). Liberal equality models dominated where sexuality was addressed at all.

Epstein ([1987]1998) has characterised liberal approaches to sexuality in the 1980s as being dominated by what he calls the 'ethnic model'. In making arguments for equality on the basis that they were a minority group, lesbians and gay men relied on an '"ethnic" self-understanding' (Epstein, [1987]1998: 140), in which those categories seemed to describe a distinct type. The consequences of this model are a tendency towards 'essentialist' views of sexuality categories, the prominence of 'identity' models and liberal equality agendas.

Essentialist views of sexuality categories rest on the idea that terms like 'lesbian' or 'gay' refer to fixed, obvious and identifiable 'types' of person. In addition, these types are seen as unchanging across both time and place, so that 'lesbians' and 'gay men' are imagined to have always existed throughout history and across all cultures. Within the social work literature, for example, McMillan (1989: 31) argued that sexuality was an 'essential ingredient' of people, while Gramick (1983: 139) suggested that homosexuality had existed within ancient Greek and Roman cultures and that it was a 'natural phenomenon'. The notion of a distinct gay or lesbian identity was present in Newman's work (1989), and in articles which considered the development of 'stable personhood'. These claimed that the political analysis of lesbian and gay oppression was a 'militant' or 'aggressive' phase, which must be resolved in order to reach a state of 'self-acceptance' (Lewis, 1984). Berger (1983: 134) referred to a 'militancy' phase, which is 'aggressive', uses 'symbols such as gay or lesbian buttons [badges], eccentric dress, or exaggerated mannerisms', but must be resolved into 'self-acceptance', 'a less defensive posture toward heterosexuals'.

There was also a marked prevalence of liberal equality models in the social work literature. Dulaney and Kelly (1982: 180) argued that:

> Gay or lesbian individuals who accept their own lifestyle and are acutely aware of the daily injustice confronting those who are not heterosexual may need help in learning the efficacy of gentle education and positive modelling in influencing people's attitudes.

McMillan (1989) said that social workers should accept the equal validity of homosexual and heterosexual lifestyles.

However, it was during the 1980s that two neologisms began to appear in the social work literature. 'Homophobia' was originally defined by Weinberg (1972) as an individual dread of, or revulsion towards, homosexuals. During the 1980s, Wisniewski and

Toomey (1987: 455) surveyed 77 social work staff and found signs of homophobia among a third, while Decrescenzo's (1984) study of 140 mental health professionals found that social workers had higher homophobia scores when compared with psychiatrists and psychologists. However, this literature treated 'homophobia' as if it were an easily detectable, and therefore preventable, state. Tievsky (1988: 58), for example, lists a series of 'signs and symptoms' to detect homophobes. This is a problem for a discourse theory of sexuality, which would see homophobia as an enacted set of practices and ideas, rather than a condition or fixed set of attitudes.

The word 'heterosexism' also came to prominence in the 1980s, and this was used to refer to a form of social relations in which 'heterosexuality is assumed to be normal, and everyone is assumed to be heterosexual' (GLC Women's Committee, 1986: 5). Thus, heterosexism was used to define the oppression of lesbians and gay men as more than just an individual fear or reaction, but rather as a system in which heterosexuality was promoted as natural, preferable and normal. This concept was used by Hillin (1985) to explain why many lesbian or gay social workers were not open about their sexuality at work, and by McMillan (1989) to show why questions of sexuality were rarely, if ever, addressed by social workers in assessments of need.

Nevertheless, 1980s' social work literature showed little sign of what was perhaps the most important debate within lesbian and gay studies of the time, the 'social construction' of sexuality. 'Social constructionism' is a broad term that covers a diverse set of ideas that share an important purpose, the rejection of the essentialist models of sexuality discussed earlier. This is summed up in Weeks' (1985: 6) statement of a social constructionist perspective:

> My starting point was the rejection of any approach which assumed the existence, across cultures and across time, of a fixed homosexual person. On the contrary, I argued then, as I argue now, that the idea that there is such a person as a 'homosexual' (or indeed a 'heterosexual') is a relatively recent phenomenon, a product of a history of 'definition and self-definition' that needs to be described and understood before its effects can be unravelled. There is no essence of homosexuality whose historical unfolding can be illuminated.

Instead of assuming a continuity to the very idea of the 'homosexual', the social constructionists pointed out that sexual acts are given different meanings at different times. Thus sexual categories, like 'bisexual', 'heterosexual', 'lesbian' or 'gay', are ways of making sense of and indeed constructing the world. Such categories perform important functions of producing and enforcing particular views of 'sexuality'.

Section 28, foster care and adoption

CASE EXAMPLE

Rajinder and Mark had been together for six years when they decided to apply to their local authority to foster a child. Their social worker, Sam, told them that no gay men had ever been approved by the panel before, and so recommended that the couple consider respite foster care for a disabled child in the first instance. Rajinder and Mark were unsure about this but went along with it because they felt they might be rejected otherwise. Sam did not talk to the couple much about their sexuality, which meant that they were ill-prepared for potential problems that might have arisen at the panel, matching, introductions or placement phases of the process.

During the 1980s, a new right-wing discourse suggested that homosexuality was being actively 'promoted' by some local authorities. The Conservatives implemented section 28 of the Local Government Act 1987–88, which prohibited the 'promotion of homosexuality' by any local authority and outlawed the 'teaching in any maintained school of the acceptability of homosexuality as a pretended family relationship'. This impinged directly on the question of lesbians and gay men as foster carers and adopters. (Section 28 was repealed in Scotland in 2000 and England/Wales in 2003.)

Skeates and Jabri's *Fostering and Adoption by Lesbians and Gay Men* (1988) devoted a chapter to what they called 'myths and stereotypes about lesbians and gay men'. These included the ideas that:

- lesbians and gay men were deviant, unable to provide correct gender role models and a sexual risk to children
- the children of lesbians and gay men would automatically become gay
- lesbians and gay men were not 'natural' parents (pp. 20–1).

Skeates and Jabri (1988: 18) referred to these ideas as 'a false set of assumptions', but a discourse approach would consider them as versions of the categories 'lesbian' and 'gay', which perform the work of asserting and maintaining hierarchical ideas about sexuality. That is, they are not just 'myths' to be replaced by a 'true' set of ideas about lesbians and gay men, but rather are part of discourses about sexuality that aim to define 'normal/abnormal' relations.

One consequence of such ideas was that many social services departments blocked or refused applications from lesbians and gay men to care for children. Accounts by lesbians and gay men who applied to local authorities in the 1980s indicate that many experienced homophobic ideas, a focus on their sexuality to the exclusion of all else, psychiatric tests and even outright rejection (Hicks and McDermott, 1999).

Practice implications for social work

Social work practitioners should think about:

- How homophobic practices are ever-present, even within social work itself.
- Ways in which they can examine how heterosexist ideas and practices operate within everyday social work, for example within assessment procedures for potential foster carers and adopters.

- The various points at which discriminatory ideas about lesbians and gay men can operate within social work processes. Within the field of foster care and adoption, for example, this might include recruitment, assessment, the views of individual family placement social workers, panels, the views and practices of childcare teams and social workers, meetings with birth parents, the legal arena and so on.
- How the 'social construction' model of sexuality can be used to challenge essentialist views of lesbians and gay men as types with fixed 'needs'.

The 1990s

Issues of sexuality continued to be debated in 1990s' social work theory, but were still absent from core texts. Even *Radical Social Work Today* (Langan and Lee, 1989) ignored sexuality. Instead, lesbian and gay concerns found a minority voice within the field of 'anti-discriminatory practice' theory, and full discussion in a series of specialist texts (Logan et al., 1996; Appleby and Anastas, 1998; Brown, 1998; Hunter et al., 1998; Mallon, 1999).

Anti-discriminatory practice became a key theory in social work during the 1990s and remains the dominant approach to sexuality. Thompson's (1993) key text, however, devoted just five pages to 'sexual identity', while giving whole chapters to 'gender and sexism', 'ethnicity and racism', 'ageism and alienation' and 'disability and social handicap'. Indeed, Thompson (1993: 33) defined anti-discriminatory practice as seeking

> to reduce, undermine or eliminate discrimination and oppression, specifically in terms of challenging sexism, racism, ageism and disablism ... and other forms of discrimination or oppression encountered in social work.

In most versions of anti-discriminatory practice, then, sexuality was marginalised or placed at the bottom of a hierarchy of oppressions. In addition, lesbians and gay men appeared to be a group separate from disabled people, women or black people, which had two effects:

- There was a tendency to forget that lesbians and gay men could also be black, disabled, women, older or working class.
- Anti-discriminatory practice did not analyse the ways in which our ideas about sexuality also draw on ideas about gender, race and so on.

A classic example here is the way in which lesbians and gay men have been understood as 'gender deviants' (Terry, 1999; Hicks, 2006, 2008b). Further, anti-discriminatory practice promoted a particular version of sexuality categories that rested largely on the notion of sexual identities. Thus 'lesbians' or 'gay men' were seen as types with 'special needs' (Thompson, 1993: 139), and social workers were encouraged to understand them better. An equality model was therefore used in which it was argued that lesbians and gay men were not deficient but 'just different' (Thompson, 1993: 139).

Other texts also employed the 'ethnic identity' model of sexuality, in which practitioners were advised to acquire 'knowledge of the history, culture, traditions and customs, value orientation, religious and spiritual orientations, art, and music, of gay and lesbian communities' (Mallon, 1999: 23). Understanding the special characteristics of lesbians and gay men in this way allowed social workers simply to employ 'lesbian- or gay-affirmative practice' (Appleby and Anastas, 1998: 396; Mallon, 1999). In fact, readers were assured that social work theory did not need to change in relation to lesbians and gay men (Appleby and Anastas, 1998: 396), and these writers promoted the view that the job of social work was to help 'different others' assimilate into mainstream society (Appleby and Anastas, 1998: 102; Mallon, 1999: 33). Overall, lesbian issues were subsumed under a general model of homosexuality that tended to focus on gay men, and there was little, if any, attention given to theories that question or resist heterosexuality including forms of lesbian feminism.

However, an interesting parallel development within lesbian and gay theory of the 1990s was work that questioned and rejected such assimilationist or liberal equality models. Vaid (1995), for example, argued that a mainstream or liberal rights approach to lesbian and gay politics, that is, asking for the right to be included in what are normative structures, would amount only to 'virtual equality'. This is because a mainstream civil rights strategy would lead only to toleration of lesbians and gay men within an otherwise unchanged or heteronormative system and the acceptance of a narrowly defined set of beliefs about lesbians and gay men – 'not deficient just different'.

Brown's work on sexuality was important because she suggested that social work knowledge was itself problematic. Brown (1998: 19) said that social work knowledge was 'never neutral', and that attention should be given to an evaluation of ideas about lesbians and gay men. She listed pathological views of lesbians found in some social work theory (1998: 68), and the absence of any serious discussion of lesbian issues within most feminist social work texts (1992: 204). Brown (1992: 201) also questioned the tendency of some social workers to treat sexuality as an 'all or nothing' issue, that is, focusing on it to the exclusion of all else when dealing with lesbian or gay clients, or instead refusing to discuss it at all. Brown did not adopt a discourse approach, but the importance of her work is in its insistence on reflexivity with regard to social work knowledge.

Lesbian and gay foster care and adoption

CASE EXAMPLE

Sue was a single lesbian who applied to adopt a child aged six years or under. Her local authority had already approved a number of lesbian adopters and had worked alongside a lesbian and gay parenting organisation to develop some practice guidelines on assessment. Sue's social worker, Helen, incorporated discussion of Sue's sexuality into the assessment as a whole, and spent time talking to her about how she viewed her lesbianism, how others viewed it, how it might be handled with various people involved in the adoption process, potential pitfalls and how Sue had dealt with homophobia and other forms of discrimination.

Brown's (1991) work on foster care and adoption argued that social workers should be helped to feel more confident in assessing lesbian and gay applicants. She pointed out that the dichotomy of 'gay rights versus children's needs' was a false one, stating that no adult has a 'right' to be a foster carer or adopter, since all must be adequately assessed and approved, but that it would be wrong to exclude people arbitrarily on the basis of sexuality. Brown (1991) also encouraged social workers to look at a range of issues specific to being lesbian or gay when assessing such applicants. This was important because some social workers had felt unable to ask lesbians or gay men specific questions about their sexuality for fear of being seen as 'discriminatory' and applying extra standards. On the contrary, most lesbian or gay applicants wanted to talk about their sexuality and how it impacted on the fostering or adoption process.

Based on interviews with lesbians and gay men who had applied to foster or adopt (Hicks, 1996), I argued that, in many cases, a position of 'tacit acceptance' was in place. Here, agencies accepted lesbian or gay carers, but on the understanding that their sexuality should be a private or discreet issue, and that they should take only the most disabled or 'hard-to-place' children, that is, lesbians and gay men were to be used only as a 'last resort'. Later I argued that risk-based objections to lesbian or gay applicants – the idea that lesbians or gay men posed risks to the gender, sexual, psychological or social development of children – were actually based on the need to reinforce traditional views of gender and the family (Hicks, 1997). I argued for assessment practices that recognised the need to address lesbian and gay sexualities explicitly, but as a part of the whole assessment, not as the sole focus.

Practice implications for social work

Social work practitioners should think about:

- The full range of theories of sexuality (Weeks, 2003), rather than relying on anti-discriminatory practice models.
- How they can question a hierarchical or additive approach to the range of oppressions.
- The need to develop a reflexive approach to social work theories of sexuality.
- The areas of everyday life particular to being lesbian or gay in contemporary societies that are important to discuss with lesbian/gay service users.
- How they can recognise that lesbians and gay men are already disadvantaged within social work systems, such as foster care or adoption, and work to challenge heterosexist practices.

The 2000s

Lesbian, gay and bisexual issues are still absent from much of the social work theory, practice and education agenda (Langley, 2001; Logan, 2001, Manthorpe, 2003; Trotter et al., 2008). While 'measures' of heterosexism indicate a liberalisation of attitudes among social work students (Brownlee et al., 2005; Camilleri and Ryan, 2006), anti-gay ideas are 'still disturbingly present' (Ben-Ari, 2001; Brownlee et al., 2005: 491). Pathological views of lesbians and gay men are promoted by various right-wing Christian organisations that have developed well-organised campaigns to oppose all forms of lesbian and gay parenting (Hicks, 2003). It is therefore possible to see that many of the arguments from earlier decades remain, even though they take new and different forms.

However, there has been something of a resurgence of interest in sexuality and social work in recent years. In addition to UK national conferences in London in 2006 and Salford in 2007 (see www.ihscr.salford.ac.uk/SCSWR/sexuality.php) and a themed edition of *Social Work Education* (2008, 27(2), Sexualities), a number of key texts have been published (Romaine/BAAF, 2003; Mallon and Betts, 2005; Fish, 2006; Morrow and Messinger, 2006; Bywater and Jones, 2007; Myers and Milner, 2007; Fannin et al., 2008; Mallon, 2008). These show the influence of social constructionist, discourse, queer and feminist theories on social work thinking regarding sexuality, as do other shorter pieces (Spivey, 2006; Hicks, 2008a, 2008c; Jeyasingham, 2008; Featherstone and Green, 2008), although the extent to which these theories are applied to social work knowledge/practice varies. Crucially, many of these texts are critical of anti-discriminatory practice approaches, questioning what Featherstone and Green (2009: 61) term 'the sterile intellectual context of social work where dogma has often ruled in relation to anti-oppressive practice'.

Rather than a sole focus on lesbian, gay, bisexual or transgender (LGBT) issues, some of these texts analyse heterosexuality, heterosexism or 'heteronormativity', defined as those social and interactional practices that establish and maintain heterosexuality as a compulsory norm. Thus there is an engagement with how 'sexuality' is enacted or achieved within everyday settings (Fish, 2006; Myers and Milner, 2007; Jeyasingham, 2008). As Jeyasingham (2008: 149) argues, we need 'more scholarship which identifies the day-to-day practices and social apparatuses through which homophobia operates in societal and social work contexts', a methodological as much as a theoretical point. The role of reflexivity – that is, a practice that accounts for how a version of knowledge is produced – is also highlighted in relation to the production of 'sexuality' within social work (Hicks, 2008a; Myers, 2008). Myers and Milner (2007: 169), for example, have drawn attention to the ways in which sexuality is theorised across a range of complex practice scenarios, in order to

> enable social workers to practise *reflexively*, that is, to consider how their actions are producing particular constructions of sex and sexuality that have consequences for people.

However, the idea of particular sexual 'types', 'cultures' and 'needs' is still present, as is the practice of replacing 'myths' with 'facts' (Holwerda, 2002; Mallon and Betts, 2005; Pugh, 2005; Fish, 2006; Morrow and Messinger, 2006; Foreman and Quinlan, 2008). In addition, liberal equality models are dominant (Hardman, 1997), and the notion that the problem lies with phobic 'attitudes' is a recurrent theme (Bayliss, 2000; Spivey, 2006; Foreman and Quinlan, 2008). Attitudes-based analyses, however, tend to see individually expressed homophobia as the problem to be addressed. But, as Jeyasingham (2008:

144–5) has argued, 'homophobia' is often seen to be located within particular 'types' – those who are 'not secure about their own sexuality', those who have been abused 'homosexually', and gay, lesbian or bisexual people who have 'internalised homophobia'. If we add to this list the 'obvious, rampant homophobe', we can see that such ideas have 'enabled homophobia to be articulated as a problem of pathological homosexuality' (Jeyasingham, 2008: 146), or as a fixed attitude held by 'deviant' individuals.

For a discursive analysis, this doesn't work because it doesn't ask how sexual categories are produced and held in hierarchies within the everyday, as a part of mundane social relations. Smith (1990), for example, argues that 'homophobia' is a generalised concept that is frequently used as a causal explanation. He says, instead of events

> being actively produced by people in concrete situations, they are said to be 'caused' by ideas such as '[homo]-phobia'... [but this] does not have a concrete grip on how things function, this kind of theorizing is not much help in effectively challenging or changing the workings of a regime. (Smith, 1990: 634)

Reliance on the 'obvious homophobe' also doesn't ask how heteronormative practices work. As Speer and Potter (2000: 562–3) argue:

> Heterosexist talk is not a straightforward emptying out of preformed, stable, homophobic attitudes by the heterosexist person, nor something one can easily identify prior to analysis ... If one were to divide the world into those individuals with heterosexist attitudes and those who are (apparently) more liberal, one would overlook the point that the complicated contours of prejudice need to be understood in their interactional particulars.

Heteronormative practices are often subtle, disputed, and may be located within ideas about relationships, family, kinship and gender (Butler, 2004; Hicks, 2008b), all of which are at the heart of social work practice.

Conclusion

After 'sexuality'

I have argued for a discourse approach in order to interrogate the ideas about sexuality promoted within social work (Hicks, 2000, 2008a, 2008c; Hicks and Watson, 2003). Foucault (1978) argued that discourses have defined and specified a range of sexual types, so much so that sexuality is now taken to be something that can reveal the 'truth' of our selves. However, in doing so, sexuality itself was constituted as 'a possible object' (p. 98), as something that appeared to have a legitimate and factual status. Instead, Foucault (1978: 105) said that 'sexuality' in fact refers to 'a historical construct'. Queer theories, too, have asserted that 'sexuality' refers not to an identity, a being or a set of descriptive labels, but is a system of knowledge that frames ideas into moral and political hierarchies (Turner, 2000). The very categories heterosexual/lesbian/gay/bisexual, for example, are claims that involve the operations of power and result in the establishment of normative frameworks. Queer theories have also asked why heterosexuality currently exists as a privileged subjectivity that has the ability to define sexual knowledge. Why, for example, does heterosexuality occupy such a 'natural' or taken-for-granted status that it is rarely commented on? Contemporary feminism, too, has challenged biologically determinist views of sexuality and the privileging of heterosexuality (Jackson and Scott, 1996).

Social work is implicated in all of this because it too is involved, through a series of complex practices and statements, in specifying sexual subjects. We have seen that the versions of sexuality promoted in social work theory are of a limited type. I have argued that, when it is addressed, sexuality is usually theorised in the terms of anti-discriminatory practice, and this results in the establishment of a series of discrete sexual types with their attendant 'needs'. The concept that 'sexuality' is actually just a set of ideas is rarely acknowledged within social work, and other sets of ideas – those found within lesbian feminism, gay liberation, queer, discourse and other social constructionist theories – have yet to make a major impact. However, we are now beginning to see the emergence of alternative ways of theorising sexuality/social work that do draw on these ways of thinking, and it will be interesting to see how they impact on knowledge, teaching and practice.

Foucault (2000: 460) reminded us that we should not search for 'a sexuality' but rather ask, 'under what conditions something can become an object for a possible knowledge'. Social work has not done much of this, but instead prefers to replace past 'myths' about sexual types with present enlightened versions. The problem with this, however, is that it retains the idea that there is an object called 'sexuality' that is possessed by individuals. In addition, it does not recognise that homophobic discourses cannot be challenged solely by the assertion of 'better truths'. This is because homophobic discourses take many forms and are part of a wider privileging of heterosexuality as 'the normal' that defies the need for rational explanation.

Instead of creating more 'accurate' versions of sexual categories, social work would do better to ask how it contributes to the legitimation of some subjects over others. This would entail moving beyond the view of 'sexuality' as describing a series of discrete types to consider not what lesbians and gay men are, but rather what they are expected to be and what they might instead become. After 'sexuality', social work might ask difficult questions about the forms of sexual knowledge that it perpetrates. Then it can begin to recognise and even contribute to the many ways that people resist heteronormative ideas and practices.

For further discussion of aspects of feminist theory, see Adams et al., 2009b, Chapter 18.

LiNked reAdinGs

www.criticalsocialwork.com The online journal, *Critical Social Work*, contains interesting pieces concerned with social justice/radical perspectives.

www.theory.org.uk Has helpful resources on queer theory, Michel Foucault, Judith Butler, gender and identity.

Brown, H.C. (1998) *Social Work and Sexuality: Working with Lesbians and Gay Men*, Basingstoke, Macmillan – now Palgrave Macmillan. Key text that outlines debates concerning skills, knowledge and values in a range of practice contexts.

Bywater, J. and Jones, R. (2007) *Sexuality and Social Work*, Exeter, Learning Matters. Qualifying social work degree-level text, which outlines key sexuality theories and applies these to various areas of practice.

Fish, J. (2006) *Heterosexism in Health and Social Care*, Basingstoke, Palgrave Macmillan. Examines a range of research-based knowledge relating to health and social care work with lesbian, gay, bisexual and transgender (LGBT) people. It examines heterosexism in practice, engages with concerns about diversity within LGBT communities, and discusses some of the author's own research in health and social welfare fields.

Hicks, S. (2008) 'Thinking through sexuality', *Journal of Social Work*, 8(1): 65–82. Expands on the ideas in this chapter, outlines a reflexive analysis of sexuality in social work, and applies this to a worked example of foster care and adoption by lesbians and gay men.

Myers, S. and Milner, J. (2007) *Sexual Issues in Social Work*, Bristol, Policy Press. Asks a number of theoretical and practical questions about a broad range of sexual issues (not just those relating to LGBT people). Provides a number of case study examples that provoke questions about the ethical dilemmas involved in social work where sexual questions arise.

Social Work Education (2008) 27(2). A special issue on 'sexualities', with particular emphasis on challenging homophobia and questioning the norms of heterosexuality.

Weeks, J. (2003) *Sexuality*, 2nd edn, London, Routledge. Clear, useful overview text that outlines a number of different approaches to sexuality theory.

Frailty and dignity in old age

7

Chapter overview

This chapter explores the meaning of frailty and dignity in old age today, with an emphasis on the human rights of older people. An example from practice explores the complexities of care from the perspectives of users, carers and professionals. The importance of good communication and working together is emphasised. Consideration is given to the skills needed by social workers when engaging with older people who may be frail and in need of help and care.

Is it possible to be old and frail, yet live in a dignified way? For some older people – those with supportive networks and enough money to pay for their care – this may be so, but for many others, in a society that favours the productive over the unproductive, it may be difficult to live a dignified life where your needs are met and you are esteemed. Unfortunately, mental frailty is stigmatising, both for the individual and their family. In *Iris*, John Bayley's (1999: 249) tribute to his partner Iris Murdoch, which describes their later years when he became her carer, he discusses how:

> These days I find myself proclaiming to others, and to myself as well: 'She seems to want to go to bed about seven' ... Who is this She who has made an appearance, and with whom others and myself are so familiar? We are familiar because we are seeing her from the outside. She has indeed become a She.

As the above quotation indicates, the relative that one knew is not there any more in quite the same way, potentially becoming a problem instead. This can be the reality for family members and also health and social care agencies, who often become involved when carers cannot cope. One could say that the honesty of this statement is a blessing, stating what others might find difficult to articulate, but at the same time, if interpreted in an oppressive way, it could mean a restriction on the rights of a person who has become frail and old.

The language we use when talking about older people reflects the society in which we live. Demeaning words are often used incidentally to refer to older people as if they are not people to be reckoned with, but peripheral to important current events. John Bayley's quotation illustrates the dehumanising of an older person when she becomes frail, in this case mentally rather than physically. Yet it would be wrong to assume that we can use the word 'frail' casually, as if there is a common understanding of the term. Frailty can mean being weak, delicate and infirm, yet the term also relates to fallibility and foibles, as in moral weakness. To be frail may mean to demand sympathy; however, it could be a term used to indicate fragility in the sense of wrongdoing or omission through weakness.

Maintaining dignity is more than keeping up appearances: it relates to self-respect. It is a significant value because it is fundamental to human rights and how individuals relate to one another. Being in control in our society is synonymous with behaving as a worthy person should, because displays of uncontrollable behaviour tend not to be culturally acceptable. Despite the fact that Western society today is made up of many cultural norms and patterns of behaviour, being out of control or losing one's dignity are still associated with a lack of personal honour: a predominant norm is breached and the offending person is characterised as having weakness of mind or character, or, at worst, is deemed to be mad. Loss of dignity, often associated with bizarre behaviour, can be scary.

Social work and social care are about helping others to manage their lives so that as far as is possible their needs are met. By 'needs' we mean not only physical ones but emotional and spiritual needs as well (Maslow, 1954). 'Need', however, is a slippery concept – it is socially constructed and will vary in different cultural contexts. In addition, those who practise social work and may be assessing older people's needs are not exempt from being influenced by the dominant values of society today, which have been expressed as 'materialism', 'individualism', 'sensualism' and 'externalism' (Wolfensberger, 1994). The impact of such predominant values can manifest itself in many ways, including the use of language, routine and mechanistic practice and, at worst, abuse. Malin et al. (1999) relate these dominant values to the notion of 'community care', illustrating how their influence can affect service users and also those who construct theory through their practice.

The pervasive influence of ageism, which is an offshoot of those predominant values mentioned above, can influence our behaviour on a conscious and subconscious level. The notion of agency, that is, being able to form intentions, to consider alternatives and to direct action, is an important principle in the care of frail older people. Moves to models of care that put recipients in the driving seat through control of individual budgets mean a degree of risk in service provision (*Observer*, 9 December 2007). Yet despite the experience of illness and disability, having self-respect and autonomy are part of human rights. The Human Rights Act 1998 means that breaches of human rights can be followed up in the UK courts. Social workers and healthcare professionals can now link their good practice to human rights in order to reinforce anti-oppressive practice.

Frailty and dignity: an example from practice

In the real world of practice, there are often no correct answers, but rather complicated dilemmas, for no individual may have the right solution. Consider the following case example.

CASE EXAMPLE

Mrs Mary Flynn is 89 years old and lives with her son David aged 66 in a maisonette on a council estate in a city. Her husband Ray died some 10 years ago. David is divorced and has no children.

Mrs Flynn is becoming forgetful: she has left saucepans on the cooker until they burn and on one occasion the fire brigade had to be called out. Last week she told a neighbour that a thief had come and stolen her pension book. Later it emerged that she had hidden the book and forgotten about it, although some money had gone missing. It is difficult to hold a conversation with her because she repeats herself and makes inappropriate remarks. One neighbour is concerned about Mrs Flynn's continual accidents with the gas cooker and refers the matter to social services, who have had some short-term contact with the Flynns in the past. Mrs Flynn has enjoyed good health most of her life but has recently developed leg ulcers that are being treated by the local community nurse.

David has been unemployed since his industrial accident in his early thirties left him with the loss of one arm, one eye and serious damage to his back, which limits his mobility. With Mrs Flynn's increasing frailty, the household has become chaotic.

David visits the GP and tells him about his mother's forgetfulness and the incident with the burning pans on the cooker. The GP visits Mrs Flynn and suggests that she is referred to a psychogeriatrician. He recommends to David that he controls his consumption of alcohol, for David is known to have a drink problem. The GP suggests to David that social services might help with his mother, but he does not make a referral because David does not want social services to call. Mrs Flynn does not mind seeing the GP but is reluctant to see anyone else, 'especially anyone from the workhouse up the road' (the local hospital has a psychiatric wing built on the site of the old workhouse).

The social worker makes a brief visit but is not warmly welcomed by David. She holds a brief conversation with Mrs Flynn, who shows some signs of distress at her own forgetfulness and inability to do the housework.

The following comments are the initial observations of those involved:

- *General practitioner* – Mrs Flynn has dementia, she has had mild Alzheimer's disease for the past few years and it has been managed so far. It is possible that she may have suffered a series of small strokes, so part of her dysfunction may be multi-infarct dementia. Her condition appears to have worsened recently. Refer to psychogeriatrician.
- *Community nurse* – Treated Mrs Flynn's leg ulcers, some improvement in healing. She may have had a slight stroke, I observed right-side weakness.
- *Social worker* – Initial visit made to Mrs Flynn who appears to be forgetful and confused. Home conditions have deteriorated since our last visit a year ago. Mrs Flynn's son David is hostile to social services intervention. A neighbour reported that David may be stealing from his mother to buy alcohol. It has been confirmed that David has a problem with alcohol dependence; this has been noted before and confirmed with the GP. Mrs Flynn appears to have difficulty in communicating her needs. A full multidisciplinary assessment is required to explore support for Mrs Flynn and prevent further deterioration.
- *Psychogeriatrician* – Completed the IO subtest and the MMSE (see below). Evidence of cognitive impairment and clouded consciousness. Clinical judgement is that patient is suffering from dementia. Patient not overagitated and no evidence of wandering. Mood appears within normal range. Monitor. No specific drug therapy required.
- *Mrs Flynn* – I am confused about what is happening; why are all these strangers calling to see me …?
- *David Flynn* – Why don't they mind their own business?

The initial diagnoses by the professionals show similarities and differences. The differences are related to professional culture; each professional's focus depends on their professional judgement based on training and past experience. However, another aspect worth considering is the use of language and the power of terminology. Each professional appears to be using language that may be important in determining outcomes and yet may be difficult for users and carers to understand. For example, the IO is an information/orientation subtest – a diagnostic tool in the form of a questionnaire commonly used to diagnose dementia. The MMSE (Mini-Mental State Examination) is a similar test. All tests vary in their sensitivity, specificity and positive predictive value (Hall et al., 1993). For some commentators, who consider dementia to be socially constructed, alternative conceptual frameworks to biological models that reinforce pathology should be adopted (Palfrey and Harding, 1997).

Communication

A key issue is communication between the various professionals involved. In this case, like so many others involving older people, when professionals make their diagnoses, they rarely communicate them to colleagues involved and, more significantly, they do not communicate them to the persons directly concerned. Mrs Flynn's reaction is not untypical: she knows something is up because of all the visits and questions she is being asked. She might also be afraid that she is going to be taken away, that others may have the power to control her life. She refers to the callers as 'strangers'. Why should she communicate details of her personal life to strangers? Why does being old and frail give people the right to intervene in your life? One could say that the frailty and dignity of Mrs Flynn is already being compromised; her frailty is exposed by the professionals involved, but she herself may not know what is wrong, so she feels afraid. The problems of communication may also reinforce David's dislike of authority and fear that his life-style may be changed.

One role of the social worker is to be alongside, to explain and answer questions from service users and carers. It is hoped that the person who arrives as a stranger to help becomes someone who can be trusted. But one person alone is not going to solve the difficulties; the case requires a team approach. Better collaboration between agencies at the diagnosis stage is greatly assisted by organisational systems that are set up to allow the appropriate transfer of information. GP practices with attached social workers and/or multidisciplinary teams comprising health and social service personnel can often assist in facilitating the transfer of information in the early stages. It is wrong to assume, however, that being in physical proximity is enough; it is vital that communication systems exist and work effectively. Being open and honest about boundary limitations and respective roles is fundamental to good communication between professionals. Payne (2000) reminds us that failures in communication become power issues because the essence of cooperation and participation is effective communication. Without communication between professionals, boundaries and roles are unclear, leading to power struggles.

Could the social worker have assisted in easing communications at this stage? Possibly: if they had access to appropriate systems of communication, recognised the need to communicate effectively and were skilled enough to help. Let us look more closely at issues of communication with sufferers of dementia. Dementia can be defined as 'the impairment of higher mental functioning, including the loss of memory, problem-solving ability, the use of learned skills, social skills and emotional control'. The consciousness of the sufferer is not impaired, although the condition is both progressive and irreversible. Communicating with people with dementia is difficult and frustrating for all concerned. A quotation from *Iris* illustrates this dilemma:

> When Iris wakes the daily grind of non communication begins ... She does not ignore me or pay no attention; she seems to be listening to a garbled message. On the radio-telephone in the army the operator would have been saying 'I am not receiving you' or 'Receiving you Strength One'. (Bayley, 1999: 242)

Hepworth (2000) discusses how, if the processes of interpersonal communication break down, the individual sense of selfhood can be seriously threatened. He gives examples of where confusion and loss of memory are described through the eyes of the person with the condition in contrast to the external perceptions of family members. Dementia is described by the sufferer not as a blanket condition but one that moves erratically, with the dementia sufferer being aware of the change in perception and the inability to exercise self-control. Acknowledging such a change in one's abilities is a difficult and frightening prospect, and all the more so if the people wanting to know about it are those perceived to be powerful professionals who could remove one's dignity, emphasising and making public one's frailty. Hepworth (2000) considers that a central feature of an interactional model of dementia care is the recognition of the role of social approval in the maintenance of self-esteem in later life. Communication that involves a link with a 'can do' rather than 'can't do' approach can assist in helping an older person with dementia to cope with the illness. Person-centred dementia care that focuses on an individualised approach is outlined by Brooker (2006). Suggestions for improving communications include counselling and therapy built around the assumption of a positive identity.

There is also the issue of communication with David, who is hostile to social work intervention. He may be difficult to communicate with for a number of reasons, possibly related to fear. He may not be ready to acknowledge that there are problems, and/or he may have difficulty relating to a female social worker; there may be a range of barriers to effective communication between the social worker and David. In this case, both Mrs Flynn and her son are frail. David, as a man of pensionable age, may be exploiting his mother who is very elderly; his frailty may be the abuse of power that he wields over his mother, which takes the form of financial abuse. However, in old age, nastiness, vengefulness and exploitation can be a two-way process, and to assume that the state of being old is aligned to virtue is a myth. Vincent (1999) outlines in detail some of the power structures that can exist in the personal politics of identity issues and goes on to link these dimensions with macro-issues relating to professionals, state welfare, financial structures and the cultural attitudes embedded in intergenerational relationships.

It is often a crisis that brings matters to a head, for this is when actions are taken and decisions are made. The case example now moves on: it is two weeks later.

◇◇◇ CaSE EXaMPLE (cont'd) ◇◇◇◇◇◇◇◇◇◇◇◇◇◇◇◇◇◇◇◇◇◇◇◇◇◇

Mrs Flynn has a fall and appears to have had a stroke; she now has significant right-side paralysis of her arm and leg, her speech is impaired and her cognitive abilities have been further weakened. She is admitted to hospital under the care of a geriatric consultant. David remains in the house alone; his drinking is getting worse. When the social worker calls at the house, he is abusive to her. After a month in hospital, Mrs Flynn's physical condition improves: she can now walk unaided. Physiotherapy has eased the paralysis in her arm and she can just about care for herself. Her dementia, however, appears to have got worse. A case discussion is held.

The various opinions of the professional staff are as follows:

- *Geriatrician* – The patient is now mobile and is being assisted by physiotherapy, which should continue at home. Patient is ready for discharge.
- *Ward sister* – Mary has been assessed in the rehabilitation unit and can just about manage herself. Medication is now sorted out.
- *Discharge liaison nurse* – Mrs Flynn is referred for discharge. I have contacted the social work department who have been to see the patient on the ward. I have also contacted the community social work office and filled in the discharge details for a section 2 notice under the Community Care (Delayed Discharges) Act 2003.
- *Hospital social worker* – I have visited Mrs Flynn on the ward. I am concerned about two main aspects of her situation. First, her mental state appears to have worsened since her stroke and, second, her home circumstances are difficult. Mrs Flynn is keen to go home. The community social work office will need to be informed of the decision if discharge is to go ahead.

Other professionals involved but not at the case discussion have also made notes:

- *Psychogeriatrician* – Visit made to ward. Mrs Flynn's condition appears to have worsened since I last saw her. Completed an abbreviated test with her and this showed a poor response. There is some evidence of behavioural disturbance. Nocturnal restlessness could be helped by temazepam. Residential care should be considered.
- *Community social worker* – Message received from duty officer that Mrs Flynn's discharge takes place today. Not enough notification was given of pending discharge, so emergency care package to be put in until full assessment completed. Mrs Flynn wants to go home and her son David says he wants her back. The case notes indicate there may be concerns that David is financially abusing his mother, but this has not been followed up owing to Mrs Flynn's hospital admission and David's lack of cooperation.
- *Physiotherapist* – Mrs Flynn tries hard to regain her mobility. She scored reasonably well on the test in the rehabilitation flat, but her mental condition restricts her ability to understand instructions.
- *Occupational therapist* – Assessment required for aids and adaptations on discharge.

These notes and comments reveal the concerns of the professional staff involved in this case. They also reveal some lack of coordination and collaboration because, unfortunately, organisations and professionals often operate in a way that does not put the service user at the centre of decision-making. The person most involved is often at the periphery and what happens is often determined by factors other than the concerns of the user. In this case, some delay in assessment from social services, pressure to use a medical bed, the lack of coordination between branches of the medical profession and lack of communication between key players such as nursing staff and social services and allied professionals are dominating factors that demonstrate the use of power. Ideally, in a situation such as this, Mrs Flynn's case could be referred to an integrated care system where her concerns could be discussed and met in a coordinated way by all those involved in her care. Such an integrated multidisciplinary system is particularly important in cases where both physical and mental disabilities exist.

Yet evidence suggests that collaboration for the care of vulnerable user groups will continue to be a problem because needs are relatively unpredictable, best practices are unclear and different groups advocate different care models or underlying professional values (Johnson et al., 2003). Partnership working envisaged by the Health Act 1999 enables locally based multidisciplinary teams to manage the care for older people with dementia. The existence of a single source of funding, single management and clearly articulated goals can help to establish such a service. A study on Health Act 1999 flexibilities showed that trust is an essential element of success (Hudson et al., 2001). Trust is a basic human need, the necessity of which should not come as a surprise, yet lack of it appears to be a major stumbling block to working effectively. It is an essential requisite for collaborative endeavour across agencies, between individual practitioners and between practitioners, service users and carers.

Yet within the health and social care system, the potential for conflict is omnipresent. The pressure to free up medical beds is a critical issue in the care of older people. Recently, policy makers have taken a hard line on hospital discharges because they wish to encourage social services to use the period following admission to assess a patient's or carer's need and arrange discharge. When notice of likely need has been given to a local authority from the hospital under section 2 Community Care (Delayed Discharges) Act 2003, the social services must then assess and, after consultation with the NHS body, determine what services they will provide for a patient or carer. Statutory requirements, if not complied with, form a trigger for payment as a delayed discharge. One problem that can be envisaged in the case of Mrs Flynn is when her needs cross boundaries; she has some physical health problems but also some mental health ones that significantly affect how her needs will be met.

The final scenario ...

CaSE EXaMPLE (cont'd)

The social worker, Pat Smith, who is also the care manager, makes arrangements for an emergency care package for when Mrs Flynn arrives home. She is discharged from hospital back home but when the social worker/care manager arrives to complete a full community care assessment, she finds complete chaos in the house. The domiciliary care agency refuses to continue with care because of the state of the house and the difficulty of communicating with Mrs Flynn. David is nowhere to be found and the neighbours think he has not been living in the house for the past week. Pat is faced with the decision about how to manage the immediate situation, because it is apparent that the conditions at home are not suitable for Mrs Flynn. Pat manages to communicate with Mrs Flynn to some degree and it appears that she is pleased to be back home but oblivious to her own vulnerability within it. She decides to negotiate with an agency to clean the house and for domiciliary care to start immediately. In the meantime, she arranges for Mrs Flynn to go to a local daycare centre until the evening, when she will return home and be assisted in getting into bed by the care agency staff. Pat intends to call the next day to find out how Mrs Flynn is coping and assess whether the services are meeting Mrs Flynn's needs.

When Pat gets to work the next day, there is an urgent message. Mrs Flynn was found wandering on the motorway in her night clothes. The police found her and took her to the police station. The out-of-hours duty team were called out and Mrs Flynn was admitted to the psychiatric wing of the local hospital as there were no residential care places available. Pat visits Mrs Flynn the next day and finds her in a sorry state. She appears to have behavioural problems and is very agitated; she has been given a tranquilliser by the hospital staff. Pat visits the Flynns' home and finds David there. He appears to be the worse for alcohol and although concerned about his mother's welfare, says he cannot cope with her at home. As Pat leaves, he says: 'Mind you, she'll hate it up there at the hospital, she used to call it the old workhouse.'

The next sections discuss the issues in the case and offer concepts and theories that explain and put into context some of the problems that emerged.

Care management and early intervention: systems and individuals

Does care management as it is practised really involve care and management? This debate was raised by Gorman and Postle (2003). It was found that very often crisis management was prevalent and organisational structures were dominated by managerialist approaches. This meant that managers' views about meeting organisational requirements predominated over meeting the needs of Mrs Flynn. This contrasts with work that maintained a balance between individual, community and societal needs. Professional decision-making is bounded by a range of factors including cost containment, dependence on family and informal carers, changing professional roles and defensive practice. The care manager, usually the social worker, has to operate in a climate of role conflict and ambiguity. In our case example, planning did not take place early enough; Mrs Flynn's case was not perceived as important enough for intervention that may have prevented breakdown. Mrs Flynn's home set-up was less than perfect, but if appropriate help had been offered and accepted earlier, she may have remained at home with David as the main carer supported by domiciliary care. Being old and frail may have influenced others' perceptions of their need in this case. Working with older people with dementia requires time, patience and skilled help; unfortunately, in this case, Mrs Flynn's needs were not put centre stage and she became a victim of 'the system'.

Older people as carers

David was a difficult person to work with; indeed, his frailty as an older person was that he had personal problems related to his industrial accident. He was unwilling to cooperate, but maybe a relationship could have been established with him to develop enough trust to allow appropriate help to be accepted. His needs were mostly ignored, because as an older man with a drink problem, he did not demand the care and attention that 'more deserving' users could receive. He was frail in the sense that he appeared morally weak. There was an indication that David might be abusing his mother by using her money to buy drink. This aspect needed careful investigation and could trigger an adult abuse inquiry as part of the whole assessment of the case.

Looking to carers' needs is an important aspect of care in the community, especially as it is becoming more commonplace for elderly children to be caring for their even older parents. Carers' rights are recognised in the Carers (Recognition and Services) Act 1995 and in the Carers and Disabled Children Act 2000. Carers can be assessed in their own right for community care services. It is, however, important to recognise that carers' needs may differ from service users' needs and there is a potential for conflict.

Coordination and collaboration between agencies, professionals and service users

Working together has become a vital part of health and social care, although it may have taken time over recent years for both agencies and their managers to recognise the importance of this. The integration of this concept into policy and legal requirements has helped to reinforce professional good practice. The pressures against collaborative effort need recognition to enable barriers to be crossed; these include economic factors translated into competition between agencies, professional tribalism and differences in the priorities of the individuals working in health and social care. Both organisational and individual strengths and weaknesses play a part in the success or failure of collaborative work (Gorman, 2000a).

To work in collaboration with service users means being aware of the values, skills and knowledge that they possess, to work as co-workers with them. Yet this is not as easy as it might seem. Research shows that older people tend not to complain and are most likely to express satisfaction (Bauld et al., 2000). They may receive a poor service and have unpleasant experiences but do not want to make a stressful situation worse by complaining about a service or lack of care that they perceive as unalterable. Poor communication, lack of respect, and failure to understand the living situations of people in advanced old age were reported to be widespread among hospital and primary healthcare staff. Staff who have a philosophy of user empowerment can help to improve practice by influencing the systems that operate and convincing their colleagues of the value of collaborative work.

Social workers need particular skills

What sort of skills did the staff involved in the Flynns' case need in order to improve outcomes for them? Research has shown that there are a number of skills required in care management with older people: these include coordination, collaboration and networking, negotiation, teamwork and conflict management. Analytical and reflective skills, especially when used in evaluative processes, are particularly necessary and these are developed with experience (Gorman, 2003). Recognising the significance of emotional labour, which is the management of feelings performed as part of paid work, affects the state of mind and/or the feelings of another person. This concept has been applied to care management work in terms of how relationship-building is often missing from work practices in favour of more mechanistic approaches to the assessment and planning of care (Gorman, 2000b). Working with service users, when translated into how Mrs Flynn and David perceived the outcomes of intervention from health and social services, becomes a critical issue related to quality of outcomes.

It is important that money for care is spent wisely and effectively, and the systems are in place to enable the movement from hospital to the community to work efficiently. However, it is important to ensure that the process of work and the use of expertise in context are recognised as equally important, because quality outcomes depend on it. Staff need to be offered professional development as part of a continuing process within health and social care organisations (Gorman and Lymbery, 2007). Recognising this need and doing something about it is a challenge for agencies involved in work with older people (Gorman and Postle, 2003). Training approaches require a great deal of thought because blanket acceptance of competency-based approaches to social work have been criticised as contradicting anti-oppressive practice (Dominelli, 1996). In the same vein, it has been argued that such approaches can be reductionist, relegating the consideration of values, critical evaluation and the deployment of frontline knowledge to second place (Adams, 1998a). The Flynns' case is a difficult one and waving a magic wand to restore Mrs Flynn's mental capabilities is an impossible dream. However, it is possible to improve the quality of Mrs Flynn's life and that of her son David. Confident and skilled professionals who are trained to negotiate and work collaboratively stand more chance of success.

Reconsidering frailty and dignity: the human rights agenda

Whether it is using a carrot or a stick, consideration of human rights by public sector organisations and those who work closely with them is now essential. Acting in an anti-oppressive way, being mindful of the potential for discrimination against older, mentally frail people and making sound judgements that can be evidenced and supported by good recording practices are what human rights are about. It is important that staff in health and social welfare encourage service users and carers to be aware of their rights. Challenges in welfare are most likely to be claims under Article 8 of the Convention for Human Rights (UN, 1950), which requires authorities to take positive measures to secure respect for private or family life. There are other Convention rights that can be the source of challenge, such as Article 6, which relates to procedural fairness. Delay in performing duties, failure to recognise a carer's needs and cases in which there was a great deal of stress and anxiety are all situations in which there could be a breach of human rights and a claim for damages against a local authority (*Bernard* v. *Enfield LBC* [2002] EWHC 449).

Conclusion

Frailty is a multifaceted concept that needs to be considered in the context of human weakness, both physical and mental. Much depends on individual perceptions: losing one's dignity can be a matter of personal perception but one that goes to the core of a person's identity – it can mean the end of the quality of life. Social work is about ambiguity and managing situations that are problematic, so often there are no right answers but there could be better outcomes.

We can make some suggestions as to how practice could have been improved in the Flynns' case:

- *Putting the user and carer at the centre of the decision-making, that is, making person-centred care a reality:* Neither Mrs Flynn nor her son were involved in decisions. Mrs Flynn could have been more involved at the earlier stages of the case and when she was ready for hospital discharge. Working with unwilling clients such as David can be difficult, but more attempts could have been made by the social worker to find out what his needs were, especially if, with help, he could undertake the role of carer.
- *Better and more effective communication with people who suffer from dementia:* Using time to communicate effectively with Mrs Flynn may have built up relationships and trust that could have led to more successful outcomes.
- *Ensuring a balance between social and medical perspectives in determining wellbeing:* Tensions between medical and social aspects of a case can become polarised because the professionals involved do not recognise the strengths and contributions of others. It is important that social workers can articulate to their colleagues the significance of the social aspects of people's lives.
- *Greater awareness of the human rights of older people and the procedures that apply to challenge abuses:* Social workers need to be aware of the potential for human rights challenges and the significance of providing evidence to back up the decisions they make.
- *Earlier multidisciplinary assessment of the needs of the user and carer:* Opportunities were missed to harness the skills of professional staff for the wellbeing of the service user and carer. Everyone involved has a responsibility to share relevant information.
- *Better partnership working between practitioners and with user agencies:* All

the professionals involved were ploughing their own furrow. The systems were not in place to enable collaboration, a basic element of which is establishing common goals. When systems are in place, they need to be utilised effectively.

■ *Professionals need to update skills and learn new ones in a context of continuing personal and professional development:* There were several skills that could have been used in this case. Negotiation is an important skill that is underused and undervalued. Coupled with effective communication and a collaborative approach, the hospital discharge could have been managed more successfully. The lack of collaborative work meant that the discharge home had little chance of success.

Nowhere in the case example did we really get to know what Mrs Flynn wanted or what her interpretations of maintaining her dignity meant. Putting the service user at the centre of planning and intervention should help, but unfortunately systems that appear to prioritise other factors still dominate in our hospitals and social services departments. Maintaining a perspective that reinforces social justice and awareness of human rights can help to bring about change in organisations. Looking to improve one's practice through self-evaluation, careful appraisal of one's own practice, reflexivity and research-mindedness is a desired approach. A word of warning, however, about the fashionable stances of welfare practice that purport to follow a policy of social inclusion, the reality of which can be engagement on our terms. Our intentions may be good, but they can be perceived by the service user as patronising. Really listening and taking advice from elders is a positive vision for the future (Simey, 2000).

We cannot always make things right, but with skilled social work intervention, we can help to ease the burdens of older people who have become frail and are in danger of losing their dignity. Becoming old should not be synonymous with a poor quality of life. The challenge for social workers with frail older people in today's work environment is to trust themselves, the service users and their health and social care colleagues much more.

For further discussion of aspects of work with older people, see Adams et al., 2009b, Chapter 32.

www.careinfo.org/dementia Practical information, news, key organisations, books, conferences and access to the *Journal of Dementia Care.*

www.dh.gov.uk/en/consultations/Liveconsultations *Transforming the Quality of Dementia Care: Consultation on a National Dementia Strategy.*

The recommended reading focuses on partnership work with other agencies in helping people with dementia and their carers and emphasises the importance of person-centred care.

Brooker, D. (2006) *Person-centred Dementia Care: Making Services Better. Bradford Dementia Group Good Practice Guides*, London, Jessica Kingsley. Contains helpful hints for practitioners.

Gorman, H. and Postle, K. (2003) *Transforming Community Care: A Distorted Vision?*, Birmingham, Venture Press. Discusses the dilemmas in sourcing and arranging community care packages for older people in their own homes, and critiques notions of empowerment.

Marshall, M. and Tibbs, M. (2006) *Social Work with People with Dementia: Partnerships, Practice and Persistence*, Bristol, BASW/Policy Press. Examines what is involved in working in partnership with and for older people with dementia.

Payne, M. (2007) 'Partnership working in the interdisciplinary agenda', in M. Lymbery and K. Postle (eds) *Social Work: A Companion to Learning*, London, Sage. Discusses why partnership is critical in health and social care.

Simey, M. (2000) 'How and where I found independence', in M. Simmons (ed.) *Getting a Life: Older People Talking*, London, Peter Owen/Help the Aged. Contains useful accounts of older people speaking for themselves.

Wilkinson, H. (ed.) (2002) *The Perspectives of People with Dementia: Research Methods and Motivations*, London, Jessica Kingsley. Examines research questions, such as giving a voice to the user with dementia.

Risk, rights and anti-discrimination work in mental health

8

This chapter discusses how disabled people and mental health service users are prevented from doing things on the grounds of potential risk. Anti-discriminatory and rights-based practice can stop this from happening unfairly, increase people's autonomy and social participation and avoid using risk-thinking as an excuse to limit opportunities.

Chapter overview

The risk to others: care staff, service users, the wider public – and cats

The risk to cats

Emma Stevens, from Blackburn, Lancashire, was turned down by the Cats' Protection League as a potential cat owner on the grounds that, being deaf, she would not be able to hear the cat if it was in distress. A spokesperson for the Cats' Protection League said she was well placed to judge as she had experience of working with deaf children. A deaf person living alone could not look after a cat – 'the cat comes first' (*Lancashire Evening Telegraph,* 24 December 2003). The deaf woman said 'I felt offended.' She planned to find a cat from another source.

The risk to care staff

Two women with physical and learning disabilities challenged East Sussex County Council's policy that staff should not get involved in manual lifting and handling. Disabled people's requirements to be helped in and out of bed, or the bath, presented a risk to the staff's backs; so policies preventing staff from manual lifting and handling were put in place. Following the case, other examples emerged, including one in which Ms Wolstenholme from Milton Keynes had slept in her wheelchair for months, apparently because staff were not permitted to lift her. Ms Wolstenholme weighed 7 stone. She stated that when five health officials visited her to decide if they could use slings or hoists to lift her, she fell. 'I asked them for help. They did not. They watched me crawling on the floor.'

In other instances, elderly relatives noted that they lifted the disabled person in and out of bed while care staff stood by. Mr Maddison of Dewsbury managed to secure home care for his wife, but writes:

> We soon found out that we were paying more than £5 an hour for a service that was completely useless because of the tasks the carers were not allowed to do. Banned tasks included lifting the patient; giving the patient a shower (even though we have a special wheelchair and shower); administering prescribed medication (over the counter stuff was OK); moving patient's position in chair or bed; opening or closing a window above head height; assisting patient with toileting. (*Daily Mail*, 16 September 2003)

The risk to service users

Wright and Easthorne (2003) found that disabled students trying to enter nursing encountered barriers based on fears for the health and safety of service users. Deaf people were assumed to be a health and safety risk as they might not be able to hear alarms. Students with dyslexia were seen as a risk in administering medication. Students with mental health problems were thought to pose a potential risk of violence. Following nurse Beverly Allitt's murder of children in her care, many NHS trusts introduced the infamous 'two-year rule', requiring anyone entering nursing or working as a nurse to have been free of psychiatric treatment for two years. This has since been lifted.

When social worker Peter van der Gucht submitted his registration details under the General Social Care Council (GSCC) social care registration system, he was approved for practice only under stringent conditions, for example regular checks and new assessments at the point of any job change. The reason was his diagnosis of bipolar disorder. This was despite the fact that, in over 17 years of successful practice, he had always managed his condition effectively, been open with his line manager and agreed an approach to take if he became unwell.

The risk to the wider public

When a woman jogger was stabbed to death in London, in 2003, Philip Johnston wrote in the *Telegraph* (10 December 2003):

> Police were astonished to find at least 30 care-in-the-community hostels, containing more than 400 ill people close to Victoria Park in Hackney where she was murdered. None of these institutions is secure. This is the legacy of one of the great scandals of modern times: the abject failure of care in the community.

These comments were made before any arrest. It seems it was not necessary to have any evidence that the murder had been committed by one of the '400 care-in-the-community patients' before interpreting the murder as a community care failure.

There still appears to be no taboo against viewing 'psychiatric patients' as guilty until proven innocent.

Some cases are more complex. Ms Brazier, who has a diagnosis of psychosis, was threatened with eviction after causing a nuisance to neighbours. This raises the question: Is it reasonable to evict someone who poses no threat, but does cause disturbance, due in part to a mental health problem?

The risk to self

Mr Paul had long-term depression. He applied for two part-time jobs with the probation service – a community service supervisor and a handyman. He was offered the handyman man post but turned down for the supervisor post on the grounds that it was thought too stressful for him. This decision was made without consulting him, his psychiatrist or the organisation with whom he had successfully been volunteering for some years.

Tom White has diabetes. At 16, he was refused permission to go on school trips in case he had a glycaemic attack.

The simultaneous risk to self and others

On 17 January 2004, the *Mirror* reported:

> Eleven friends were ordered to get off a packed holiday flight seconds before take-off – because they were deaf. The pilot claimed the group was a liability to the safety of the plane. One passenger said 'The pilot thought that because we were deaf we would not be able to follow emergency instructions'. The humiliated passengers are now seeking compensation from easyJet.

In 2003, Anthony Ford-Shubrook, who has cerebral palsy, got the GCSEs he needed to study information technology (IT) at the only sixth-form college in his area offering the courses of his choice. But the IT department was on the first floor and there was no lift. His parents offered to buy a 'climbing' wheelchair. The college refused him entry, as the wheelchair would be a health and safety risk – to Anthony and other students.

Discussion: is risk approached fairly?

Some academic commentators have argued that an ever-increasing focus on risk makes us excessively risk averse. Children spend all their time sitting at home or being driven from one place to another, for fear of the danger of the streets. Government demands for risk assessment and accountability at a micro-level distort the activities of public services, de-emphasising positive and imaginative developments in favour of defensive practice to avoid disaster. For example, Rose (1998: 180) argues that society has become overpreoccupied with preventing dangers:

> Some go as far as to claim that we live in a 'risk society', which is no longer structured by belief in progress and concerns over the distribution of 'goods' (wealth, health, life chances and so on), but rather is saturated with fear and foreboding, and structured by concerns over the distribution of 'bads' or dangers.

O'Neill (2002) refers to the increasingly centralised policies concerned with risk management. It is undeniable that, in some circumstances, risk-thinking is used unfairly in relation to disabled people, including people with mental health problems. There are instances of institutionalised, not individual, unfairness, for example no lifting policies in local authorities. The following three important themes run through the examples confirmed by research, case law and health and social care practice.

Impairment as a fixed problem

The tendency of decision makers to see an impairment as a fixed problem – posing risks – rather than thinking first how to resolve the apparent problem has been reported in numerous consultations and surveys of the experiences of disabled people (Barnes, 1991; Campbell and Oliver, 1996; DRC, 2004, 2007a). To give one example, 60 per cent of deaf people report that they find primary care inaccessible (Knight et al., 2002), because they do not know when their appointment comes up or cannot communicate with the GP. If, however, the appointments are shown on a visual screen and GPs learn to speak directly to someone who lip-reads or work with British Sign Language interpreters, what seemed a fixed problem can disappear. Imagination is required rather than a reflex response that 'this is not possible'. The findings of a Disability Rights Commission (DRC, 2006a) formal investigation into health inequalities experienced by people with mental health problems and/or learning disabilities included that people with long-term mental health problems were significantly more likely than other citizens to get 'killer' diseases (heart disease, respiratory illness, diabetes, breast cancer, bowel cancer), they were more likely to get them young, and to die of them faster. This was partly because of major barriers to healthcare, for example difficulty in making appointments by phone at fixed times, or waiting in a waiting room; and 'diagnostic overshadowing', whereby clinicians saw and treated the mental health condition but overlooked physical disorders. Despite these barriers, the investigation found that health service providers saw the 'problem' as residing in the individual. As the researchers put it:

> In almost all interviews with primary care staff we heard about patients from these groups who don't follow advice as given, don't attend for appointments and who can't cope with the implications of the advice they have been given. There did not seem to be any strategies in place to support these groups to follow any advice or guidance they might have been given. (Samele et al., 2006)

A DVD made as part of this investigation (DRC, 2006b) shows a range of straight-forward, reasonable adjustments that can overcome the service barriers, for example enabling someone who is anxious waiting in a waiting room to wait in their car and be called by mobile phone when the appointment comes up, or training of clinicians by mental health service users to help overcome diagnostic overshadowing.

In relation to the other examples above, if the IT department is moved to the ground floor, a wheelchair user can study the A levels of his choice. If hospitals have flashing lights as alarms as well as sirens, or arrangements in place that colleagues will alert deaf people to the emergency, then deaf people can practise in nursing without danger. If someone is unable to travel in the rush hour due to panic attacks, the answer is not to refuse them the job but to explore whether the hours can be changed or some home working permitted. This is simple good practice under the Disability Discrimination Act (DDA) 1995, which requires employers and service providers to make reasonable adjustments, so that disabled people are not treated 'less favourably'.

Judgements about potential risk to others

Judgements about potential risk to others are used to disadvantage disabled people – especially those with psychiatric disabilities – in ways that would never be considered acceptable in relation to non-disabled people. It has often been noted that a mental health service user can be compulsorily detained for a level of risk of violence, which – if it were applied to young men who drink alcohol – would mean thousands of young men detained in advance of committing any crime (Sayce, 1995). There is no actuarial basis for allowing preventive detention in advance of crime for people with psychiatric disabilities and no one else. Moreover, when a mental health service user is deemed a 'high risk of violence', for example because they have allegedly hit someone, they have not had the opportunity to be tried in a court of law. They might be innocent but have no way to prove it.

Although 'community care' has facilitated greater autonomy for people with psychiatric disabilities and is preferred by them to institutional care (Leff et al., 1996), it is often considered a 'failure'. Frank Dobson, when secretary of state for health, famously stated that 'community care has failed', seemingly on the grounds of a number of high-profile homicides during the 1990s. This assessment ignores the important evidence that the proportion of homicides committed by people with mental disorders actually went down steadily over the period of deinstitutionalisation – from about 35 per cent in 1957 to 11.5 per cent in 1995, according to Home Office figures (Taylor and Gunn, 1999). Evidence that could be used to reach fair judgements can be ignored in favour of populist reactions. These feed into policies that appear to expect health and social care staff to reduce risk virtually to nil. This is extremely hard to achieve without a significant encroachment on human rights.

Mental health law itself – including the Mental Health Act 2007 – discriminates against psychiatric service users, in allowing them (but not other citizens) to be treated without consent even when they are legally 'capable' of making decisions for themselves. Organisations including the Disability Rights Commission (DRC, 2002) argued instead that a threshold of 'capacity' should be used, with only those demonstrably lacking capacity being treated without consent:

> Suppose I have two patients, one with schizophrenia and one with cancer. Both patients recognise that they are ill, that their illnesses can be treated and that there would be consequences to not receiving treatment. They both have the same level of understanding of their illness and the proposed treatment – in legal terms they are both capable. The patient with cancer may refuse my treatment and if I go ahead with it I will be committing an assault. But I will have a legal duty to impose treatment on the patient with schizophrenia ... If my patient has both conditions he will be able to refuse treatment for the cancer but not for the schizophrenia. This is unfair, absurd and makes the mentally ill lesser citizens. (Dr Tony Zigmund, Royal College of Psychiatrists, writing in the *Independent*, 30 June 2002)

These patterns of unfair judgements about risk to others mean that social goods – community living, parenting, work – can be jeopardised (Sayce, 2000). When the government introduced its Independent Living Strategy in 2008, some commentators raised the spectre that with more individuals potentially controlling their own care budgets, they might misspend them (on holidays, prostitutes, drugs and so on) and damage the reputation of national and local politicians. Others, more moderately, noted that the benefits of increased control for large numbers would be likely to outweigh the risk of a small level of fraudulent use and that politicians could be supported to take considered risks by non-governmental organisations committed to choice and control.

The notion of risk to self

The notion of risk to self can be just as pernicious as the risk to others. Corrigan et al. (2001) found that what they called the 'stigma of benevolence' towards people with mental health problems was as much associated with discriminatory public attitudes – including authoritarian responses and a desire for social distance – as was the assumption that people were a risk to others. Protecting 'vulnerable' people from harm – although well intentioned – can be stifling. The 1970s' disabled people's movement began in Britain when people with physical impairments living in residential homes broke the rules that kept them safely inside after the typically early institutional supper and wheeled themselves to the pub (Campbell and Oliver, 1996).

Attempts to prevent mental health service users from taking up stressful jobs – as happened with Mr Paul above – are widespread. One study found that of people with mental health problems who were working, about 40 per cent had been told by mental health workers that they would never work again (Rinaldi and Hill, 2000). A 1995 MORI survey found that the public was most likely to accept people with mental illness as road sweepers, actors, comedians or farm workers and least likely to accept them as doctors, child minders, police officers or nurses. It seems that madness co-exists in the public mind with the most menial and the most creative jobs – but not with jobs requiring responsibility. In reality, many decision makers have had mental health problems. The attitude that mental illness is incompatible with responsibility may, however, help to explain why people with mental health problems so often work at levels below their qualifications and capacity, if they are working at all.

People with mental health problems are less likely to be in work than any other group of disabled people, partly because of extreme employer prejudice. A 2001 evaluation of the government's ONE programme (DWP, 2001), designed to increase employment opportunities for people excluded from the labour market, found that despite acute labour shortages, only 37 per cent of employers said they would in future take on people with mental illness. This compared to 62 per cent who would take on physically disabled people, 78 per cent long-term unemployed people and 88 per cent lone parents.

A joint study by the DRC and the Health and Safety Executive found that health and safety are sometimes used as a 'false excuse' not to employ disabled people. A review of case law concludes that stereotyped views, wrong decisions and excessively cautious risk assessments may all act as unnecessary, but still sometimes lawful, barriers, so long as they do not give rise to decisions so perverse as to fall outside the range of responses open to a reasonable employer (DRC/HSE, 2003). Case law shows that employers are particularly likely to use health and safety justifications when defending against charges of discrimination brought by people with psychiatric disabilities (DRC, 2003).

This brief review shows that risk is not applied neutrally to disabled people. Disabled people are seen through a lens of risk.

The lens of risk

There is evidence of systemic patterns of discrimination in decision-making based on risk in Britain – across fields including employment, education, transport and health and social services. Assumptions about the risk to self and others go untested, often they are exaggerated and then applied unfairly, in ways that restrict people's autonomy and in some cases their human rights.

People with psychiatric disabilities are viewed as particularly high risk to others, but also as risks to themselves. They might be unable to cope, or a job may be too stressful for them. The discourse of risk is the justification for severe constraint on social participation.

Within the risk-dominated stereotypes, there is precious little attention to the (very high) risk of social exclusion. In reality, a concentration on risk in terms of violence and vulnerability leads to social exclusion, as people's autonomy is denied and the wider public's tendency to desire social distance is magnified. A mark of respect towards mental health service users would be to stop subjecting this group to a different set of assumptions and rules on risk than that which applies to other citizens. Without risk, there can be no autonomy, no social participation and no achievement.

Clinically, Repper and Perkins (2003) have noted that risk is essential for recovery – for resuming roles and attaining hope. No one can do anything without risk of failure, they argue. Every new relationship means the risk of rejection, every job application means the risk of not getting it, every outing means the risk of being run down by a bus. But without risk, there is also no hope – confidence is eroded and opportunities limited. It is the job of mental health workers to support people in taking risks – not systematically avoiding them. Shepherd et al. (2008) note that people have the right to take some types of risk. Encouraging very low risk often means low expectations, which, they say, can become a self-fulfilling prophesy.

What can be done to challenge discriminatory approaches to risk?

Some of the individuals in the examples at the beginning of this chapter have – or could have – challenged discrimination or human rights abuses under existing legislation.

Peter van der Gucht challenged the GSCC and won. Moreover, the DRC under-took a formal investigation into fitness standards used to guard entry to (and exit from) the professions of social work, nursing and teaching. They concluded that the fitness standards could be used to discriminate and recommended scrapping them (DRC, 2007b). In 2007, the GSCC agreed and, in 2008, government was seeking ways to amend primary legislation to achieve this in relation to social work. This should mean that a diagnosis alone should not create a barrier to professional practice. Rather, the decision would have to be made on a case-by-case basis as to whether the person could actually do the job, with adjustments if required.

Tom White argued that it was discriminatory to stop him going on school trips, particularly without doing an individualised assessment of the risks. He took a case under the DDA 1995 and won. This sent a message to schools and colleges that blanket bans – on the basis of assumptions or stereotypes – are not acceptable. The key is to assess individually and make adjustments – such as providing extra support – where necessary. The failure to do so is discriminatory and is illegal.

Mr Paul took a DDA case and won. The Employment Appeal Tribunal ruled that the employer could have scrutinised the occupational health assessment with more care, obtained specialist advice from Mr Paul's consultant, spoken further with Mr Paul himself and looked at adjustments to the job to enable Mr Paul to do it. Again a blanket ban on the basis of diagnosis – and the assumption that depression meant he could not do this job – was not acceptable. It was discriminatory. The probation service was instructed to provide Mr Paul with the next available suitable vacancy and he therefore obtained the work he wanted, as a community service supervisor.

It would be possible for a deaf person to challenge being rejected as a cat owner – on the grounds that she appears to have been treated 'less favourably' by a provider of services, arguably without justification. It is not yet possible for deaf people to challenge being thrown off an aeroplane, as transport is not yet covered by the DDA, although the government is committed to plugging this legal loophole.

There is a pattern in these judgements: health and safety 'justifications' for refusing someone a job, an education or a service cannot be based on assumptions or stereotypes. There has to be an individual assessment and it has to meet certain standards, for example employers have to take some care over it, and look at whether reasonable adjustments could enable the person to do the job.

The Disability Rights Commission (DRC, 2003) pointed out weaknesses and limitations in the DDA 1995, especially in relation to mental health service users, who – although they make up 23 per cent of those using this law in the employment sphere – are somewhat less likely to win at tribunal than other groups of disabled people. As a result, the Disability Rights Commission urged government to strengthen the Act. The following recommendations are particularly important for people with psychiatric disabilities:

- No questions about disability in recruitment except in highly specified circumstances. This would prevent, for example, an employer from doing an occupational health check before deciding which person to appoint to a job and rejecting the person with a history of depression. Government rejected legislating on this, although the DRC promoted it as good practice and the Equality and Human Rights Commission (EHRC) reiterated that commitment in 2008. The EHRC, created under the Equality Act 2006, brought together the remit of the DRC, the Commission for Racial Equality and the Equal Opportunities Commission in 2007, with additional responsibilities for sexual orientation, age, religion/belief and human rights.
- Improved definitions of disability, to better cover people with psychiatric impairments, for example a definition of 'day-to-day activities' that reflected problems in social interaction, and self-harm, on a par with problems in walking or seeing. Proposed single equality legislation in 2008–09 presents a potential opportunity to address this.
- Removal of the requirement that a mental health problem must be 'clinically well recognised' to count as a disability: this did not apply to physical impairments and therefore introduces discrimination into the face of law itself. In 2005, the government legislated to remove this discriminatory requirement.

Formal investigations can be undertaken under the DDA – establishing systemic patterns of discrimination in particular organisations or sectors and requiring action to tackle it. And in 2006, the government introduced a disability equality public sector duty – requiring the public sector actively to promote equality of opportunity, rather than waiting for discrimination and tackling it only after the event. The DDA is becoming a strong lever to encourage changes in policies and practices, without even going to court or a tribunal, to ensure that organisations do not discriminate against people with mental health problems or other disabled people.

The Human Rights Act (HRA) 1998 can also be used by practitioners to challenge the unfair application of risk-thinking to disabled people. The two disabled women who encountered East Sussex County Council's 'no lifting' policy took the council to judicial review and the judgement encouraged reviews of policy in other areas. The judge ruled that the dignity and independence of disabled people is so important that some manual lifting is an inherent and inescapable feature of the task for which care workers are employed. An approach is required that attends to staff health and safety – which can be addressed through training and agreed protocols – and the independence and dignity of disabled people.

Challenging the stereotypes that underpin unfair risk-thinking in mental health

Legally driven remedies alone are not enough. It is also important to change the stereotypes that underpin discrimination (Sayce, 2003, 2008; Read et al., 2006; Sayce and Curran, 2007), not least because people go beyond mere compliance to best practice when they understand the point of doing so.

The *National Service Framework for Mental Health* (DH, 1999) opens with an introduction from the then secretary of state that talks promisingly about 'combating discrimination' and 'promoting positive images of mental ill health'. But it goes on to talk of people with mental health problems in two groups: the minority who are 'a nuisance and a danger' and the larger group who are 'vulnerable', 'presenting no threat to anyone but themselves'. It is worth noting that this description is utterly permeated by risk-thinking: if people are not a risk to others, then they are a risk to themselves.

The academic literature on how to reduce discriminatory attitudes towards people with mental health problems shows that it is necessary to go beyond seeing people as a risk to self or others and instead break the link with both violence and incompetence. Discrimination, or stigma, has four components (Link and Phelan, 2001):

1 Distinguishing between, and labelling, human differences
2 Linking the labelled persons to undesirable characteristics
3 Separating 'them' (the labelled persons) from 'us'
4 Culminating in status loss and discrimination that lead to unequal outcomes or life chances.

There is a particularly strong evidence base for how to interrupt component 3 – by stopping separating 'them' from 'us'. Attitudes improve as a result of contact or familiarisation with a person/people with experience of mental health problems (Corrigan and Penn, 1999; Alexander and Link, 2003; Thornicroft, 2006; Sayce and Curran, 2007). Opposition to mental health facilities disappears once the facilities open and neighbours 'see service users as people' (Repper et al., 1997). Contact appears to reduce fear of the 'other' and increase empathy. Contact affects attitudes whether or not the contact is voluntary (Desforges et al., 1991; Corrigan et al., 2001). Contact can be retrospective or prospective, in other words, engineering contact as an anti-discrimination intervention promises to be effective (Couture and Penn, 2003).

It is vital that contact is between people as equals. Other key factors are that people should be brought together in situations where stereotypes are likely to be disconfirmed, where there is intergroup cooperation, where participants can get to know each other and where wider social norms support equality (Desforges et al., 1991; Corrigan and Penn, 1999; Hewstone, 2003). Where people with psychiatric disabilities have ongoing significant roles as employees, bosses or teachers – or are trainers, with status – this is likely to impact positively on the attitudes of those around them.

Inclusion itself is a powerful way of changing non-disabled people's beliefs. British research finds that the group with the highest DDA awareness and the most inclusive attitudes about disability are people who 'know someone who is disabled at work' (DRC, 2002b). Inclusive schools also influence non-disabled children to hold more accepting attitudes towards disabled children (Gray, 2002).

A key challenge is thus to make it safer for disabled people to assert the right to participate. The other significant body of evidence relates to the messages that are used to interrupt component 2 in the stigmatising process – linking the person to undesirable characteristics. When setting out to replace undesirable with more desirable associations, evidence shows that it is essential to test whether the new proposed characteristic actually is viewed as positive by people with psychiatric impairments and the intended audience. It is all too easy to replace one stereotype with another.

One type of message that 'works' is one that disrupts the link between mental ill health and violence (Penn et al., 1999; Read and Law, 1999). This matches the finding that the association between dangerousness and mental illness is 'the core' of stigma (Link et al., 1999). People who associate mental illness with violence are most likely to hold discriminatory attitudes (Link et al., 1997) and where educational interventions break the link with violence, discriminatory attitudes wane. The more the message is spread that mental health service users are generally not violent the better. Another promising message focuses on the contribution of mental health service users as employees, community leaders and so on. It is likely to be helpful to convey examples of mental health service users who contribute. In Britain, the charity Rethink achieved a shift in public attitude through its campaign in Norwich in 2006, through positive profiles of people with mental health problems and by mounting a statue of Winston Churchill in a straitjacket, in order to ridicule the idea of restricting the opportunities of talented people with mental health problems. In 2008, evidence-based approaches were used in a major campaign led by Mind, Rethink, Mental Health Media and the Institute of Psychiatry.

Beyond these areas, evidence for the effectiveness of particular messages is much less clear-cut. It is troubling that many anti-stigma campaigns worldwide are using, or even relying on, messages for which there is no clear evidence base. One of the commonest is the message that 'mental illness is an illness like any other' (or is a brain disease). There is no body of research that supports the effectiveness of this 'illness' message, or any message focusing on the causes of mental health problems. Causes are not the point when it comes to combating discrimination. The illness message does not disrupt the link between mental illness and violence. In popular culture, 'sickness' co-exists readily with evil – as 'sick monster' tabloid headlines attest. The disease model also does not break the link between mental illness and incompetence and it can reinforce it (Read and Harre, 2001; Sayce, 2004; Read et al., 2006).

Illness also means one is excused from social roles which may be exactly what the individual does not want. There is a powerful need to create images of possibility that go beyond the two models put forward in the National Service Framework – of mental health service users as either dangerous or a risk to themselves. The new images of possibility are needed by people with psychiatric disabilities themselves, and the staff who work with them, and decision makers like employers, and the wider public.

It is not possible to overthrow discriminatory attitudes as long as people are seen through the lens of risk. Instead, people with psychiatric impairments need to be viewed as equal citizens who can and do contribute. Where risk needs to be assessed, that is one activity, not something that should define people as individuals or dictate society's response to them. Mental health service users are far more than a bundle of risks.

Implications for social workers and other mental health professionals

Mental health practitioners, including social workers, need to:

1   Gain an understanding of how people with psychiatric disabilities, and disabled people more broadly, can be subjected to unfair risk assessments across different life domains, for example employment, education, housing, health and social services. Accounts of disabled people's own lives provide a very different focus, one that goes far beyond a focus on risk to looking at people's hopes, disappointments and the barriers they face to realising their aspirations (Leete, 1989; Deegan, 1994; Repper and Perkins, 2003). Often these barriers take the form of other people's attitudes, including – at times – the attitudes of those providing services to them. It is important to think about the opportunities in people's lives and how barriers might be overcome and not to get sucked into thinking only about risk, which can restrict opportunity and even wipe hope out of the dialogue altogether. Hope is essential to recovery. Mental health practitioners can help to foster it (Shepherd et al., 2008).

2   Think through how people with psychiatric disabilities can be supported to take risks. For example, who will encourage the person if they go for a job and ensure support is in place in the recruitment process and the employment itself if needed? Who will remain encouraging whether they get the job or not and support them in taking further risks rather than giving up?

3   Inform people with psychiatric disabilities of their rights under the DDA and the HRA and enable people to understand that they can negotiate for adjustments. For example, if you are working or seeking work, you can ask for a 'reasonable adjustment' ranging from time off for appointments with a mental health worker to some change in the hours or specific job tasks. For further details of the type of adjustments that can be sought – in employment and beyond – see the Employers Forum on Disability (1998) and Sayce and Boardman (2003).

The Royal Association for Disability and Rehabilitation's publication *Doing Work Differently* (RADAR, 2007) – written by and for people living with any kind of ill health (mental or physical), injury or disability – offers encouragement by describing what many other people have found helpful; evaluation showed that this peer-based material made people feel less alone, more able to talk about hidden conditions and more confident to begin taking action to keep or get a job. People need to know that they have rights to negotiate for adjustments, what they can negotiate for and to complain if they are not provided.

4 Inspire people with what is possible. People do not have to settle for the unimaginative view that because you have mental health problems, you are 'unable' to do all types of things. Just as deaf people can look after cats (see above), so people with psychiatric disabilities can work, achieve educationally and raise families, if the right adjustments are put in place. Role models can be useful – not just the 'creative' ones like Stephen Fry or Vincent van Gogh (since the public already believes madness is acceptable in comics and artists) and not just menial roles but also people achieving in a range of responsible positions. In *Not Just Stacking Shelves*, Rinaldi et al. (2006) show how community mental health teams supported people with significant mental health problems to work in jobs ranging from events management to accountancy and hairdressing.

5 Aim to ensure that in mental health practice, risk does not distort decisions or the quality of relationships. For example, if the individual wants to raise their child, it is good practice to judge parenting abilities just as a non-disabled person's abilities might be judged, that is, without discrimination, and also explore what supports might enable them to be a good enough parent. This should happen before making any long-term decisions on whether the child can safely stay with this parent. The approach should be fair: not expecting more of this person just because they are a mental health service user, and not making assumptions based, however unintentionally, on stereotypes of dangerousness or incompetence. Try to estimate risk accurately – not exaggerate it – and balance risk against opportunities and the desirability of social participation and valued social roles (such as parent). It is worth noting that under the 2005 DDA legislation, public authorities' decisions are covered by the DDA, so the requirement not to discriminate needs formally to be addressed alongside the best interests of the child.

6 Be aware of the tensions between an anti-discriminatory approach and certain legal or policy requirements, for example discriminatory elements of the Mental Health Act 2007 or, following the death of Victoria Climbié, greater requirements to track parenting by people with mental health problems than other citizens. Where possible, within legal constraints, ensure that you avoid discrimination. Feed back to managers or policy makers where this tension is most problematic.

7 Familiarise yourself with the evidence on risk. For example, employment is far better for your mental health than unemployment (Warner, 1985; Link et al., 1997; DWP, 2008). Do not assume that the stress of work will be damaging – being unemployed is likely to be far worse for a person's mental health. Not having control at work is stressful – so the more junior jobs are usually more stressful. Do not fall into the trap of assuming a more responsible job will be particularly stressful – the reverse is more likely to be true. Do not feed into people's low expectations by

discouraging people with psychiatric disabilities from roles that might be 'stressful' – let them decide and support them to take risks if they wish to.

8 Consider the 'risks' for the person of being kept in a safe cocoon, with no risk, no job, no major activities and no life at all. Remember that risk assessment can dominate dangerously and lead to risk-averse, overcautious behaviour, by clinicians and disabled people alike. Do not let assessment of risk seep through all aspects of a helping relationship. Do not let risk obscure opportunities. In doing a risk assessment, keep it in proportion – risk is only one aspect of the person's life. Overdoing risk aversion can make the life not worth living at all.

9 Involve people with psychiatric disabilities in thinking about risk. For example, many people who sometimes feel angry or violent recognise their own triggers. Others know when they are becoming unwell and may be likely to neglect themselves. Talk with service users about risk assessment and how best to respond when triggers happen or the person is becoming unwell. Writing a risk assessment without reference to the person is not usually a good idea.

10 Become an advocate for the huge national priority to reduce discrimination. Familiarise yourself with the evidence on what works to change attitudes, make the law work and raise awareness in others. Talk about the DDA, the HRA, single equality law, the need for people with psychiatric disabilities to know and use their rights, the need to support disabled people in challenging discrimination and negotiating for rights. And talk about needing to replace old stereotypes with genuinely new messages – not illness and incompetence, not violence, but contribution and opportunity.

11 Work for the goal of users and survivors of mental health services leading programmes to reduce discrimination. Discrimination is only effectively challenged when power is addressed. This means users and survivors of mental health services taking positions of power, leading change initiatives.

Conclusion

Risk has become a powerful driver of both policy discourse and practice and it is used in discriminatory ways to restrict opportunities and recovery for people with psychiatric disabilities. There are promising ways of challenging these forms of discrimination and risk aversion, including:

- using the Disability Discrimination Act and Human Rights Act to change systems for the better
- disabled people securing their rights
- replacing old stereotypes with hopeful messages of social participation and equality.

Mental health professionals have a critical role in achieving change on this basis, operating as allies to people with psychiatric disabilities who need to set the agenda and be in the lead.

For further discussion of approaches to mental health practice, see Adams et al., 2009b, Chapter 29.

www.radar.org.uk The Royal Association for Disability and Rehabilitation is run by disabled people.

www.equalityhumanrights.com The Equality and Human Rights Commission has the mission of eliminating discrimination, promoting equality and protecting human rights.

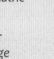

Deegan, P.E. (1994) 'Recovery: the lived experience of rehabilitation', in L. Spaniol and M. Koehler (eds) *The Experience of Recovery*, Boston, Center for Psychiatric Rehabilitation. Useful illustrations of the recovery approach in practice.

DWP (Department for Work and Pensions) (2008) *Working for a Healthier Tomorrow: Dame Carol Black's Review of the Health of Britain's Working Age Population*, London, TSO. Summarises the benefits of work to people's health and family life.

Link, B.G. and Phelan, J.C. (2001) 'On the nature and consequences of stigma', *Annual Review of Sociology*, 27: 363–85. Relevant analysis of the character and impact of stigmatisation.

Repper, J.M. and Perkins, R.E. (2003) *Social Inclusion, Recovery and Mental Health Practice*, London, Ballière Tindall. Contains useful discussion of relevant practice issues.

Sayce, L. (2000) *From Psychiatric Patient to Citizen: Overcoming Discrimination and Social Exclusion*, Basingstoke, Macmillan – now Palgrave Macmillan. Critical discussion that helps to highlight barriers to inclusion and ways of overcoming them.

9

Social work with asylum seekers and others subject to immigration control

Chapter overview

This chapter focuses on the changing role of social work in relation to asylum seekers and others subject to immigration control. It considers tensions and ethical issues with reference to examples of, and implications for, good critical practice.

We have been familiar for some time now with scare stories and panic-stricken headlines about asylum seekers. These stories present predominantly male images of asylum seekers as feckless, bogus, criminal, terrorist, illegal and diseased. At this particular historical point, we are also in the midst of a dangerous escalation in the brutality of these messages. The global concern with terrorism, which has constructed the Muslim as the dangerous interloper in the West, is having a profound influence on the lived experience of many within our communities, some of whom are asylum seekers, many of whom made much earlier journeys before such a label was constructed. One of the consequences of this bombardment is the dehumanising of those forced to leave their home, homeland, family, love, support, shared language, culture and identity. We can then accept without flinching a system of immigration controls and an asylum infrastructure that revels in its purpose – to exclude, deter, separate and impoverish. The question at the centre of this chapter is whether social work itself has become so enmeshed in that culture of suspicion that we have lost sight of some of our central principles, namely, human dignity and worth, social justice and service to humanity (BASW, 2002).

My personal journey regarding these issues began over 10 years ago when I was a probation officer in an inner-city borough. I was to be shaken out of my naivety, ignorance and complacency when a black prisoner I was working with was served with a deportation notice. 'That can't be right', I thought, 'he's lived here for 14 years, has a wife and children who were born here, has a job, a mortgage, a community.' Mr X was in fact serving a five-year prison sentence for importation of heroin and while the court did not recommend deportation at the point of sentencing, he was subsequently served with a notice of intent to deport mid-sentence on 'conducive to public good' grounds. Later I came to understand the significance of these processes and will return to them shortly. I had not, of course, received any training on anything close to these issues during my social work course and spent subsequent months considering more thoughtfully what exactly the response of a worker in such circumstances should be. Mr X was eventually deported, leaving a divided family, fatherless children and a distraught wife and mother behind. I came to learn that in the UK, just like most other rich parts of the globe, there are many long-term residents who are not 'illegal', who are settled within communities, but who do not enjoy full citizenship rights, which has consequences when they break the rules. This 'lesser' status confirms the position of these predominantly black residents as 'other', as 'outsider', and creates a particular and inferior relationship with the state, and, more significantly for our purposes, with the local and welfare state of which social work is a part.

A history of discrimination

While it is essential that we explore here the particular position of asylum seekers in a separate and inferior welfare system and the knock-on effects for them as users of social work services, I start with the above example to illustrate that there is a much wider community of residents in the UK who are excluded from equal access to both citizenship rights and welfare, as a result of their immigration status. From my experience of working with practitioners and students alike, it is necessary to contextualise contemporary immigration policies and practices in order to understand their role and purpose. In integrating immigration and asylum matters into the curriculum of a social work degree, it has been the grounding of students in the history and ideology of immigration that has created the foundation for understanding the law, policy and practice in relation to those subject to immigration controls.

While the movement of people around the globe is part of human history, the control of that movement is very much a modern phenomenon (see Hayter, 2000). In the UK, this has a track record of around a century. At each of the key moments in that history, calls for restrictions have been posed in racist terms, marked by the Aliens Act 1905:

> It was the poor Eastern European Jew who was to become the focus for control and in the run up to the first piece of immigration control in 1905, 'alien' became synonymous with 'Jew'. (Hayes, 2002: 31)

Black and Asian Commonwealth immigration came under scrutiny after the Second World War. Culminating in the 1962 Commonwealth Immigrants Act, anti-immigration lobbying was based on an open hostility to 'coloureds':

> In the last forty years the main objects of anti-immigrant racism in Britain and elsewhere have been, and are, people of African and Asian origin. (Hayter, 2000: 4)

Contemporary constructions of asylum seekers also rely heavily on racist stereotypes. As Liz Fekete from the Institute of Race Relations states: 'Government policies and practices aimed at asylum seekers have educated a whole nation into racism' (*Guard-*

ian, 2001). A historical framework allows for the unpacking of this seemingly inherent connection between immigration control and racism:

> Although controls formally discriminate on grounds of nationality, racism has fundamentally informed the construction of immigration controls. The ideological justification for control has been a racialised nationalism, and the practice of control by the state has been directed at racialised groups. (Mynott, 2002: 13)

Nowadays, we use words like 'asylum seeker', 'refugee', 'economic migrant' and in the past words like 'immigrant' or 'alien'. These different words do not necessarily represent different types of people, they simply reflect the changing political purposes to which the categories have been put across time and space. Today's asylum seeker may well have been previously constructed as an immigrant. A glance at the current 'top 10' countries producing asylum seekers to the UK – Eritrea, Afghanistan, Iran, China, Somalia, Zimbabwe, Pakistan, Iraq, Nigeria and India – reveals a number of former British Colonies (see Bennett et al., 2007). Waves of immigration restrictions since the 1960s have changed the status of former colonial subjects, turning many who had a strong allegiance to 'Mother England' into nothing more than 'aliens':

- The Commonwealth Immigrants Act 1962, which took away automatic rights of entry to Commonwealth citizens by introducing work vouchers
- The Commonwealth Immigrants Act 1968, which systematically removed citizenship rights overnight to UK passport holders, unless they, a parent or a grandparent had been born, adopted or naturalised in the UK
- The Immigration Act 1971, which created 'patrials', who were largely white and had been born in the UK or had parents or grandparents who were, and 'non-patrials'. This effectively ended immigration for settlement for people from the Caribbean, the Indian subcontinent and Africa
- The British Nationality Act 1981, which, among other things, abolished automatic rights to citizenship to those born on British soil, establishing the bloodline as the key factor.

Since the 1980s, migration for settlement has been difficult to obtain, as we have changed the goalposts and increasingly restricted entry. This process has continued in most of the richer parts of the world, leaving a divided globe with very few means by which the poor can enter the richer, safer territory (see Marfleet, 2006). It is also important to understand that attacks on settlement are attacks on family reconstruction. The richer parts of the globe will always need labour, different skills for different times, but what we don't want is to pick up the tab for the broader social costs of settlement – education, health, social security, social housing and so on.

Obstructions to family unity are institutionalised now, to the extent that many long-term residents find it difficult to unite their families, even for short-term visits and holidays. Our colleagues at work, students and social work service users have differing access to family networks. The significance of this should not go unnoticed in a profession that looks predominantly to that institution, the family, to find solutions to problems. I was struck by the enormity of this recently when a student, who happens to be an asylum seeker, experienced the death of her father in her homeland. Distanced from his death, she was also distanced from family support and the rituals we associate with bereavement. It was enormously difficult for her to access those rituals here, they were and are specific to her country and culture. Working with those subject to immigration control, we are already in an arena dominated by loss. It seems to me that listening to those stories can inform our own practice enormously and usefully challenge the complacency with which we construct 'family' in our professional arena.

The current focus, then, is on asylum seekers and the debate is posed in terms of genuineness. What is clear from those asylum statistics is that the countries dominating the list are in crisis. Despite the relentless media machine's presentation of asylum seekers as scroungers (see Refugee Council, 2002), it is global crisis that forces people across boundaries and within that context, it is meaningless to differentiate between a flight from crippling destitution, war or persecution. The 'economic migrant' may be constructed as bogus, but with few legitimate routes to survival open, it may be that leaving family is the only way to support them.

Controlling welfare

Throughout all this is a common thread, a concern with ensuring that the resources of the nation are not spent on the wrong people. 'Outsiders' are, of course, by their nature, the wrong people:

> Who those 'outsiders' are remains the product of racism, but no longer a racism simply targeted at black people, it now encompasses new layers of the world's poor and dispossessed. (Hayes and Humphries, 2004: 13)

So, while immigration controls have concerned themselves with who gets in, their other central purpose has been control over those who do and the conditions under which they live. The social cost of these newcomers is always presented in entirely negative terms, with scant attention to the taxes, labour and skills contributed by them. It is this powerful and distorted ideology around social cost – which runs throughout the history of immigration control – that has forced the drive to oppressive internal control of non-citizens. It has been astonishingly easy for the Far Right to make best use of this because the foundations for the argument are already there. Protecting the public purse from abuse from the outside is a popular position for most mainstream politicians on the Left and Right of the political spectrum. It encapsulates an acceptance of certain taken-for-granted ideas, for example that belonging to a nation should bring some security and support and being outside it should not.

One of the most powerful media representations of asylum seekers is that they are the ones unfairly accessing public resources and are coming precisely to do so (see Fell and Hayes, 2007). It is not simply the Far Right who struggle to see humanity globally and are influenced by an idea of nation, which makes it appear natural for us to restrict resources to our own. In my experience of working in higher education, black, white and Asian students alike have a sense of allegiance to other UK citizens when they are pitted against the needs of new arrivals. The idea of contributing in order to have rights to welfare is connected and equally powerful.

In fact, those outside 'nation' have also always been constructed as outside 'welfare'. The centrality of nationality for claims upon welfare existed long before large-scale black migration to the UK and is rooted in the very purpose of welfare, which is precisely to improve the quality of our nation, in particular in relation to other competing nations (Cohen, 2001, 2003). Those calling for the control over the entry of largely Jews, escaping persecution in Eastern Europe at the turn of the last century, stood side by side with welfare reformers in this. The enormously influential welfare programme of 1906–14, introduced by the Liberal government, included the Old Age Pensions Act 1908 and the National Insurance Act 1911. Both Acts contained residency and citizenship requirements, ensuring that Jewish entrants had no access to the provisions contained within them, because:

> it might be that crowds of foreigners of the age of 45 or 50 might come over here in the hope that, having resided in this country for the required time, they might get a pension. (Arthur Fell MP in 1908, cited in Cohen, 2003: 91)

From the beginning, immigration control was constructed as a mechanism for deciding who would be beneficial to the British nation and who might be a burden. The Aliens Act 1905 only applied to those in third-class travelling conditions, that is, the poor. The Act allowed for refusal of entry where an alien immigrant was considered to be undesirable. The most common reasons for undesirability were:

> ■ If he cannot show that he has in his possession or is in a position to obtain the means of decently supporting himself and his dependents; or
>
> ■ If he is a lunatic or an idiot, or owing to any disease or infirmity appears likely to become a charge upon the rates or otherwise a detriment to the public. (Aliens Act 1905, cited in Englander, 1994: 279)

Decisions about undesirability focused predominantly on who might be costly, both socially and economically. If families could not support themselves without access to public monies, they simply could not come in. This concept has remained in immigration control since and there is a powerful reminder of this in the current immigration rules, which prevent entry to anyone likely to have 'recourse to public funds' (see Seddon, 2006). This illustrates the strong link between immigration control and the delivery of welfare and illuminates one of the central purposes of immigration controls – to target and control welfare spending. The state then uses a dual approach, first, by creating immigration controls at borders and internally that debar those who might require assistance and, second, by building arrangements into welfare to exclude the outsider.

Postwar welfare

In the five years immediately following the Second World War, commonly associated with the development of a comprehensive welfare state, welfare was seen as part of a hopeful new world where ordinary people could look forward optimistically to universal healthcare, social security, education, and affordable and good quality housing (see Thane, 1996; Timmins, 1996). These improvements created a sense that the

> postwar Labour Government had established something qualitatively new: a new approach to the use of the power of the state consciously in the interests of social justice for the mass of the population: a welfare state. (Thane, 1996: 249)

This period also coincided with a period of mass migration, which was encouraged in order to help in this era of economic and social reconstruction. These predominantly black immigrants, unlike the Jews before them, did have citizenship rights as Commonwealth subjects, as well as a strong emotional and ideological connection with 'Mother England'. However, this group were treated not as citizens at all but as short-term labour, migrant workers who, it was assumed, would return home to their families and not require the benefits of long-term settlement. Only when they began to present for services did the question of entitlement emerge. There is evidence in the areas of allocation of council housing, access to free healthcare and in claims for social security of inappropriate refusals and exclusions and common requests for passports falling mainly on black claimants (see also Ginsburg, 1989; Cohen and Hayes, 1998):

> What developed during this period was a system in which discrete and separate agencies of the state were advised or encouraged to play a part in the enforcement of immigration controls. (Gordon and Newnham, 1985: 70)

These authors pinpoint here the shift to the inclusion of not only the police and immigration officials policing immigration, but also workers in welfare. This should be a major cause for concern for social workers and related professionals as this process has escalated since. As the immigration legislation in the 1960s, 70s and 80s, described earlier, reconstructed just who the citizen was, the need to 'gatekeep' access to state welfare resources has intensified. What the above examples illustrate is that layers of long-term residents, some with citizenship rights and some without, find themselves having to account for their status when they are at the point of accessing services. The full implications of this for social work are dealt with below.

It is also important to consider that anyone without citizenship with the right of abode is subject to the immigration rules and at their centre is the issue of maintenance and accommodation. Just as Jewish refugees at the turn of the twentieth century had to prove that they could support themselves and their families without needing the relief provided by parishes or charities, applicants wishing to stay or join family now must show that they 'will be maintained and accommodated adequately without recourse to public funds' (Seddon, 2006: 308–18). The list of things considered public funds is an ever-increasing one and currently includes income support, job seekers allowance, housing benefit, council tax benefit, working families tax credit, local authority housing, child benefit, disabled persons tax credit, attendance allowance, severe disablement allowance, invalid care allowance and disability living allowance (Cohen, 2001: 49).

Here we see the absolute centrality of protecting public resources within immigration control. To underline this, long-term residents of the UK, many of whom in the past would have had citizenship rights, must satisfy these conditions if they are to reunite their families or stay long term. The government has come to understand the key role of agencies outside the Immigration and Nationality Directorate (now Border and Immigration Agency) in gathering information concerning immigration status, explicitly now making welfare agencies accountable for

> identifying claimants who may be ineligible for a benefit or service by virtue of their immigration status; and to encourage local authorities to pass information to the IND about suspected immigration offenders. (Home Office, 1996)

Entering the asylum

As described earlier, 40 years of legislation, which has restricted rights of entry, even for those with previous citizenship rights, have left few avenues for entry open. Seeking asylum from war, persecution, famine and other consequences of global crises has become the remaining route of entry. The asylum seeker, then, is a modern construct, as migration for settlement has become all but impossible. All focus is now on asylum, with little reference to others subject to immigration control as described above. Nevertheless, the language and ideas from previous periods have been taken forward into the contemporary construction of the asylum seeker. They are seen only as poor, burdensome and socially costly. The velocity and force with which this ideology has been constructed has gained such momentum that it has been possible to go much further than previously. No more tinkering at the edges of welfare restriction, but the creation of a completely separate and inferior system. The Immigration and Asylum Act 1999 removed entitlement to a range of non-contributory, family and disability benefits to this group, extended the use of vouchers, and created a system of compulsory dispersal (Fell and Hayes, 2007: 129–31). A centralised agency, the National Asylum Support Service (NASS) was created. NASS entered into arrangements with both voluntary organisations and local authorities regarding arrangements for asylum seekers in dispersal areas. Subsistence was by way of money or vouchers to the value of 70 per cent of basic income support. Asylum seekers continue to live well below the level considered as subsistence. Housing was organised via a consortia of local authorities and voluntary organisations to accommodate the asylum seekers being dispersed to zones on a 'no choice' basis.

What we now have, therefore, unashamedly, is a 'welfare' scheme, deliberately separate and inferior, making no attempt to offer even subsistence-level support and which manages and moves human beings without offering any choice or indeed any consideration of individual need:

> The 1999 Act has systematically excluded asylum seekers from many aspects of mainstream life and forcibly located them in poverty stricken areas in substandard housing in often hostile communities. (Fell and Hayes, 2007: 130)

As a profession, social work is now part of the machinery administering this system, a system that discriminates, excludes and fuels a climate of hostility. The Nationality, Immigration and Asylum Act 2002 further underlined a government strategy fuelling popular nationalism and hostility to asylum seekers. The requirement for applicants to pass an English test and the introduction of a citizenship ceremony involving an oath of allegiance illuminate the government's thinking. As learning English is often a priority for asylum seekers themselves, it would be easy to see this policy in entirely benevolent terms. In debates on the imposition of English testing, it is instructive to ask groups who can speak more than one language. In my experience, it will almost always be predominantly non-white participants who can, adding a further dimension to the debate. Asylum seekers have far higher language skills and educational qualifications than the average UK citizen (*Guardian,* 2001), illustrating that we seem unable to focus on strengths and continue to present the group as deficient. Of most significance to us in social work is the notorious section 55 of the 2002 Act, which established the denial of any support from certain categories of asylum seeker. For the first time, we have a category of people even outside the basic safety net of national assistance who are completely destitute. From 2002, we began to see widespread destitution of single asylum seekers and a voluntary sector now burdened with the task of feeding and clothing people.

In 2004, the Asylum and Immigration (Treatment of Claimants) Act further controlled and penalised those entering 'unlawfully', which may mean simply not having all the right papers. It also created a one-tier appeal system and even established controls on the circumstances under which persons subject to immigration control can marry. The most important part of the Act, however, adds 'asylum seeker with family' (s. 9) to the list of those who can become ineligible for NASS support. Section 9 caused considerable concern in the social work profession, with the realisation that children in such destitute families may need to be removed for their protection. Section 9 was piloted in a number of areas, the situation being that families who failed to take steps to comply with removal directions would have all support withdrawn. In reality, few families left the UK, a higher proportion going underground (Refugee Council, 2006, in Fell and Hayes, 2007). It is to the credit of the profession that there was a strong response including lobbying by the British Association of Social Workers and the Association of Directors of Social Services. Particular families hit the headlines and local campaigns involving communities and social workers served to highlight the injustice of section 9 and the undermining of basic childcare principles in our work.

Asylum has been thrust centre stage in social work and avoidance is no longer an option. In other ways, the shift in the role of local authorities in the management of asylum seekers has had further significance for social work, for example in the community care arena. Many care in the community functions depend on immigration status, with exclusions for those 'subject to immigration control'. Research by Harris and Roberts (2002) shows the consequences for disabled asylum seekers of not accessing mainstream services. In reality, if an asylum seeker's needs arise because of anything other than 'destitution', for example disability, physical or mental ill health or old age, they do have an entitlement to assistance. Harris and Roberts point to the need for community care assessments to be done to ensure full access to a range of benefits and services. It has taken Appeal Court rulings to 'persuade' local authorities of their responsibilities (*Community Care*, 2002). Refugee Council (2005) research has shown how social services departments have been failing to provide help to asylum seekers being discharged from hospital because of financial considerations and found only a third of asylum seekers in its sample who had entitlement to community care assessments actually received one.

Accessing suitable healthcare remains problematic for asylum seekers (Burnett and Fassil, 2002). Worryingly, many asylum seekers are healthy on arrival and their health deteriorates as a consequence of dispersal, poverty and poor housing. Many do, unfortunately, have physical and mental health conditions as a result of the situations from which they escaped. The popular debate concerning asylum and health, though, has again not focused on need, but resources. Exaggerated claims regarding the burden on the NHS, outlined in the Refugee Council's (2002) analysis of press myths, replay the debates in previous periods outlined before. Asylum seekers are not only seen as responsible for bringing in disease, but are seen to get preferential access to resources. Current plans to remove entitlement to free healthcare for failed asylum seekers will only add to the horror of destitution and draw other workers in welfare into policing the potential users of their services.

Implications for social work

The experience of restricted rights and poor access to welfare for long-term residents subject to immigration control has for decades gone largely unnoticed in social work. While the restrictions on access to housing, health, education and benefits have impacted greatly on people's lives, social work has intervened only minimally. We have also seemingly not noticed that many of our service users in this category are living in divided families, which has consequences in so many ways. What has forced the issue onto the professional agenda has been this separating out of the category 'asylum seeker', compulsory dispersal and the scale of the enforced destitution. There is now an inescapable reality, as social work is faced with individuals and families with enormous needs, sometimes in geographical areas without an infrastructure or history of support to such groups. The work is now emerging in and across a full range of social work contexts with varied levels of preparation, practically, ethically or emotionally.

In attempting to improve service delivery to asylum seekers and others subject to immigration control, the context of hostility, racism and grinding poverty has to be acknowledged. For our purposes, the question is how far social work as a profession has become uncritical of these arrangements and complicit in their delivery. Social work seems to have largely occupied itself with concerns over gatekeeping resources rather than responding to need (see Hayes and Humphries, 2004). The issue of asylum is now asking questions of the social work profession and its role, function and values, but this can also be seen as a challenge and an opportunity to reflect and retrieve something from an alternative perspective for those concerned to work within a profession committed to supporting the poor and the oppressed and willing to offer challenges to the social order.

There is evidence of widespread uncertainty, confusion and abstention within social work teams concerning this work. A key theme, which has emerged time and time again, concerns contention around responsibility between mainstream teams and asylum teams. The idea that 'the other team do that' is exacerbated by the conflicting status of asylum seekers. Asylum seekers are not just that, they might also be children, families, old, disabled and a range of other things, which contribute to them being passed from pillar to post. More worryingly, it appears that workers have been steeped in the negative culture described above and have absorbed these stereotypes, which contribute to a deserving/undeserving dichotomy (Sales and Hek, 2004). Given that they are working in a culture that prioritises resource control and involves decisions about desirability and deservedness, this should be of some concern. Hostility towards asylum seekers within social service offices, with teams in conflict with voluntary/ community refugee organisations, is certainly a situation we need to take stock of.

The voluntary sector is not immune from these difficulties. As the sector has to chase money and resources for future survival, it is not surprising that monies have been accepted with conditions. Conditions concerning surveillance, control and cooperation with the Home Office are not uncommon now for organisations working with asylum seekers and refugees. In addition, involvement in a system that allocates accommodation and money means withdrawing that when the end of the asylum process arrives. It seems to me that we have had very few conversations as a profession about our role at that end of the process. The majority of these service users will not be moving on with the security of refugee status, they are moving on to destitution. This is not to say that workers will not struggle with sending individuals off into the abyss, but to acknowledge that this is a long way off our vision of the role and function of social work. In such circumstances, we become at risk of constructing a culture of suspicion and blame to justify the unjustifiable.

Social workers' involvement in the internal control of immigration is of most significance. Being required to identify immigration status in order to ascertain eligibility raises serious ethical questions and colludes in the racist questioning of service users. Research within a London asylum team by Sales and Hek (2004) indicates that asylum seekers understood clearly the role of state employees and were unlikely to trust them completely. Given many of their personal histories, this is an extremely worrying place for social workers to be. In organising the first national conference for social workers on immigration and asylum in 2004, I was asked by a group of young unaccompanied asylum seekers if they could provide a workshop. Their unsolicited offer was to focus on their experiences – not of the Home Office, the police, or immigration officials but of social workers.

Conclusion

Positive ways forward

As a profession, social work has had a history of work with the poor and oppressed and historically has grappled with its dual care and control functions (Humphries, 2004a). It is better placed than many other professions within social care to take on this challenge because it still holds up social justice and respect for individuals as core values. The social arrangements we have established for asylum seekers increase need and risk. These are familiar concepts to social workers – there is a knowledge base around risk conditions that should be used to argue against current arrangements on both an individual and political level. The conditions in which we are placing asylum seekers are precisely those we know to contribute to risk – poverty, isolation and hostility.

For qualified workers, there are models of good practice to look to. Save the Children's research on unaccompanied children (Stanley, 2001) called for section 20 assessments under the Children Act, rather than section 17, to ensure a full package of appropriate accommodation and support. The Refugee Council's (2005) more recent research shows some progress has been made in securing section 20 support for unaccompanied asylum-seeking children. There is still disparity between areas and the courts are still needed to persuade some local authorities to fulfil their commitments, particularly in relation to leaving care services. However, there is no doubt, as a profession, that there has been much more attention to good practice in work with this group (see Kohli, 2007). But we must continue to be vigilant. Government plans are looking to specialist social workers in specialist teams providing services like age assessments (Home Office, 2007). At first glance, this seems attractive, particularly using skilled practitioners to assess age, rather than have invasive medical tests performed on children. Unfortunately, there is a naivety to this when the age assessment frameworks are so clearly immigration led and are conducted within a climate of disbelief concerning those seeking safety. Also mooted is care planning that incorporates 'preparation for return', taking social work into new terrain fraught with ethical tensions.

When decisions are made and the asylum process is over, there remains the question of campaigning. How far is it legitimate to become involved in campaigns for, alongside or on behalf of service users? In the UK, there is a long history of anti-deportation campaigns, which have included social workers, doctors and teachers, who have been influential in some success stories (see Gibbons, 1999). Irrespective of the individual outcome, campaigns also serve to highlight the inhumanity of immigration laws and offer an alternative set of ideas to the powerful media presentation of the issue.

Similarly, there is a need for thoughtful consideration of aspects of the work from which the profession might withdraw. Being within systems that are fundamentally discriminatory and oppressive needs to be a focus for this debate. Social work has at times stood up against racism and been influential in noting discriminatory practices, and although this has become a weakened position, we have the opportunity now to refocus that discussion. These conversations about refusal and withdrawal can present as abstract and naive. Non-compliance/non-cooperation is certainly confrontational and requires union support, but the alternative is simply to collapse into informing the Home Office concerning immigration status, interrogating service users concerning their status before offering services, enforcing homelessness and withdrawing financial support at the end of the asylum process.

Immigration and asylum law and policy can be a daunting arena for social workers. We are likely to have been poorly equipped in our training pre- and post-qualification and feel a sense of impotence concerning how to intervene. The development of good practice, though, is always possible, and to return to the original case example, workers can become equipped with good skills of intervention. My first experience with Mr X and family taught me that understanding the law, policies and procedures is the necessary first step. I learned that there are two possible routes to deportation for non-UK citizens committing criminal offences, one at the point of sentencing on the criminal matters and one during imprisonment on 'conducive to public good' grounds. Understanding this can help in preparation for both the criminal court case and report-writing and also in preparing and supporting the defendant and family. I learned that certain offences were more of a trigger than others, for example drugs offences, which can also inform your work with the defendant. In Mr X's appeal against the deportation, I was able to produce a report to describe his place in his family and community. While in this case the outcomes were negative, I became aware that social workers and probation officers could be putting their report-writing skills to good use in immigration appeals and tribunals if encouraged to do so (see Brown, 2004).

I also learned the limits of individual casework and in Manchester in the years that followed a collection of practitioners began to explore and develop the professional role in relation to mainly black prisoners and deportation. This culminated in the construction and delivery of training materials and a user-led voluntary organisation offering support to families in this situation. In addition, the organisation led and supported anti-deportation campaigns locally, some of which were successful in challenging removal. What this example illustrates is that we can improve our individual interventions with this service user group, but we also need to look beyond the casework to developing collective professional and community-based responses to oppressive immigration systems.

For further discussion of tensions between social work intervention and empowerment, see Adams et al., 2009a, Chapter 19.

Cohen, S. (2001) *Immigration Controls, the Family and the Welfare State*, London, Jessica Kingsley. Cohen is one of the first authors to critique the increasingly close relationship between immigration controls and the welfare state. This book is helpful in offering case studies in numerous areas of practice, offering good practice solutions, as well as raising the political, ideological and ethical tensions therein. The book is informed by his extensive work as an immigration lawyer in an inner-city area of Manchester.

Fell, P. and Hayes, D. (2007) *What Are They Doing Here? A Critical Guide to Asylum and Immigration*, Birmingham, Venture Press. Aimed at the specialist professional working with asylum seekers and the numerous non-specialists who increasingly find themselves confronted with this work in social work and social care, the book offers a dictionary-style guide to relevant topics. Accessible in its practical solutions and legal information, but also challenging in its critique of current asylum policy.

Hayes, D. and Humphries, B. (eds) (2004) *Social Work, Immigration and Asylum: Debates, Dilemmas and Ethical Issues for Social Work and Social Care Practice*, London, Jessica Kingsley. Important as the first text to consider the practical, ethical and political challenges of this area of work for social workers, acknowledging the changing role and function of social work practice and the drift to collusion in internal immigration control. Draws on the experiences of practitioners in a variety of settings, and although out of date on some practical issues, the ethical and political tensions outlined remain crucial.

Kohli, R. (2007) *Social Work with Unaccompanied Asylum Seeking Children*, Basingstoke, Palgrave Macmillan. This is the most comprehensive and up-to-date resource on unaccompanied asylum-seeking children – probably the issue that has dominated social work practice the most. Uses case study material and draws on international research to offer a good practice guide to this growing area of social work practice.

Marfleet, P. (2006) *Refugees in a Global Era*, Basingstoke, Palgrave Macmillan. Critical reading for anyone seeking to understand the global context creating waves of migrants. This book considers displacement, flight and search for asylum and the conflicts and contradictions inherent in the global system. Offers an authoritative analysis of migration in the age of globalisation and the constructed nature of the 'refugee' in the West.

Sales, R. (2007) *Understanding Immigration and Refugee Policy: Contradictions and Continuities*, Bristol, Policy Press. Provides an overview of the key concepts and issues in global migration and immigration and asylum policy. Based on documentary sources and primary research, it focuses on Britain within an international and European context. One of the few texts bold enough to question whether immigration controls can be justified on ethical or practical grounds.

Legal and illicit drug use 10

This chapter considers current concerns relating to social work and illicit drugs, focusing on the debates surrounding changing patterns of illicit drug use and related attitudes in the UK, and recent developments in government policy and drug service provision.

Chapter overview

The social work response to what research evidence on illicit drug taking suggests is a major issue for the social work profession and continues to be a cause for concern (Galvani, 2007; Paylor, 2008a, 2009). Particular attention is paid to the implications for social workers of multi-agency collaboration between drug workers and the criminal justice profession, through a consideration of the complexities of multi-agency collaboration responding to local and national agendas, against a backdrop of rapidly changing public attitudes and behaviour.

Contextual factors

The past 20 years have seen rapid socioeconomic, technological and cultural changes in the UK, exemplified in the field of illicit drugs. Social workers are operating within and have to respond to this world of change: in patterns of availability, consumption, wider attitudinal change of both drug users and non-users and, in terms of policy, enforcement and service provision at the local, national and international level. An international shift from the American-led prohibitionist 'war on drugs' policies to a European-influenced new managerialism (Dorn and Lee, 1999) has to be set against the growing critique of a UK legal framework that has changed little in the past 35 years. The key piece of legislation governing psychoactive drugs is the Misuse of Drugs Act 1971, which came into force in 1973. This legislation created a structure whereby psychoactive substances were classified from Class A to C according to the specified drugs' perceived potential for dependency and relative harmfulness (for individuals and society), and their medicinal usage was governed by their segregation into Schedules 1–5 according to their perceived clinical value and consequent availability for use. Schedule 1 controlled drugs include heroin, ecstasy and cocaine and are deemed to have no medicinal value, while Schedule 5 drugs can be purchased over the counter at a pharmacy without prescription and include well-known cough mixtures and painkillers. The classification of individual drugs also determines the severity of penalties for offenders convicted under the Misuse of Drugs Act 1971. Subsequent modifications to the Misuse of Drugs Act have most usually been either to add new drugs to those considered to have the potential for misuse (such as the addition of gammahydroxybutyrate (GHB) and four types of anabolic steroids to the list of Class C drugs under the Misuse of Drugs Act in 2002, psilocin in all its forms in 2005 and ketamine in 2006) or to reclassify specific drugs according to a perceived increased or decreased risk of misuse and/or harmfulness (such as the depenalisation of cannabis from Class B to Class C in 2004 and the increased classification of methamphetamine from Class B to Class A in 2007). However, as Shiner (2003) has noted, such minor modifications do not affect the overall thrust of the Misuse of Drugs Act, which remains framed within a medical model of drug misuse. Indeed, the medical profession has had a significant input into British drug policy throughout the last century, from the Rolleston Committee of 1924–26 and the subsequent establishment of drug controls to the 'British system' of heroin prescribing prevalent from the 1920s to the 1960s (Berridge, [1981]1999).

Drug-related attitudes, patterns of availability and the use of drugs controlled under the Misuse of Drugs Act 1971 have changed enormously since its introduction. Levels of availability, experimentation and the use of illicit drugs increased rapidly throughout the 1990s and now appear to be declining slightly from these unprecedented levels. If we look at the broad trends across the 1990s, we can see from the official statistics that drugs offenders have quadrupled from approximately 26,000 in 1987 to 106,000 in 2004 (Mwenda, 2005). Although official statistics are in part inevitably a reflection of police targeting and enforcement policy and practice, this escalation in illicit psychoactive drugs is supported by national figures on experimentation available from alternative sources such as self-report surveys. The British Crime Survey, a national annual household survey administered by the Home Office that includes a small number of questions on self-reported drug use, also indicates increased experimentation and use of illicit drugs across the 1990s. Among young adults aged 16–24, rates of lifetime prevalence of illicit drug use increased throughout the 1990s from 43 per cent in the 1994 British Crime Survey peaking at 54 per cent in the 1998 British Crime Survey, then slowly falling down to 45 per cent in 2005/06 (Roe and Man, 2006). Past year use of any illicit drug by young adults also increased throughout the 1990s to a peak of 32 per cent in 1998 and has since fallen to 25 per cent in 2005/06 (Roe and Man, 2006). We might suspect, however, that a general national survey based only on private households such as the British Crime Survey might underestimate the levels of experimentation and use of drugs for a range of methodological reasons. Specifically focused, sensitively administered self-report studies of drug use have found higher levels of experimentation and use of illicit drugs than national household surveys: with the national schools survey conducted by Balding (2001) finding rising levels of drug use among school pupils across the 1990s.

Two large regional longitudinal studies of teenage drug use across the 1990s also found considerably higher levels of drug use than the British Crime Survey, alongside almost blanket access and availability of illicit drugs to young people by their late teens. A longitudinal study of young people in the northwest of England found that by the age of 18, over nine in ten young people reported having been in 'offer' situations where drugs were available to them either free or for money, nearly two-thirds of them reported having tried drugs at least once in their lifetime and over a quarter could be considered regular drug users (Parker et al., 1998). A separate longitudinal study of young people in the north of England found not dissimilar levels of self-reported experimentation and drug use (Aldridge et al., 1999). The body of empirical research from these (and other) studies by these authors led to their development of the 'normalisation' thesis (see Parker et al., 1998), which suggests that there has been both a quantitative and equally significant qualitative shift in relation to recreational drug use in the UK since the early 1990s, with significant changes in the degree of knowledge and understanding of illicit drugs and related behaviours by both users and non-users, the acknowledgement of the existence of such behaviour and the broader actual and symbolic role of drugs in the sociocultural terrain. Of further significance for those working in the field of drugs is that these longitudinal studies found that gender, ethnicity and socioeconomic background were no longer significant predictors of, or protectors from, illicit drug use, with levels of experimentation spreading across the social spectrum, thus challenging the conventional images of drug users. This is not to suggest that there is no longer any relationship between social exclusion and drug use. As Gilman (2000: 23) has noted: 'drug *use* may well be an equal opportunity recruiter. Drug *addiction* is highly discriminatory'(emphases added). Thus the notion of 'recreational' drug use – as distinct from 'problematic' drug use – has come to the fore in the public domain in recent years, adding a new political and professional relevance for social work.

CASE EXAMPLE

Social services is contacted regarding a young woman of 15 whose school non-attendance is linked to suspected family problems. Alongside sporadic attendance, the pupil is frequently late for school and her performance and concentration are poor when she does attend, but her parents seem unconcerned when these issues are raised with them. In discussion with the school head, parents and a social worker about where the young woman goes during the daytime, it comes to light that the young woman, along with two school friends from the same school, spends her time at a friend's house whose parents work during the week. While the details of these visits are explored with the three young women, cannabis use by the group is revealed as occurring on a regular basis during the day, both on and off school premises. The three pupils are temporarily suspended while the head conducts a full investigation according to school policy on drug use.

Research and policy

The growing overall level of availability and experimentation with illicit drugs across the 1990s has been accompanied by an increasingly diverse repertoire of pharmacological possibilities, a willingness to experiment with a range of legal, illicit and prescription drugs to achieve altered states of intoxication and an involvement in drugs that has touched schools, families, friendship networks, pubs, clubs and workplaces across the country and across the social spectrum (see Measham, 2004). Contemporary drug use is scattered across a kaleidoscope of possibilities, which range from dependent and daily usage to occasional and casual usage, resulting in professional imperatives to define what counts as problematic consumption to warrant or justify agency intervention. Simplistic characterisations of drug users as 'junkies', 'ravers' and 'dope heads' are no longer possible. Furthermore, the increased number of young men and women of childbearing age experimenting with illicit drugs well into their twenties and beyond will result in more drug-using parents (see, for example, ACMD, 2003, 2007), as well as more drug-using social workers (see, for example, Measham, 2002; Parker et al., 2002). For social workers this means that their professional intervention may well relate not to whether or not drug involvement exists in a particular case but the complexities of the assessment process and their own subjective experiences drawn from personal contact with drugs. As Harbin and Murphy (2000: 6) note in relation to parental drug use and childcare:

> The crucial dilemma during the assessment process is … what types/levels/ complexities of substance misuse, in what kind of family systems, will lead to significant harm or impairment, to which types of children? Conversely, what types of substance misuse, in what kind of family systems, will lead to minimal harm to children? Furthermore what types of professional interventions will help reduce this harmful impact on children?

At a time of increased drug use in the UK, we have also seen a move towards a more child-centred approach in child welfare. The Children Act 1989 (and re-emphasised in the 2004 Children Act) specified that agencies should aim to work in partnership with parents in childcare cases: with an assumption throughout the Act that children are best looked after by their parents, it follows that active involvement by parents is recommended to facilitate the process. The Act expects professionals to involve parents in plans for children; it also expects those parents to have the child's best interests in mind. Thus parental responsibility is seen by the Act to be more than a definition of rights. The concept of partnership with drug-using parents and the 'no order' principle (that is, the courts should make no order unless it is in the interest of the child to do so) mean that social workers have begun to look beyond the consumption of a substance to the development of an understanding about the wider context of that consumption, including the recognition that it is not enough to label all drug-using parents as bad, nor is it enough to say that drug use puts the child at risk. Thus social workers are required to develop an understanding of whether and how drug use might put a child at risk and also develop an understanding of how they can work with drug-using parents to reduce that risk.

The Framework for the Assessment of Children in Need and their Families (DH, 2000b) provides the recommended guidance for social workers undertaking an assessment. It suggests looking at three domains:

- the child's developmental needs
- family and environmental factors
- parenting capacity.

The SCODA guidelines (Standing Conference on Drug Abuse – now Drug Scope) on drug-using parents, first published in 1987 and recently updated and revised, offer an important guide to work with drug-using parents, focusing as they do on the concept of 'good enough parenting'. Is the parenting good enough despite the drug use? How can staff work with parents to reduce harm and help to make their parenting good enough? For social work practice, this means:

- Developing an understanding of drugs and their effects on people
- Having an understanding of the context of drug use
- Knowing about the range of support services available for people who use alcohol and drugs
- Developing an understanding of the nature of drug problems to avoid placing unnecessary pressure on parents
- Developing an understanding of harm minimisation in relation to substance use, so that realistic goals can be set and worked towards with the parents.

As Gilman (2000: 23) has warned, social workers need 'to be wary of a tendency to overreact to recreational drug use and underreact to problematic drug use'.

The spectrum of drug involvement has expanded not just in relation to the use of illicit drugs but also in relation to the supply of drugs and here too there can be a danger of overreaction by welfare and criminal justice agencies. Contemporary government drug policy is underpinned by a polarisation of users and suppliers, in the face of a growing body of research on the complexities of the retail drug trade in the UK and the hierarchies of the manufacture and supply chains that implicate the majority of drug users (Dorn et al., 1992; Parker, 2001). Research suggests that many users will obtain their supplies by buying in bulk for economies of scale, sometimes combining resources with other users to save time, money and risk in drug transactions, or users may buy drugs to sell on to friends or acquaintances to subsidise their own consumption. While technically supplying others according to British legislation, the lowest levels of the retail trade are quite different to the middle market and top-level distributors outlined in the work of Pearson and Hobbs (2001), leading to the Runciman Report recommendation – alongside the suggested depenalisation of cannabis, ecstasy and LSD – of a new drug offence that recognises low level supply between friends which may not necessarily be for financial gain (Police Foundation, 1999).

It may well be that social work professionals come into contact with clients with criminal convictions for the possession, manufacture and supply of illicit drugs from across the range of possible levels of involvement. With 67 per cent of drug offenders in the UK having been cautioned or convicted of the unlawful possession of cannabis for personal use, and 62 per cent of herbal cannabis seizures and 48 per cent of cannabis resin seizures involving amounts under one gram in weight, however, we can see that the majority of the 100,000 plus people caught up in the criminal justice system each year are at the lower end of the spectrum of drug involvement (Mwenda, 2005). Such convictions may have significant implications for educational and employment opportunities, parenting and so forth, and yet, given the high levels of experimentation with illicit drugs and the high level of continuing police activity in relation to this experimentation, the convictions themselves may provide no indication of the scale of drug involvement. For social work researchers and practitioners, as for wider society, the challenge is to identify and intervene when illicit drug use becomes problematic for the users, their families, friends and communities, in a climate where definitions of problematic drug use are historically, socially and culturally context specific (Harbin and Murphy, 2000). Problem drug use is more usefully considered across a spectrum of possible patterns and consequences of use – physical, psychological and social – rather than as a simple dichotomy of problematic versus recreational usage, with the concept of drug careers helpful to a consideration of appropriate interventions (Measham et al., 1998; Heather and Robertson, 2003).

◇◇◇◇ CASE EXAMPLE (cont'd) ◇◇◇◇◇◇◇◇◇◇◇◇◇◇◇◇◇◇◇◇◇◇◇◇◇◇◇◇◇◇◇◇◇◇◇

If we return to the head's investigation of the three 15-year-old young women, a key question considered by the school is the source of supply for the cannabis being smoked by the pupils during school hours. The three young women revealed that they regularly pooled their part-time earnings for one of them to buy £20 bags of herbal cannabis or 'grass' from a friend of a friend, raising the issue of social supply to peers. Given that the young woman in question admits to technically supplying cannabis, a controlled drug under the 1971 Misuse of Drugs Act, to her school friends, the head has no choice but to implement the school policy on the supply of drugs and permanently exclude this pupil from the school, while reinstating her two friends who are not believed to have supplied the drug to fellow pupils. This example is repeated across the UK, where pupils buy an illicit drug without realising the grave consequences of seemingly rational consumption patterns and bulk purchasing between friends. The pupil's parents launch an appeal to the school governors at the perceived overreaction to their daughter's cannabis use and the disparity in treatment of the three pupils. In the meantime, the young woman remains at home and receives no formal education, compounding her earlier unauthorised absences from school and missing a significant portion of her GCSE classes. The social worker explores the 'liberal' attitude of the parents to both their daughter's cannabis use and her non-attendance at school, discovering the parents' recreational use of cocaine and ecstasy at weekends. The parents consider it preferable that their daughter is smoking cannabis in the safety of a friend's house to drinking alcohol on the streets with some other teenagers, or taking dance drugs in clubs. Given that cannabis is no longer an arrestable offence and the parents consider it to be relatively 'harmless', in both legal and health terms, they do not share the school's concerns about their daughter's drug use. The parents also view their own drug use as equally unproblematic, despite its admitted impact on family life, both financially with the considerable amount of money they are spending on Class A drugs, and emotionally with their 'comedowns' at the end of a weekend partying. While the parents' drug use could not be considered daily, dependent or chaotic, it raises the issue of 'good enough' parenting and 'bad enough' drug use for intervention by the case worker.

Agency responses and practice issues

There has been a fundamental change in agency policy towards intervention since the emergence of HIV/AIDS in the mid-1980s. Concerns that injecting drug users who continued to inject – and therefore, by implication, could also be continuing to share injecting equipment – might be instrumental in spreading the infection led to a change in political and agency priorities. Prior to the emergence of HIV/AIDS, most agencies had seen their client base consisting primarily of those who had decided to modify, or abandon altogether, their use of drugs, with a smaller number who had not yet reached that decision being offered soup kitchens, day shelters and detached work provision. Subsequently, the priority shifted to make and maintain contact with those drug users (often deeply suspicious of specialist drug services) who were at greatest risk of continuing to share needles, in other words, those who had little or no intention of stopping.

With harm minimisation strategies established in the mid-1980s and the forecasted HIV/AIDS epidemic averted, although figures are beginning to rise and the issue of the levels of hepatitis C infection continue to be ignored (Paylor and Orgel, 2004), recent policy has moved away from a primary focus on public health, at least at the national level. UK drug policy emphasises utilising the criminal justice system to target drug-using offenders and exploiting the legislation to coerce suitable candidates into treatment. Previously, the criminal justice system had been used to tackle drug use punitively, by increasing the associated costs, with the aim of deterrence (Hough, 1996). In current drug policy, the criminal justice system is instead viewed as a mechanism for diverting offenders towards appropriate treatment interventions, with the secondary aim of reducing drug-related crime (Pearson, 1999; Hughes et al., 2001; McSweeney et al., 2006).

A wide range of initiatives has been piloted and introduced at all stages of the criminal justice process to facilitate implementation of the drugs strategy (Paylor, 2008b). First, arrest referral schemes were launched in 1999 and are now operational in many police custody suites across England and Wales (Mair, 2002). Arrest referral schemes involve drug-misusing offenders being referred to a drug worker who encourages them to take up an appropriate treatment programme. Involvement with the scheme is voluntary and it is not an alternative to prosecution or due process. They aim to exploit the opportunity provided by arrest to encourage problem drug users to access treatment services. Schemes vary in their content, from the provision of information about drugs services to the opportunity for arrestees to be assessed by a drug worker based in the custody suite. Offenders can then be referred on to specialist drug treatment services (Edmunds et al., 1998). Statistics from the Arrest Referral National Monitoring Programme on the arrest referral scheme in England and Wales, collected between October 2000 and September 2001, show that 48,810 individuals were interviewed by arrest referral workers in England and Wales and 58 per cent of all arrestees interviewed were voluntarily referred to a specialist drug treatment service (Sondhi et al., 2002).

Second, the Crime and Disorder Act 1998 brought an alternative form of intervention within the criminal justice system, in the form of drug treatment and testing orders (DTTOs), introduced as part of the government's attempt to break the links between problem drug use and persistent acquisitive crime. DTTOs and their successor, drug rehabilitation requirement, are community sentences that enable a court to order an individual who is 'dependent on or has a propensity to misuse drugs' to undergo an intensive treatment and rehabilitation programme for a period of between six months and three years, which includes weekly drug testing, counselling, groupwork and contact with a probation officer (Hales, 2002). DTTOs were subsequently extended to include a less intensive treatment and rehabilitation programme for offenders with less serious offending and drug use.

Finally, the prison service set out a programme for tackling drug use among prison populations (HM Prison Service, 1998). A major strand of this was the establishment of CARAT (counselling, assessment, referral, advice and throughcare) schemes, which are now operational in every prison in England (Hamer, 2002). The aim of these schemes is to assess prisoners who have problems associated with their drug use and ensure that appropriate treatment services are available to them. CARAT workers might therefore generate referrals to detoxification programmes, prison-based therapeutic communities or community drugs services where an individual is approaching release (Hughes et al., 2001). As a result, there has been an unprecedented increase in recent years in the number of drug workers employed within criminal justice settings and a parallel increase in the number of offenders accessing community-based drugs services (Harman and Paylor, 2002).

The drug interventions programme (DIP) is the latest part of the government's strategy for tackling drugs. The delivery of the DIP at a local level is through drug action teams using criminal justice integrated teams (CJITs) (Home Office, 2005b). Social workers occupy key worker roles within CJITs, with responsibility for agreeing care plans, motivational engagement, referring to other agencies and linking with other services (NTA, 2005).

The involvement of criminal justice agencies with drug agencies has required significant cultural shifts on both sides (Rumgay, 2000). The move towards a partnership of the statutory and voluntary sector drug agencies with those in the criminal justice system has been hindered by differences in their objectives, values, organisational culture and operational systems. Organisational goals and values have often developed over significant timescales and define an organisation's identity and purpose. They impact on practice at every level and can be resistant to change (Gibbs, 2001a). In the case of drug agencies and criminal justice agencies, a number of their fundamental values and objectives appear to be opposed. This potential incompatibility may be a barrier to effective partnership and has implications for social workers working in the field (Rumgay, 2003).

Consider, for example, the different value placed by each on the right of the individual drug user to choose whether to access treatment. Drug agencies typically provide treatment services that users access voluntarily. This approach has been adopted for both ethical and practical reasons. First, compulsion into treatment poses ethical dilemmas that challenge the value base shared by many voluntary sector drug agencies, that is, the belief that it is an individual's right to choose whether or not to access treatment, at what point in time and what type of treatment (Newburn, 1999).

Second, in terms of effectiveness, it is widely believed by drug workers that individuals who are coerced into treatment are less motivated to change and treatment is less likely to be effective (van Brussel, 1998). In contrast, criminal justice agencies are, by their nature, agencies of control and have the ability to coerce offenders into accessing treatment services. Even where coercion is not explicit, that is, offenders do not have to decide directly between punishment and engaging in drug treatment, offenders may feel under pressure to access treatment services. Turnbull et al. (2000: 6) expand on this with reference to arrest referral schemes, highlighting 'the pressures on arrestees to demonstrate compliance and to show the intention of "turning over a new leaf" in advance of court'. It should be noted, however, that clear distinctions between 'choice' and 'coercion' may be abstract and illusive, with some drug users perceiving a degree of implicit coercion into treatment anyway, whether from relatives, work colleagues, agency staff or even wider society (Paylor, 2008b).

Since the turn of the twenty-first century, UK drug policy has identified as a strategic aim the coercion of drug-using offenders into treatment services, further emphasised in the new drug strategy (Home Office, 2008). For drug workers, the implication is that they will be required to adapt some of their methods of practice to enable them to work effectively in partnership with criminal justice agencies and this will be vital to drug agencies, given the growing government focus of funding in this area. An example of this is the effect that partnership working is likely to have on the organisational policies of drug agencies regarding confidentiality. Where treatment is entered into voluntarily, the primary obligation of a drug agency is to the service user and client confidentiality is assured. Where an offender is coerced into drug treatment through measures in the criminal justice system, however, the treatment provider is additionally held accountable to the referring agency and may be required to share information regarding the service user with relevant criminal justice professionals (Hough, 1996). Such cultural differences in the goals of voluntary drug agencies and those of agencies within the criminal justice system evidently have the potential to cause conflict over the way in which treatment is provided to drug users. Drug workers operating within and alongside the criminal justice system may find that their role is constrained or they are forced to modify their practice, as a result of conflicting or divergent objectives.

The primary roles of voluntary sector drug agencies vary significantly to those within the criminal justice system. Typically, drug services aim to support and empower individual drug users, while the primary function of the criminal justice system is law enforcement and protection of the public. Although in reality agencies have multiple and overlapping functions, there is likely to be a divergence in opinions regarding the priority that should be accorded to each (Edmunds et al., 1999). This is illustrated by the change in emphasis of different treatment outcomes that has occurred, with the pendulum swinging between a public health and criminal justice-driven national drug policy. Since the 1980s, voluntary sector drug agencies have embraced a wide range of treatment goals, ranging from abstinence at one end of the spectrum to the reduction of drug-related harm at the other. However, although harm reduction strategies have been widely accepted and often prioritised at the local level in community health and welfare services for drug users, they do not fit readily within the context of national government policy and the criminal justice system, where the criminal and control aspects of drug use are viewed as paramount (Keene, 1997). This has resulted in tensions between national criminal justice-driven drug policy and the local public health agenda, for example when recommendations for harm reduction strategies in prison environments were rejected on the basis that they could be viewed as the criminal justice system condoning illicit drug use (Hough, 1996).

In addition to the scope for role conflict between criminal justice agencies and voluntary sector drug agencies, there is the potential for problems to arise from differences in their organisational structure and working practices. Criminal justice agencies are statutory agencies, with clearly defined, hierarchical structures of accountability. In contrast, drug treatment services are often, although not exclusively, small and localised, and typically adopt more flexible organisational and management arrangements (Edmunds et al., 1999). In the UK, drug services tended to develop in response to localised needs, with a notable absence of any 'national standard' for evaluating their effectiveness before the arrival of the National Treatment Agency (NTA). The NTA is a special health authority, created by the government in 2001, to provide national guidance on model treatment services in England. It has yet to fulfil that remit but caution needs to be expressed here. As McGrail (2003: 7) points out: 'good policies can be hampered by "one size fits all" models of implementation because local services work best with local delivery'.

Edmunds et al. (1999) also identify that differences in working style between these two types of organisation can be a barrier to effective partnership working. Specifically, they highlight the procedure-led approach adopted by probation officers and contrast this with the client-centred approach that drug workers more usually employ. Difficulties can arise for drug workers employed within a criminal justice context if criminal justice agencies expect or require them to align to their own working practices. For drug workers to be able to operate effectively in partnership with criminal justice agencies, drug services cannot simply be viewed as 'add-ons' to criminal justice services. There is clearly a need for drug workers and those employed by the criminal justice system to develop joint service provision initiatives, rather than one agency taking a 'control' role and the other forced to align with them. The recent developments in drug policy and the emphasis that has been placed on the criminal justice system as a vehicle for directing drug-using offenders into treatment make clear the government's intention that drug agencies and criminal justice agencies will continue to work in partnership into the foreseeable future.

One of the key objectives for successful partnership working is clarity in the roles of the different agencies involved. Turnbull et al. (2000: 83) identify the need for:

> a clear division of labour which exploits the strengths of each discipline, but also allows for collaboration on key decision-making areas such as the assessment process and treatment plan.

For partnership between agencies to be successful, it is vital that good working relationships are developed (Paylor, 2009). The implementation of the Children Act 2004 and the policy developments that accompany the new legislation herald major changes in the structure and presentation of children's services (Jones et al., 2005). The new children's agenda highlights the potential impact that good partnerships between agencies can have on the services they offer to children and parents (Tunstill et al., 2007).

The importance of working together sets the backdrop for the Children Acts of 1989 and 2004 and can be seen as vital to achieve an effective outcome for families: interagency collaboration and communication are essential to effective working. The absence of interagency collaboration causes a breakdown in communication, delays in service delivery and general confusion and dissatisfaction with service users (Weinstein et al., 2003). Taylor and Kroll (2004: 1122) highlight practitioners' worries regarding the 'different agendas' and 'at times ... polarisation', which can occur within adult and children's services, which has sometimes 'significantly affected the assessment process'.

Consistent messages concerning factors that help and hinder interagency communication within child and family services are well documented (Moran et al., 2006; Mason, 2006). Different treatment systems that seek to address these issues are often not integrated (Stanley, 2007). The fact that these problems can be detrimental for a child's wellbeing shows the need for children's and adult's services to work together. Unfortunately, it is still the case that this does not often happen (Stanley, 2007).

In the case of liaison between drug workers and criminal justice agencies, there is a need for clarification of the responsibilities and role limitations of each party, particularly with respect to issues where there is the potential for conflict in objectives or practice. Take, for example, the issue of enforcement. Where drug treatment is provided within a criminal justice context, offenders may be reluctant to talk openly and honestly about their drug use and associated lifestyle, and drug workers may need to maintain a level of independence from criminal justice services in order to work effectively with clients. However, if the limitations to this independence in terms of information-sharing and confidentiality have not been established and agreed with the appropriate criminal justice agency beforehand, there is the potential for inconsistency in practice and for criminal justice workers to view drug workers as inappropriately collaborating with offenders, resulting in feelings of non-cooperation on both sides.

Newburn (1999) also identifies the need to clarify roles to ensure that the work of criminal justice workers and drug workers does not overlap significantly. This is particularly relevant in the case of offenders serving community sentences under probation supervision. Drug workers may work with clients in a holistic way, looking at a range of issues rather than focusing solely on an individual's drug use.

Interagency rivalry has been identified as a potential barrier to effective partnership between drug workers and criminal justice professionals, that is, the situation where there is concern by workers in one agency that a traditional area of service provision is being encroached upon by another agency (Edmunds et al., 1999). In a study of probation programmes for drug-using offenders, Rumgay and Cowan (1998: 130) recognised that

> the quality of relationships between partners appeared to be linked to the extent to which probation officers perceived substance misuse workers as enhancing or threatening their direct work with clients.

They noted that a frequent difficulty faced by drug workers in their study was that few or no referrals resulted where relationships with probation teams were poor. Thus the effectiveness of drug workers in a criminal justice context is highly dependent upon the efficacy of the partnership between them and criminal justice professionals. A major implication for drug workers is that to function effectively in this environment they need to allocate a significant proportion of their time to 'public relations' work and fostering positive working relationships with potential referrers (Rumgay and Cowan, 1998).

With the shift towards utilising the criminal justice service as a means of directing drug-using offenders to treatment services, it is vital that there is adequate service provision for this population, within both criminal justice and community settings, to enable drug workers to manage the associated increases in caseload. Many community drug treatment services are already operating at capacity or are oversubscribed, and pressure to accept more referrals from the criminal justice system may mean that drug workers are asked to prioritise criminal justice referrals at the expense of those referring themselves voluntarily, who may well have equally significant drug problems but have not been in contact with the criminal justice system. Clearly, the forced redistribution of existing resources would pose an ethical dilemma to drug workers. In their research, Edmunds et al. (1999) noted a tendency for referral workers to develop caseloads of clients with whom they were meeting regularly, due to a lack of appropriate drug services to refer clients on to. Without adequate service provision, the effect of the shift towards a criminal justice-led drug policy will be to place more burdens on drug workers, with consequences for the quality of service.

In addition, it is important that the services available to drug users are appropriate to their needs and not constrained by the criminal justice context of their commission and/or delivery. There is evidence to suggest that different types of treatment may vary in their effectiveness for different individuals (Hough, 1996). There is a need for the range of drug services available to offenders to be expanded, a process that will require more drug workers to work specifically within a criminal justice context. In addition, services provided by drug workers in community treatment agencies will need to be flexible enough to meet the requirements of referring criminal justice agencies. Finally, drug services across all settings need to be better integrated to ensure that appropriate treatment is available to clients moving in and out of the criminal justice system. As Hough (1996: 4) has noted: 'coercing a drug misuser into inappropriate treatment can arguably be regarded as a miscarriage of justice'.

Clearly there is a long way to go. CARAT teams operating in prisons have a specific throughcare function, but to date there is little evidence that this is being effectively put into practice. Although often optimistic about their intentions to stop using drugs, Edmunds et al. (1999) found that over half the prisoners in their study used drugs on the day of their release. With this statistic in mind, it is vital that effective links are forged between criminal justice drug workers and those working in community settings, to ensure that clients receive continuity of care. With research suggesting that high levels of positive drug tests, programme non-completion and reoffending are common within drug treatment programmes (NAO, 2004), the challenge of delivering high-quality and effective community services to drug users remains.

Conclusion

The increased experimentation, use and trafficking in a growing repertoire of illicit drugs in the UK in the past few years means that more social workers will be coming into contact with drug-involved clients and their families. Current drug policies envisage partnership between voluntary sector drug agencies and criminal justice agencies as an essential tool in achieving policy objectives, which include the protection of communities from drug-related crime and access to appropriate treatment services for all problem drug users. However, the strategic shift from a primary focus on public health issues to a criminal justice-driven drug policy, at least at the national level, has had considerable implications for those working with drug users. This chapter has identified a number of potential obstacles to interagency and intersystem collaboration, in terms of differences in organisational values, objectives and practices. If recent policy developments are to be of value in tackling problematic drug use, it is vital that professionals within drug agencies and criminal justice agencies work together to address and overcome these barriers, to prevent the primary aim of partnerships from being obstructed. Perhaps a more fundamental issue, however, is whether the key objectives of UK drug policy, such as the reduction of drug use and drug-related crime, are deliverable, or whether it is more important for policy to focus on meeting the needs of drug users, their families and the wider community, including drug-using offenders.

For further discussion of aspects of the law, see Adams et al., 2009a, Chapter 8.

www.homeoffice.gov.uk Provides, for free, the latest official statistics and government-funded research on drugs, crime and the criminal justice system in England and Wales, as well as the official statistics on drug seizures and offenders, and the self-report survey of adult drug use administered as part of the annual British Crime Survey. Also contains research reports of a large number of government-funded studies of relevance to social work researchers and practitioners.

Brownlee, N. *This is Alcohol*; Constable, N. *This is Cocaine*; Farrington, K. *This is Nicotine*; Thomas, G. *This is Ecstasy*; Brownlee, N. *This is Cannabis*; Ashton, R. *This is Heroin*. The current Sanctuary series of six books, published in 2002, is lively, informative and accessible and specifically aimed at those with a general interest in drugs, including drug users. Each book provides a historical and cultural overview of the individual drug, alongside health information and contemporary policy and treatment issues. Available from mainstream bookshops.

Goodman, A. (2007) *Social Work with Drug and Substance Misusers*, Exeter, Learning Matters; Barton, A. (2003) *Illicit Drugs: Use and Control*, London, Routledge; Manning, P. (ed.) (2007) *Drugs and Popular Culture: Drugs, Media and Identity in Contemporary Society*, Cullompton, Willan Publishing. Three good introductory texts.

Gossop, M. (2000) *Living with Drugs*, 5th edn, Aldershot, Ashgate. Classic introductory textbook.

Peele, S. (1985) *The Meaning of Addiction: Compulsive Experience and its Interpretation*, Lexington, Lexington; Orford, J. (2001) *Excessive Appetites: A Psychological View of Addictions*, 2nd edn, Chichester, Wiley; Booth Davies, J. (1997) *The Myth of Addiction*, 2nd edn, Amsterdam: Harwood. Three stimulating and quite different critiques of traditional disease models of 'addiction'. All three make robust challenges to classic, common-sense and medical models of addiction that social workers may come up against when working in the field. In addition, Prochaska and DiClemente's (1994) 'Cycle of change' is an approach that seeks to educate and empower the user by concentrating on the identification of triggers, insight into high-risk situations, the development of relapse prevention strategies and positive self-talk. This approach emphasises client choice and client responsibility. Motivational interviewing techniques (van Bilsen, 1986) have been widely used with much success in this area.

South, N. (ed.) (1999) *Drugs: Cultures, Controls and Everyday Life*, London, Sage. For the social work researcher, an excellent collection of essays by key researchers in the field, providing a good overview of the research and debate surrounding drugs in the UK. Includes chapters on gender, 'race', dance drugs, government policy and drugs in sport. Is complemented by the special editions on drugs of two journals: the *British Journal of Criminology* (1999) **39**(4), and *Probation Journal* (2004).

Part 2

MANAGEMENT, LEADERSHIP AND CHANGE

Management refers to the process of organising our work effectively. Leadership enables an organisation to engage with its employees and help to provide direction and motivation. Organisational change refers to the process of altering how organisations help practitioners to manage better. This second part of the book examines the major aspects of management and leadership that social workers are likely to encounter in their practice, in their own team and organisation, and in work with other partners and organisations.

We begin with a critical consideration of the relationship between management and managerialism (Chapter 11). The practitioner needs to consider how to balance different priorities in order to manage their workload (Chapter 12). The requirement to develop various forms of partnership adds to the complexity of the task of management (Chapter 13). Not least, it has implications for managers themselves in terms of how they prioritise and lead (Chapter 14). At a day-to-day level, students and practitioners rely on supervisors for professional support, and supervision has much to offer practitioners too (Chapter 15). Different degrees of uncertainty and risk need to be balanced in the process of decision-making (Chapter 16), in which budgetary and financial considerations often are prominent (Chapter 17). The last two chapters of this section look first at how best to assure quality of services and outcomes and, second, what the issues are in working in complex and ever-changing service delivery organisations.

Management and managerialism

11

Management in social work involves a clash between control by an organisation and freedom of professional action. Managerialism seeks to control through rational management processes, while good management involves taking up important issues, responding effectively to them to help practice and its organisational setting make progress.

Chapter overview

Introducing management and managerialism

Management is part of the practice of working in organisations and this chapter builds on Chapter 9 in *Social Work: Themes, Issues and Critical Debates* (Adams et al. 2009a). Social work takes place in agencies and social workers are accountable to the policies of those agencies; management is the process of organising that accountability. As students approach the end of their course and begin to take on personal responsibility for their practice, they must integrate it with the aims and processes of the organisation in which they work. Management faces us starkly with the conflicts of critical practice in social work, because it involves a clash between control and freedom. In this chapter, I examine how a practitioner might integrate critical practice with their organisational responsibilities. The organisational base of social work means that practitioners do not have the freedom of independent discretion in decision-making that we associate with some professions, such as medicine, the law and the Church, so are they also not free to be critical? I argue here that being critical is necessary in management in order to achieve an integrative social work.

Many practitioners focus only on the controlling element of management, ignoring its other aspects. Management is often about controlling an agency and its employees in order to provide services within the resources and policies laid down by political decisions or pressed on us by economic forces. There are current concerns about managerialism or 'businessology' (Harris, 2003a), in which managers focus on achieving compliance with organisational policies using numerical targets rather than encouraging flexible responses to clients' and carers' needs, using the language and techniques of business rather than encouraging professional judgement (Harris, 2003b).

'Good' management, therefore, seems to be about control on behalf of the 'powers that be' rather than 'powers for change'. If all this is so, should the critical social worker simply dismiss management as irrelevant to, or should they attack it as inherently opposed to, critical practice? One resolution of this issue is to create areas of freedom for critical thinking within the boundaries of controlling management forces, for example by a team leader supporting feminist practice within a local government agency. However, this only creates some areas of critical practice within an oppressive structure, rather than influencing the structure itself, it supports critical practice for some clients, while maintaining unequal resources for others who do not have access to this area of freedom.

Critical practice, therefore, needs to incorporate the duality that good service requires control and freedom. The presence of both enables social workers to question critically colleagues who might exercise excessive freedom and discretion, and the availability of critical freedom permits social workers to question excessive control. As we saw in Chapter 1, integrative social work has to incorporate such dualities into practice to respond to the complex lives that clients lead and the need to incorporate social work agencies into the network of organisations that serve clients and their families.

Management is clearly not social work, yet there are demands that social work must embrace management. We see this in ideas such as 'case management', 'care management' or 'managerialism' (Clarke et al., 2000; Payne, 2009) in social work organisations. Managerialism promotes techniques such as 'quality assurance' or 'performance indicators', in which predetermined requirements are set by the powerful, rather than encouraging flexible responses to the needs and wishes of the powerless. Yet the powerful would say that just such a flexible response is what they want.

◇◇◇◇ CaSE EXaMPLE ◇◇◇◇◇◇◇◇◇◇◇◇◇◇◇◇◇◇◇◇◇◇◇◇◇◇◇◇◇◇◇◇◇◇

Management and Mrs McLeod

Mrs McLeod, an elderly, somewhat disabled and lonely woman in her early eighties, illustrates how different understandings of management can seem irrelevant to good critical practice. As greater age restricted her horizons, she had had a limited community care assessment and received meals on wheels from a local voluntary organisation and a home help service from a private operator contracted by the social services department. A few months later, she broke her collarbone in a fall and went into hospital for treatment, receiving physiotherapy, nursing care and a further assessment for adaptations to her old-fashioned cottage. Volunteers redecorated before she moved back home.

When Maria, a social worker acting as a care manager, visited on referral from her GP several months later, she found a community care 'case' typical of many thousands. By this time, a district nurse was visiting weekly to help with her physical care. Talking over the situation, Maria found that Mrs McLeod's son and daughter lived with their teenage families in different towns, visiting on family occasions and taking her out sometimes. Only a nephew who lived a few streets away dropped in regularly of an evening. His mother, Mrs McLeod's sister, had died a few months ago, just before Mrs McLeod's fall and hospital stay, and this had brought to the front of her mind the ache of the loss of her husband through cancer almost 20 years ago, which had been dulled by time.

Neither the twice-weekly visits to the Age Concern day centre that Maria arranged, nor the cheerful rota of drivers who took her there really abated Mrs McLeod's loneliness and depression. The GP said that medication for depression was 'over the top', when Maria inquired. On the social services department's priorities, Mrs McLeod was a long way from a residential care home place, which she quite liked the idea of, because there would be people around to talk to. She quite liked talking things over with Maria, but was coping well enough not to justify casework help for her depression and unresolved bereavement.

So, Mrs McLeod carried on 'managing' in a rather forlorn and unsatisfying final phase of her life. Maria was a care 'manager', implementing her department's priorities and fulfilling the objectives of community care. Her 'managers' were pleased by a sensitive and thoughtful assessment, which met government objectives and performance indicators by maintaining Mrs McLeod in the community. They noted the effective liaison with health service provision, the delivery of a complex range of services from different sources. It was all very well 'managed', yet these human needs might be better met, and this is so in many of the situations we deal with. Many children drift into residential care, many mentally ill people cannot make full use of their skills, many people with learning difficulties are excluded from social integration, many disabled people cannot take the fullest control of their lives.

If we are critical, therefore, our current service does not entirely satisfy us. By 'manage', we imply that we do just well enough, or that we juggle successfully with constrained resources and inadequate services. On the other hand, without managing, it might be worse. We sometimes meet social workers whose practice does not impress, and we hope that some manager is keeping them up to standard.

What we mean by management, what it means to be a manager in social work and what it means to incorporate a concern for management within social work raise complex issues. As always with critical practice, the first step in this chapter is to sort out the different aspects of meaning. This is the purpose of the next section, where I develop a practical model of management, which social workers may find useful. In the following section, I examine some basic theoretical positions within management, because I find that these help to establish the ideas we can use in critical practice.

The meaning of management

The word 'management' comes from the Latin word ', meaning 'hand' (I am grateful to Lydia Meryll for this insight). Perhaps it implies that to manage is to 'handle', to cope, to get things done; perhaps to 'give a hand', to help things happen; perhaps to 'lay your hands on', to grasp and take action. All these aspects of meaning are present in Mrs McLeod's case.

Levels and skills of management

These meanings of management imply different levels of management action. In Figure 11.1, I call the 'coping' level 'management as taking up'. By this, I mean that the fundamental requirement of doing anything is to confront it, try to understand its implications and work on it. Avoiding, forgetting or missing things that we need to work on is the opposite of good management. We often criticise managers, for example, when they will not confront a colleague who is not pulling their weight, because we suspect this will lead to greater problems later on. By not confronting her grief about her husband, Mrs McLeod is putting herself at risk of adverse bereavement reactions later on; by not taking this up, Maria is not managing the full situation that Mrs McLeod faces.

The next 'giving a hand' level in Figure 11.1, I have called 'management as taking hold'. In order to work on a problem, we have first to gain a grasp of its implications and then participate actively in doing something about it. Good management means not leaping in without clear aims, thinking whether someone else is the right person to refer a problem to and helping them to take the right action. We criticise managers if they delegate the tough jobs and then make themselves scarce. We feel that Mrs McLeod's care is merely adequate, rather than good, because Maria is not able to pick up on the more complex interpersonal work that might be done.

I have called the third 'taking in hand' level in Figure 11.1 'management as taking forward'. 'Doing things' is not enough, because good management means making good use of resources and developing our work strategically. Good management means thinking out our aims and planning the coordination of services. We criticise managers if they decide to create a new day centre and get clients' responses to the way they want it to run, and then find out that there are not enough resources to offer anything at all. This is because they should have suspected that they would raise expectations that they cannot fulfil. We are unhappy about the services in Mrs McLeod's care because they do not meet the full range of needs that we can envisage, and society, through political decisions, is not prepared to go far enough to meet needs that we can identify.

Each of these levels of management is involved in many tasks that we undertake: we have to take them up, take hold and take them forward. The left-hand side of Figure 11.1 describes the skills that are important at each of these levels of management. 'Taking up' requires engagement, 'taking hold' requires understanding and 'taking forward' requires us to take action in a purposive way. Each of these levels of work runs into each other. Being prepared to become engaged sets us off to make sure that we have understood all the implications of what we are about to do (taking up) and this means getting involved with the issues and exploring the problem more deeply (taking hold). As we do this, we begin to build up a conception of possible aims and strategies, and, very often, investigating the issues will start to resolve the questions that we are trying to deal with (taking forward).

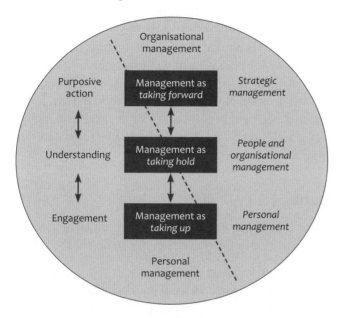

Figure 11.1 Levels of personal and organisation management

Personal and organisational management

All these levels of management include two elements: personal management and organisational management. Personal management is about keeping ourselves organised and efficient through good decision-making, record-keeping, time or workload management. This is relevant to everyone in ordinary life, how Mrs McLeod organises her life, for example. Remembering what it takes to run a household, or buy a car, reminds us that everything involves personal management. We can transfer everyday experience in personal management to work and use management techniques we learn at work in everyday life.

Organisational management is about getting the organisation to work to meet its service aims. It involves things such as supervision, which in practice develops from the student supervision discussed in Adams et al. (2009a, Ch. 21) to incorporate a practitioner's personal development and learning needs with organisational requirements, partnership working (Chapter 13), strategic management and leadership (Chapter 14), quality management (Chapter 18) and reorganising agencies (Chapter 19). The higher levels of management will involve more organisational management, while the lower levels will involve more personal management.

The comments on the right-hand side of Figure 11.1 suggest that this is also true when we look at the structure of organisations. People working at the lower levels will be mainly organising themselves, so their jobs will involve a greater proportion of personal management, whereas people in middle management will probably be organising other people and resources for most of their time, while people in senior management will be mainly working on strategy. People at the lower levels will have to be strategic and purposeful about their work, while people at the top will need to organise their time and make decisions effectively, so that the skills and management levels will still apply to everyone. However, senior management will usually involve a higher proportion of strategic than personal management, and practitioners' work usually the opposite. So, discussing reorganising agencies in Chapter 19, a strategic activity, Jones takes into account personal responses among staff and clients, while the care planning process (see Adams et al., 2009b, Ch. 28) is not only a personal activity for clients but also raises implications for managers.

Ideas about management

Social work management involves three basic distinctions between different sorts of management activity, which are represented in the chapters in this section of the book:

- Between policy, public administration and management
- Between rational, human relations and organic views of management
- Between task, individual and group.

Policy, public administration and management

The first distinction is partly about lines of study and development of ideas and knowledge. The development and study of policy is concerned with how governments determine the direction and form of the actions to take in public affairs. Public administration is the process of organising and administering such services. Management derives more from the business and commercial world and is concerned with how to plan and organise the production and delivery of services and goods. This is relevant to public service and social services because social care is a service, and can use ideas about service delivery from the private sector. This has led to a greater use of ideas and language from business (Harris, 2003b). For example, some agencies refer to clients as 'customers' to emphasise the service ethos they want to encourage in their staff. However, such linguistic changes often sit uncomfortably with a public service ethos of responsibility to elected government for good service to citizens who are helped because they are part of society, not because they have paid for the service, as a customer might do in a shop.

The academic traditions of study in each of these areas have different origins and lines of development, but they overlap and influence each other to some extent. They also have different focuses. For example, a policy focus looks at the processes of, and factors involved in, making policy decisions, while public administration and management are more concerned with how decisions are carried out. Policy issues would suggest what services we should offer Mrs McLeod and whether they should all be in the public sector, or be part of a 'mixed economy of care' covering public, voluntary and private sectors. Public administration and management would be more concerned with, say, how services should be coordinated. Each of these traditions also has different underlying assumptions. For Mrs McLeod, public administration would want to know about the accountability of the different services, to local government or the NHS, for example. Management would be more concerned with whether the workers are well coordinated and motivated to provide a good service; this neglects the role of democratic government for providing services for the benefit of all citizens on behalf of everyone who is part of society.

The first two parts of this book demonstrate that all these aspects need to be integrated together. Part 1 shows that how we think about the issues we face and the values we want to implement in a service crucially affect what we do. Similarly, Part 2 shows us that social work requires a detailed critical analysis of the complexities that clients and their families face, so that simply delivering a service is inadequate; clients and carers need to participate as partners in the social work processes explored in Part 2 of Adams et al. (2009a). Returning to Mrs McLeod, we are dissatisfied with the social services policy that does not seek to deal with the bleakness of her existence and we are dissatisfied with the limited character of a social work that simply organises services rather than engaging with stimulating her dreary lifestyle. To practise management within both policy and social work contexts requires management to interact with policy choices and social work opportunities. It is no use organising things well, if the organisation does not achieve the policy objectives and does not allow social workers to take up the opportunities to practise their craft with clients.

Rational, human relations and organic management

The second distinction is between rational, human relations and organic management. Scientific management focuses on management as a way of structuring organisations and the tasks they undertake, controlling the people within them so that the objectives of the organisation are met. Looking critically at this, however, I discussed 'organisations' and 'tasks' without acknowledging that organisations do not actually exist – they are collections of people. Consequently, tasks can only exist as thought out and done by people. Human relations management proposes that relationships between people carrying out tasks within the organisation are crucial to the success with which objectives are met. It emphasises aspects of the organisation such as 'culture' – the collective identity of members of the organisation and formal and informal groups within it.

Taking the importance of culture further, organic ideas of management are particularly relevant to smaller organisations based on expertise, rather than controlling work or people. In an organic organisation, people work collaboratively, share leadership and focus on allowing knowledge and skill to be expressed and used flexibly. An example is Wenger's

(1998) communities of practice. He argues that people working together develop shared practices and within a mutually supportive process of self- and group education.

These approaches represent a range of styles of organisation, between the controlling and liberating aspects of management. For example, supervision in rational management involves designing appropriate tasks, checking they are performed as required and paying more for better performance, while human relations management focuses on improving the skills and education of employees in order to improve services, and organic management encourages shared personal development. Quality management in the rational view is about the effective definition, planning and sequencing of tasks, while in the human relations view, it is more concerned with involving people in organising their work effectively. Organic management involves questioning what kinds of qualities might be developed. In some respects, these approaches to management are appropriate for different kinds of tasks. For example, rational management might be suitable for more routine, repeated and mechanised tasks involved in factory assembly lines. Human relations management, on the other hand, might be more suitable for more creative, less repetitive and more service-oriented tasks.

Integrative management practice needs to incorporate all these elements. The nature of work in many societies is changing, moving towards less routine activities requiring people to think creatively and flexibly, which might suggest that rational management approaches are less relevant in management nowadays. The nature of social work suggests that a human relations style of management is appropriate, because of its varied nature and human interaction, which seems to need effective motivation of staff, who need a high degree of discretion; in small-scale social work organisations, organic management might be more appropriate, particularly if they seek to develop innovative practice. However, rational management control is not only oppressive and human relations management is not only liberating. In the case of care management in adult social care, for example, practitioners assess and process a range of information that is similar in most cases and come up with consistent decisions that clients and carers can accept as fair. Fairness and consistency are important to members of the public, and a more rational approach is therefore a valid contribution. For example:

- Child protection work implies a consistent attention to detail and checking of information.
- Managing risk for someone who is mentally ill and may harm themselves also requires careful planning.
- Running a residential care home or day centre contains many programmed details.
- Supervising a student or staff member well means keeping careful records and checking information.

Many aspects of social work, then, are susceptible to the processes of rational management and they provide for equality and justice. However, taking this too far would damage the flexibility and responsiveness that many social work tasks seem to require. The question for the critical social worker is where the boundary between programmed and flexible approaches lies, and how the two approaches interact.

The distinction between rational, human relations and organic management helps us to judge the appropriate style of management for our daily activities and work organisation. When are you becoming too programmed, too controlled by the system? When are you using so much discretion and flexibility that you may act unfairly to different clients who have rights to similar treatment?

Task, individual and group

The third distinction is between task, individual and group (Adair, 1986). Clearly, there are tasks to be performed. Organisations and managers need to be clear about what these are. Part of management is defining the work and getting it done. Then there are people who will be doing the jobs and organisations and managers need to think about what they need to do the jobs well. Part of this is the individual practitioner: finding the right people, supporting, training and supervising them. What they need to do the job may be concrete, for example a chair, a desk and a computer. Or they may be fairly esoteric, as for example where managers consider strategically whether to switch assessments from paperwork to computers and what training and support are needed to achieve the move, or whether to use more social and less healthcare or psychological knowledge.

The third aspect is the group. People in organisations are by definition in groups because an organisation implies more than one person. Therefore, managers have to consider how the groups help or hinder individuals in carrying out their tasks. This may be quite concrete, such as organising systems for workflow from, say, the intake to the long-term teams. I have seen staff groups where this contributed to serious conflicts and, in one case, a strike. It is a classic problem in social services (Buckle, 1981), because the culture of such teams tends to differ. Intake teams focus on finishing off pieces of work quickly. Long-term teams sometimes think that work that needed more extensive activity was closed by intake teams, depriving them of work. On the other hand, intake teams sometimes think that long-term teams are rather precious about their therapeutic work and maintain high workloads, preventing them from taking on new cases and adding to the pressure on the intake team, which has to carry the case until it can be taken on long term or close it inappropriately.

Because much social work is multiprofessional, there are also networks of other professions or organisations to deal with. Moreover, social work clients are part of family, community and social networks, whose interests and concerns social workers have to deal with. I call reaching out and drawing in such networks of professional, family and community care 'open teamwork' (Payne, 2000). The need to do this is a powerful support in critical management. For example, in Chapter 19, Jones centres the issue of reorganising agencies as a problem of strategic organisation, looking at the needs of an agency. It would be equally possible to examine the problem of reorganisation by centring on the point of view of service clients and workers. In this way, we may look at the freedoms and controls needed from a variety of points of view. Decentralisation may benefit clients by making workers more accessible, but disadvantage them by separating specialist help from general community provision. As Jones makes clear,

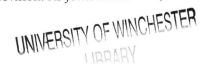

there is no single complete answer, but a range of opportunities and disadvantages. Problems must be compensated for, in this example by organising effective links between community offices and specialist workers.

Managers are helped in making these people-related decisions by understanding the programmed systems and the organisational structures they participate in and the policies, practices and values that come from the agency's decision-making processes and the professional values incorporated into the organisation. All these things interact to help us to work with the person, task and group or network; that is the focus of our action as a manager. However, choices made among the distinctions discussed here construct our managerial practice and form what we do, how we do it and its effect on the people who we manage, our services and the people we serve.

Service management and the people served

Social work is a service, not the manufacture of a product. Many Western societies are increasingly becoming 'service societies', in which providing services and the social structures and behaviours involved in this are more important than the class and organisational structures of traditional manufacturing industry. Services are reflexive, that is, how the person served thinks and behaves affects how the worker can do their work and how the manager can organise the service, and how the worker and manager think and behave affects how the person served can make use of the service. For example, if Mrs McLeod is so depressed that she will not do anything for herself, Maria, her worker, will have difficulty in making her assessment and will have to organise services to respond to this. If Maria is brusque and unsympathetic, she may have difficulty in getting Mrs McLeod's nephew to do more than make the occasional visit.

Therefore, a crucial element of management in social work is how we manage the relationship between the service and the people served, whether we see them as citizens, clients, consumers, service users or customers. It is an important focus of critical practice because it embodies how we manage issues of oppression and empowerment. To the social policy and public administration traditions, citizenship is an important issue, because citizenship confers rights to participation, for example through voting and political accountability, that balance the potential oppression that comes from dependence.

I suggested above that to be a citizen is, in one way, more than to be a customer. A customer is entitled to what they are willing to pay for and standards of service that may be legally defined but are often only set by the service provider. Mrs McLeod is a customer when buying groceries in her local shop, but in receiving social and health services, she is a citizen. A citizen has rights to service, whether or not they can pay and arising from the humanity they have in common with service providers. To manage services as though Mrs McLeod is a customer who cannot pay and so receives services by the goodwill of society fails to perceive her rights as a sister human being and in particular fails to respond to her participation in society and as a voter. However, in another way, she may be excluded from services by a commonplace perception that older people, having had a good life, are less important than children or, being slow and frail, are irritating. So, she may benefit from an organisation that has inculcated among its staff a business-derived 'customer care' approach, which would overcome some of the ill effects of these exclusionary attitudes. A worker's official and legal authority in some aspects of social work does not prevent them being open to influence and a client's direction and self-determination in many other aspects of the worker–client relationship and in their lives. The fact that Maria must assess Mrs McLeod for services, in a way that is partly legally defined, does not prevent her from respecting and responding to Mrs McLeod's preferences and attitudes.

Obviously, clients are 'users' of services, as Mrs McLeod is, and the role of the social worker is sometimes in relation to services. However, social work also develops positive helping relationships with clients; they do not just 'use services'. We saw that Mrs McLeod would benefit from a conception of social work like this. Carers have also become more important in social work thinking. An important social movement emphasises the role that carers play in providing for social need in all societies. Legislation and official guidance have sought to give them rights to contribute to assessments of services appropriate to the person they care for and to have their own position assessed (CSCI, 2006). However, looking at their position critically, their whole being should not be defined by the caring role; they are themselves citizens and members of wider communities. Therefore, they have a political role in social provision that transcends the limited role of 'carer'.

The language we use about the people we serve implies the approach we take to the management of our service, our political conception of its nature and our attitude to the people involved. Whether it is oppressive and regulatory or enhancing and empowering is disclosed by the language of our management approach. We can use this language to understand the nuances of people's perception of their position and our role. This is also true of our colleagues. Thus, an emphasis on 'businessology' discloses a managerialist assumption about the appropriate way of managing an organisation. Similarly, a language of health ('patient') or education ('student/pupil') might disclose a medical or educational model of clients' needs.

Organisational structure and culture

Much management thinking concerns how the organisation is structured (the traditional focus) and its culture and style (a more modern focus). This aspect of management is about accountability. When we think about structure, we are asking ourselves: 'How do I understand how I fit into this collection of people?' When we think about culture, we are asking: 'In what historical and social traditions do I relate to these people and how do they relate to me?' In a cultural view, our work is not bounded by the organisation. Instead:

- It relates to clients.
- It derives from social interactions and policies.

■   It interacts with others' activities in our multiprofessional and community networks.

Traditionally, we ask these questions about the organisation internally. In recent years, however, management has also been concerned to see how these issues affect the organisation's relationship with people outside the organisation. This concern is both with 'partnerships' with other organisations involved in the network of activities, and with 'customer care', that is, how the organisation responds to the people it serves. Clear and positive relationships with customers and 'suppliers', such as people who refer clients to us, ease the work of an organisation, provided they are pursued genuinely, rather than as a veneer of responsiveness – Lymbery and Millward pursue this approach in Chapter 13.

'New public management' emerged in the 1990s. It is a managerialist conception of management within the public sector, treating the public organisation as the organiser, enabler and promoter of services, rather than always being the direct provider (Clarke et al., 2000; Askeland and Payne, 2008). It seeks to disperse power over service decisions, replacing it with public control over the resources that pay for the services rather than the services themselves. This control is exercised through setting targets and performance indicators to achieve compliance with policy objectives. Sometimes central government sets the targets and indicators mainly for local government, but the same conception informs contracts where local public authorities commission voluntary and private organisations to provide services.

This is important for social work management because social workers have become the assessors for new public management service provision. Their major relationship with the public is on behalf of managerialist approaches to their role and practice. However, it is possible to see organisations in a different way, so that while managerialism exerts surveillance and control, it also supports variety and alternatives. Rather than seeing the organisation as a machine, in which accountabilities are structured in linear ways, we can see organisations as systems of interacting groups, with many different cultures, relationships and influences (Bilson and Ross, 1999).

Newman (1996) suggests that organisational culture is not always (or perhaps never) an integrated whole, closed to outsiders and outside influences and consensual in its decision-making. Culture may be a site of contested values, practices and symbols. It may be analysed and changed. A concern of modern management practice is to focus change where there are contested values and practices. In Mrs McLeod's case, the central conflict between the managerialist care management objectives of her managers and the practice possibilities open to Maria is a site of contested values and practices between the open possibilities of social work and the closed assumptions of centralised managerialism. However, within managerialism, there are also elements in tension. Identifying and presenting Mrs McLeod's needs effectively within the organisation offers opportunities for Maria to build on the importance of clients' views in the managerial model of organisational practice.

Seeing organisations more flexibly, so that models of influence are possible that provide alternative sources of power for workers, clients and carers, can help workers to find ways to gain leverage on behalf of clients. This is the aim of the personalisation policy, which has developed from the development of direct payments and independent budgeting approaches to care management in adult social care (see Adams et al., 2009a, Ch. 24). Instead of the care manager assessing clients and carers and organising services for them, a partnership between client, carer and care manager creates a shared plan, which is costed. Services are then organised by the client or carer, perhaps aided by a user-led agency. The practitioner becomes an advocate, supporter and facilitator in 'self-directed care'. The objective is to encourage the interplay of influence.

The personalisation policy thus recognises that organisations are not monolithic – having a single, powerful centre – but contain contending cultures, a variety of centres of influence, and opportunities for external influence to move them. This offers a focus for critical thinking about organisations. Thinking critically leads on to finding alternative modes and sites of action within and outside the organisation. Thus, again, we may see the same management approaches as containing control and opportunities for creativity on behalf of clients.

Work, management and social divisions

It may seem obvious that management is about work, but sometimes this is not considered. Everything about management connects with being in work. As soon as activities are carried out in an organisation, more than one person must be involved, because organisations are by definition a collectivity of people. Organisations require division of labour, responsibility and accountability among the people who work in the organisation. It also means that the people in the organisation must devise ways of ensuring that the organisation works together in some way.

The first point is that management takes place in relation to employment. Personal management involves organising our lives to report for work on time, wearing appropriate clothing, being efficient in keeping appointments with clients and using our skills to answer the telephone or emails appropriately. Organisational management lays certain responsibilities on the organisation and us. Among implied conditions of employment contracts in the UK are that we must cooperate with our colleagues, obey reasonable instructions and work as required. The organisation has a responsibility for organising and planning the work appropriately and protecting our health and safety while we are doing it. Buildings must be planned and laid out, heated and lit, furnished and equipped. Salaries and wages must be paid.

The second point is that work carries obligations, because we are paid and therefore are accountable to those who pay us for the work we do. This may involve doing things we do not want to do. It may also require us to account for our time to others, through the hierarchical system of an organisation.

The third point is that employment has social and psychological consequences. It provides personal support and validation and structures our time. Being part of important social structures, employment can also reflect and incorporate power relations and social divisions within wider society. Thus, many organisations face problems in offering equal opportunities for employment and advancement to employees. Employing organisations may be just as oppressive as other social structures within the societies in which we live, because they take their form and practices from other social structures and must interact with them. Women workers, workers from minority ethnic groups and disabled workers are disadvantaged in employment and so less able to use their shared experience with clients as part of their practice (White, 1995).

Conclusion

Management is a practice, just as social work is a practice. Flowing from this point, critical thinking in management is just as relevant to management practice as to social work practice. Critical practice requires understanding context: the social structures and relationships within which the practice takes place. It also requires understanding meanings: what we mean by management and its different elements and how other people's meanings interact with our own. Does 'managing' mean 'coping' to Mrs McLeod, 'taking hold' to Maria's manager, 'taking forward' to Maria? How do these different meanings matter to the others? What do we do about them?

The succeeding chapters in this part take this forward. They examine some important aspects of personal management and organisational management, the context in which they arise and how they may be carried out. Each in its own way raises questions about how aspects of management may be understood in different ways. In doing so, they put forward their own positions about the aspect considered. However, there are always opportunities for the reader to examine critically the material presented, using the principle of this chapter, that management practice always incorporates both control and freedom. For example, many chapters focus on finding ways of increasing freedom from the constraint of conventional assumptions about their topic.

Inevitably, in the complexity of the tasks undertaken in modern organisations, professions and communities, different aspects of management will be contested. The accountability to her employer in her work role may constrain or liberate Maria's accountability to Mrs McLeod and her family and community as a citizen and human being, and her accountability to the values of a profession that requires critical and creative practice. Management means taking hold, taking on and taking forward those contests, those accountabilities.

 For further discussion of aspects of accountability, see Adams et al., 2009b, Chapter 3.

Coulshed, V., Mullender, A. Jones, D.N. and Thompson, N. (2006) *Management in Social Work*, 3rd edn, BASW/Basingstoke, Palgrave Macmillan. Useful book thoughtfully covering the main practical issues in social work management.

Hughes, M. and Wearing, M. (2007) *Organisations and Management in Social Work*, London, Sage. Good broad general introduction to understanding organisations and management.

Seden, J. and Reynolds, J. (eds) *Managing Care in Practice*, London, Routledge. Useful collection of articles on a wide range of topics relevant to social care.

12 Managing the workload

Chapter overview

This chapter briefly reviews the systems that have been utilised in social work agencies to help manage workloads but, in doing so, it highlights a number of competing dilemmas in such schemes. The goal of critical practitioners is to find creative rather than mechanistic ways of managing these.

At its simplest, managing workloads requires ways of receiving, allocating and supervising the work undertaken within a social work agency. The aim is to ensure that tasks are performed effectively and that there are appropriate resources to undertake the work. Critical practitioners will not only become aware of the limitations of mechanistic attempts to quantify and organise work, but will also be alert to the different management theories and organisational values that can be reflected within them. They will understand that managing the workload is integrally tied to meanings of social work and the value bases on which it operates.

(Mis)managing the workload?

CASE EXAMPLE

A worker in an adult services team has had an unusually high number of referrals allocated to her in the week before she is due to go on leave. On her last day, she has a number of assessment schedules to complete in order to finalise care packages for people she has already seen. This is a slow process, as she has to ensure that all the data are fed accurately into the computer. Also, local performance guidelines demand that the documentation is completed within a certain number of working days. Finally, she is aware of pressure on the provider agencies and she wants to ensure that the requirements of the individual packages are met as fully as possible.

However, she has to give priority to undertaking the assessment of Ms P, an 89-year-old woman who has been referred by neighbours to the emergency duty team during the night. Action needs to be taken, not only because Ms P appears to be at risk, but also because this is not the first time that the neighbours have been disturbed by her behaviour and they are threatening to go to the local press. Previous workers have described her as a fiercely independent woman who wants nothing to do with social services. When the worker visits Ms P on this occasion, she finds her in a distressed state. She is malnourished and it is difficult to assess whether her incoherence and disorientation are due to lack of food, or whether there are more substantial physical and mental health problems. Therefore the worker decides to set up a multidisciplinary assessment. While her presence is not absolutely necessary at this meeting, she becomes aware that she is the only person who, in the short time she has spent with her, has developed a rapport with Ms P and can give support and provide advocacy for her.

In the light of the various pressures on her, the worker makes the decision that she will have to cancel her leave to ensure that the needs of Ms P are properly identified, and that the other assessments are fully completed to secure the necessary services.

Some weeks later, the worker has to take sick leave because of illness, which her GP diagnosed as being stress related. Her personnel records show that for the past three years she has not taken her statutory leave entitlement.

This situation could have been handled differently. The worker could have routinised her tasks by spending less time with Ms P or deciding to be less conscientious about the paperwork (Moffat, 1999). She could have consulted with her team leader/manager at the time that the case of Ms P was allocated to her and shared her concerns about her workload. The agency could have had an effective workload management scheme, which would ensure that the worker had a manageable workload, or that there were systems for dealing with cases at times of overload.

These possible alternatives illustrate that managing the workload has implications for all levels of the organisation. At the macro-level, ensuring systems for allocating work to individuals and balancing workloads between workers are an important part of the health and safety responsibilities of an organisation. This was evidenced by the decision of an industrial tribunal in 1994 to uphold a claim by a social worker that repeated stress-related mental health problems were caused by the failure of his employing social services department to monitor and allocate workloads appropriately. Research demonstrates that one cause of stress in workers in social services is role ambiguity: being exposed to conflicting demands, being expected to do things that are not part of the job and/or being unable to do things that are part of the job (Balloch et al., 1998). In the case of Ms P, such conflicting demands are exacerbated by a lack of time to undertake the tasks allocated.

At the micro-level, the individual worker has to make crucial decisions about competing needs, either between individual service users for whom they have responsibility, or between the needs of those on their caseload and their own needs (or those of any of their dependants). Such decisions reflect the freedom that the autonomous professional values. But if the consequences are overwork, sickness and a resultant poor service, the value of such freedom may have to be questioned.

Workload, values and practice

Attention to issues of stress, worker safety and support are aspects of a more supportive culture, which sees individuals as part of the 'human resources' necessary for the organisation to perform its responsibilities, but also questions what those responsibilities are. Is a system of workload management designed to give a service, irrespective of the quality of the service? Is it in place to ensure high-quality service to those whose needs are seen to be paramount, or are more deserving? Does it represent a welfare system that acknowledges the responsibility of the state to provide for the needs of all those who are not able to provide for themselves? Or is it designed to calculate the cost of each activity, and then analyse its value? These are some of the questions raised for the critical practitioner.

Decisions about workload impact on practice. Jordan (1989) has argued that practitioners have to make ethical choices on a daily basis. They have to make decisions about whether they are responsible for providing absolutely, or achieving the greatest good for the greatest number. But, as the case of Ms P illustrates, such decisions may be taken out of the hands of the worker if the political pressures are so great that an immediate response is required.

Equally, managing the workload and rationing resources are about balancing risk. Official inquiries into childcare cases illustrate that if a worker makes a professional assessment not to offer services, or not to intervene, it is often the individual worker who bears the consequences if the assessment is incorrect. Just as importantly, in situations where those in need of services are deluding or demonstrating aggression, the worker can be put at risk by having to refuse services. Effective management recognises organisational responsibility.

Organisational responsibilities

Within the literature on workload (Vickery, 1977; Glastonbury et al., 1987; SCIE, 2003), there has been emphasis on organisational perspectives, including:

- How are decisions made about controlling the flow of work into an agency?
- What measures can be taken to ensure the equitable distribution of workloads between workers?
- What constitutes a workload, and what are contributory pressures, for example performance indicators, record-keeping and so on?

- Who decides what to prioritise, and when?
- How can the different needs of individuals (users or workers) be addressed in the systems that are introduced?
- What factors should be considered in deciding the appropriate level of an individual's workload?

This reflects the fact that systems adopted by social work organisations to manage workloads have favoured principles of workload measurement, which involve attempts to quantify the work that has to be undertaken and ensure some kind of equitable distribution of this work between workers. Among the most sophisticated have been those developed by the probation service. Regular audits of work undertaken were used by the National Association of Probation Officers to calculate, on the basis of monthly statistics, the allocation of particular pieces of work to individual workers and negotiate staffing levels (Orme, 1995). The first practice guide produced by the Social Care Institute for Excellence (SCIE, 2003) was about managing practice, and contains a useful section on workload, with case studies. This proposes that important factors in managing workload are complexity, risk and travel. It also draws attention to the importance of managing the workload of the team, as well as individuals.

Workload measurement

The probation system used time per task as an analysis of the work to be done and workloads were measured against an agreed total of hours per working month. Such calculations are not uncommon, but the units of measurement can differ in order to reflect different aspects of the work (Bradley, 1987), although basically these units ultimately equate to time.

Practitioners consider measurement systems flawed. Calculations are criticised for not including all the aspects of the work to be done. For example, in our scenario, the increasing paperwork associated with community care assessments needs to be reflected in any calculation of the overall workload. Also, if the worker chose to meet the neighbours to try and appease them and learn more about Ms P's behaviour, would that be a legitimate piece of work to be calculated in her workload?

Other criticisms of measurement systems are that they take no account of the quality of service that might be given (Orme, 1995). Questions are raised about whether measurements on a time per task basis can accurately reflect the complexity of social work tasks, when the focus is on micro-functions, such as the number of reports to be written in a given period or the number of people seen, rather than the purpose of the social worker being involved in the first place. Tasks such as assessment can lead to decisions that deprive people of their liberty. Alternatively, they may conclude that no intervention is necessary, which in community care assessments, such as that required in the case of Ms P, could lead to neglect and death. Such processes require time over and above task completion, that is, thinking time. The arguments are that they should be allowed appropriate weightings to allow professionals to make an informed judgement.

Having said that, some form of measurement is necessary in order to attempt to ensure equity of allocation between workers and, as the industrial tribunal decision highlighted, provide some protection for workers. Also, in the mixed economy of service delivery, workload measurement has contractual implications.

Workloads and markets

The introduction of the market into welfare has brought different emphases to workload management. Service providers have to calculate the resources necessary to undertake identified tasks in order to make realistic estimates of the cost of providing the services. Commissioners have to assess the tenders for service, giving consideration to cost and quality.

Additionally, in a culture of best value (see Chapter 19) and philosophies of total quality management (see Chapter 18), organisations are concerned about performance. In the case of Ms P, the worker was involved as a care manager in the statutory sector, and as such had to be concerned about response times and be aware of the effect of her action or inaction on the public opinion of the organisation. For workers in provider agencies in the voluntary and private sectors, their performance may also affect the success of future tenders and their own employment prospects. The workload calculations made in the original tender will dictate the time they have to provide a quality service.

The interplay of purchasers and providers is therefore focused on the assessment, which becomes the blueprint (Orme and Glastonbury, 1994). At the organisational level, the problem is how to manage a system that can appropriately discern between how realistic the original assessment was and how accurate was the measurement of resources required to meet the need. It is the individual worker who has to operate at these margins, ensuring that the work is done, but not compromising their value systems. However, if they are successful, the outcome may be more contracts, where the expectations are even higher and more is expected of them. If they do not achieve what is required, the service user might suffer, or the worker may be held responsible.

Workload management

At the organisational level, therefore, workload issues are complex. Resources are allocated according to a variety of indicators. These may be certain populations in a particular area, or predictions based on past incidence of, for example, mental ill health. Budgets are allocated according to formulae that include raw data, predictions based on research evidence and political expediency. Statistical data are collected and used to make broadbrush decisions about the allocation of resources, but this is not always enough. In large organisations, different sets of data are often not cross-referenced. So, for example, a social services committee may at one meeting consider data about numbers of referrals, time lapses before cases are seen, number and cost of care packages and average number of cases per worker. At another meeting, it may have data on staff sickness levels (or absenteeism as it is pejoratively called), or make decisions about holding posts vacant in order to balance the budgets. If these sets of data are not integrated, there is little sense of the conditions in which workers are operating. The potential of management information systems to cross-reference such data is great and has to be part of management responsibility.

Equally, decisions about what happens if demand exceeds supply have to be made at the organisational level. Ideally, the response to excess demand would be to deal with the causal factors that created the need, for example poverty, housing and so on, or allocate more resources in order to meet the demand. However, these depend on policies at governmental level. Alternatives include setting workload ceilings, rationing, prioritising or the creation of waiting lists as a means of ensuring that those in extreme need are dealt with, and that workers who provide services are not overloaded.

However, when such policies are introduced, the responsibility for operationalising them again falls to frontline workers. Those in assessment and emergency duty teams, in particular, faced with someone in distress, either at their own misfortune or at the condition of a relative, friend or neighbour, find it difficult to refuse services. The pressure to respond is great, even if this means that there will be fewer resources either in terms of hospital beds, daycare places or indeed the worker's own time to give to others who might come along in greater need.

Individual responsibilities

Whatever macro-systems are introduced, therefore, they have implications for the frontline worker. The basic tenet of social work, respect for persons, has to operate in all service provision. The individual worker's dilemma in a system of rationing is how to reflect such an ethic when having to refuse requests and not meet need.

Equally significant are the decisions about how time is spent. If a worker spends time with an individual, it may be possible to identify resources that maintain the person in their own home and avoid them becoming part of the welfare system. This might not always be the most streamlined intervention, but it may be more effective for the individual who otherwise might have to give up their right to privacy and autonomy by becoming a client or user. However, the consequence for the worker in the case of Ms P of setting up an appropriate and professional multidisciplinary assessment was that she had to forego her own leave because, in the light of competing pressures, there was not enough time available.

Allocation of time is therefore crucial, but frontline workers' criticisms of measurement systems were that they are retrospective, giving opportunity for relief once overload in workload has been identified (Glastonbury et al., 1987). This does not have to be the case, especially now that computers can input, analyse and give graphical representation of data within minutes. However, such systems are dependent on workers being prepared to input the data and the systems being sensitive to the nuances of the task they have to perform.

Management responsibilities

Computerisation brings further challenges. The introduction of measurement systems may be seen to give workers protection and ensure the quality of service to users. More effective management could ensure that when there was unexpected demand, as in the case of Ms P, the work could be dealt with in other ways, either diverted to other sources of help or emergency staff recruited. However, in order to achieve this, workers would have to experience greater accountability, informing the supervisor exactly how time was being spent, justifying the work that was being done and why it was being done. All forms of overview of a worker's activities can represent a form of surveillance of the individual's work, and surveillance has been integrally related to issues of power (Foucault, 1972).

To achieve measurement, there have to be exercises that log detailed activities to achieve a baseline (Orme, 1995). In imposing measurement, there are expectations of normative practice that might not allow for individual differences. The positives of such systems therefore depend on the management culture. It is also unhelpful if, as a result of analysis, the worker is made responsible either for the cause of the overwork because they 'took too much time' or 'got too involved', or for the solution, by multitasking, streamlining their systems or undergoing training in time management.

While there has to be an element of self-management, and advice on how to cope with demands is important and helpful, what is crucial is the context (Coulshed et al., 2006). For example, where workload schemes have been used systematically and transparently, workers have welcomed the acknowledgement that they were doing 'too much', that they were working over their allocation. This was enough to relieve their stress and enabled them to keep going (Glastonbury et al., 1987). More importantly, it provided everyone with crucial information, which enabled them as a team to look at where the pressures were coming from and identify what could be done to relieve them. It is regrettable that the code of practice for social care employers, published by the General Social Care Council in the UK, does not explicitly lay a responsibility on employers to ensure that resources are adequate to meet workload and the demands placed on social workers. Instead, the code focuses on performance management and the personal responsibility of practitioners (GSCC, 2004).

At the individual level, systems such as case review involve the allocation of work accompanied by close supervision by a manager. Ongoing supervision of allocated cases involves feedback and discussion, which is part of ongoing professional development. It can offer support in decisions about the amount of time to be spent with cases and managerial accountability for rationing decisions and ongoing risk assessment. It can also provide information that can be fed into the organisational systems about the demands of particular work, or about the patterns of need that are emerging. Why, for example, did the worker in the case of Ms P have an unexpected demand before her leave? Was it because she had left some tasks to the last minute or because there were local circumstances that were unpredictable?

Simply advocating management involvement is not an easy solution. Healy (2000) warns that managerialist attempts to control, which might also relieve some of the pressures, often emphasise authoritarian and hierarchical power. The suggestion that everything can be measured, and in measuring can be quantified and controlled, is seen as part of rationalist, modernist assumptions associated with Weberian notions of formalised, hierarchical models of bureaucracy that are not always relevant to social work (Coulshed et al., 2006). Such management styles have been seen to be oppressive. For example, they can be phallocentric because they are 'not the way of women' (Healy, 2000: 91), or impact negatively on workers who, because of culture, gender or disability, do things differently (Hough, 1999).

Critical practice

It is not necessary to reject all attempts at managing workload as part of a negative managerialist agenda. As has been said, worker protection and efficient operations are important aspects of positive management, leading to effective service delivery. Understanding and critically analysing the systems that are introduced helps workers to understand how different personal, professional and organisational identities are constructed by different managerial discourses (Hough, 1999). Positive practice involves localised activities, which include networking, strategic alliances to allow for reflection on workday lives and the impact on workers' construction of their identity in the workplace (Hough, 1999: 51). Such reflection can involve individual users reflecting on how needs can be best met, workers reflecting on the way in which policies are implemented, and the impact of these on workers and service users. Active listening, feedback and achieving egalitarian relationships can support systems of workload management that are more discursive and interactional and will be more acceptable and fruitful than mechanical systems of measuring input and output.

Such interactional systems allow workers to exercise their rights and power by collective responses. They require that workers be consulted about the workload systems that are used, and the detail of the calculation. In the past, such activities might have been coordinated by trade unions or professional associations, now they are more likely to operate at the local level, where the specific conditions can influence the systems that are set up, but it is still necessary to network at national or UK level. Accurate information about workloads that reflects both the time and level of expertise necessary in social work interventions should inform policy decisions about funding, staffing levels and qualifications.

The disadvantage is that effective systems take time, a scarce commodity within social work resources. However, if time is not taken, the quality of services will be compromised and resources, including human resources, will be wasted. In social work, this can have life-threatening consequences – for users and workers.

For further discussion of the organisational context, see Adams et al., 2009a, Chapter 9.

www.scie-peoplemanagement.org.uk/resource/docPreview.
asp?docID=126 SCIE People Management provides continually updated
guidance on a range of managerial issues, including workload and priority
management.

Bilson, A. and Ross, S. (1999) *Social Work Management and Practice*, 2nd edn,
London, Jessica Kingsley. Uses systems theory to analyse social work
management.

Coulshed, V., Mullender, A., Jones, D. and Thompson, N. (2001) *Management in
Social Work*, 3rd edn, Basingstoke, Palgrave Macmillan. Provides an excellent
overview of the themes and issues relating to managing social work generally,
with specific sections on workload.

Orme, J. (1995) *Workloads: Measurement and Management*, Aldershot, Avebury/
CEDR, University of Southampton. Describes a research project undertaken with
probation officers and explores in detail the complexities of trying to operate
and refine workload measurement systems.

Payne, M. (2000) *Teamwork in Multiprofessional Care*, Basingstoke, Palgrave –
now Palgrave Macmillan. Explores how teams in care services can use
networking and team-building to strengthen their practice, with practical guidance on team-building and team-building activities – all necessary when
managing workloads.

Partnership working   13

This chapter focuses on the subject of interprofessional practice in social work. It discusses the political and professional obstacles to such collaboration, arguing that the needs of service users require such work. It concludes by identifying the attributes likely to make interprofessional work successful.

Chapter overview

Effective partnership working has been a major issue in successive government documents since the late 1990s; indeed, it has been suggested that the promotion of interprofessional working has been at the heart of UK government policy (Clarke and Glendinning, 2002). Certainly it has been catapulted to the centre of the social work enterprise, as interprofessional working is one of the elements of the core curriculum for social work courses (DH, 2002a). There is little doubt of the justice of the proposition that essentially justifies this: many of the problems of human existence with which social workers are confronted can only properly be resolved by different agencies and professions acting in concert (Challis et al., 2006). As a consequence, it is often impossible for an individual social worker to provide an adequate response to the needs of service users and their families if they work in isolation from other professionals. Therefore, the social worker does not practise in a vacuum and is often dependent on other professions to enable a satisfactory outcome for the service user.

However, despite the political conviction that effective partnership working can help to resolve social problems (Clarke and Glendinning, 2002), the conceptual and practical difficulties that might obstruct such practice are often not fully appreciated. In addition, the evidence that such working improves outcomes for people is not strong (Brown et al., 2003; Davey et al., 2005). This chapter first explores these issues, focusing on the political context before examining the core dimensions of professionalism. The majority of the chapter, however, will focus on the attributes that social workers must demonstrate if they are to develop into successful practitioners in the environment of interprofessional practice. After all, even the most sophisticated understanding of this context will not in itself improve practice; for such an eventuality, a social worker will need to engage in careful thought about a number of issues, and then work out how to put them into effect. The chapter will therefore focus on these general topics, as we believe that the principles that underpin partnership working – and the characteristics of effective practice – are common across all the various settings within which social workers operate. The chapter therefore starts with structural considerations, then considers a series of professional matters and finally focuses on practice; this replicates the analytical approach of Beattie (1994).

Partnership working: the political context

It is important first to recognise that effective partnership working does not just require understanding of how well individual professions can work together, it also presupposes that different agencies are prepared to undertake such cooperative working (Payne, 2007). Because of this, it is vital to understand the political salience of interprofessionalism in contemporary social policy. Although the British New Labour government did accelerate the pace of change, it would be incorrect to suppose that the preceding decades had contained no indications of an interest in, and need for, improved systems of partnership working (see Loxley, 1997 for a summary of the many documents that called for this). Indeed, as various contributors to Leathard (2003) indicate, there has been substantial literature on the subject for several decades. However, it is the particular significance of the concept to the Labour administration that needs to be fully understood in order to make sense of its rapid rise to centre stage in the development of welfare.

As noted above, this originates from the understanding that many social problems cannot effectively be addressed by any organisation or profession acting in isolation from others. From the late 1990s onwards, most official policy documents have promoted the importance of collaborative working as a means to improve the delivery of welfare. For example, the White Paper *Modernising Social Services* (DH, 1998) devoted an entire chapter to the subject, making improved partnership working a key element of welfare services, while *The NHS Plan* (DH, 2000c) also dedicated a chapter to improving the relationship between healthcare and social care. Similarly, one of the main elements of the Green Paper *Every Child Matters* (DfES, 2003) was its argument that improved interprofessional working was required if we were to avoid a repeat of the tragic events that characterised the Victoria Climbié case.

For service users, the benefit of this is simple: the better organisations and professionals work together, the more likelihood there is of a genuinely 'seamless' service. However, while the various organisations involved in partnership working may have much to gain from such an emphasis, they also may have something to lose. (This essential point is elided in much official literature.) Although much writing focuses on the benefits of improved collaboration, there appears to be considerably less official understanding of the second point. For example, there is relatively little consideration of the fact that the different organisations involved in collaborative working might well have incompatible priorities for the use of financial resources, and that this will affect the nature of interprofessional work (Lymbery, 2006).

While we suggest that this typifies all practice within social work, we will exemplify our argument in relation to the care of older people. This has been the subject of detailed prior analysis on which we draw for this chapter. For example, issues around the boundaries between health and social care were extensively explored by Bridgen and Lewis (1999). Adopting a historical perspective, they judged that although the relative decline in the provision of health-funded services for older people was accompanied by an increased need for local authority services, the small budgetary increases that were available to local authorities were inadequate in relation to this scale of need. Given the budgetary limitations that have existed for healthcare and social care, they argue that the postwar years have therefore been characterised by attempts by both services to transfer responsibility for older people – an enterprise where healthcare has been markedly more successful than social care (Bridgen and Lewis, 1999; see also Lewis, 2001). The financial imperatives that governed the implementation of community care policies in the 1990s originated in a similar shift; the change in supplementary benefit regulations ensured a rapid movement of people and resources from the NHS into residential and nursing homes (Lewis and Glennerster, 1996), which were often located in the private sector – where the services provided have come to be the responsibility of social care. The root cause of this problem, as far as older people are concerned, is the lack of precision in the separation between health needs and social care needs that characterised the foundation of the NHS (Lewis, 2001). In reality, there have always been people whose needs are located somewhere between healthcare and social care and who are therefore capable of being defined as the responsibility of either body. As a result, while the separation between healthcare and social care appears to be straightforward, its complexity becomes apparent on closer examination; consequently, space is opened up for different organisations to manipulate it (Means and Smith, 1998).

Thus some of the key factors that helped to create the 'Berlin Wall' – to which reference was made in the White Paper (DH, 1998) – between healthcare and social care in relation to older people were present in the very formation of the NHS in the 1940s; to see this as primarily the result of professional rivalries – which is what could be surmised from a reading of various government publications – represents a considerable oversimplification (Lymbery, 2006). As a result, the espousal of partnership working as a universal remedy to improve practice must be viewed with a degree of scepticism:

> The administrative and financial dimensions of the health/social care divide have become entrenched. It is therefore little wonder that practitioners as well as government have tended to fall back on a third form of solution that addresses the professional divide by some form of collaborative working. By itself, this approach is unlikely to prove sufficient; battles over responsibilities would continue. (Bridgen and Lewis, 1999: 119–20)

While this analysis has focused on the issues relating to older people, a similar line of argument would be applicable for many other service user groups – indeed, they have general applicability in relation to adult social care, as repeated attempts by government to clarify the respective organisations' responsibility in relation to continuing care makes clear (Mandelstam, 2005). In their research on this theme, Abbott and Lewis (2002) have noted the continuing salience of a combination of financial and structural issues on the provision of effective continuing care. They stress that the boundaries between healthcare and social care remain major obstacles to the stimulation of effective joint working arrangements. However, they also suggest that where there are closer working relationships between healthcare and social care organisations, there may also be fewer problems in implementing continuing care. We will explore the implications of this in a later section. It is important to stress that the upshot of our analysis is not that effective interprofessional working is simply impossible and therefore an unwise aspiration; however, it is equally important to recognise that these substantial structural problems may obstruct the capacity of professionals to work together effectively.

Dimensions of professionalism

As we have seen, to see the construction of the 'Berlin Wall' as primarily the result of professional rivalries would be an oversimplification of a complex issue; nevertheless, it remains vital to understand the nature of some of the professional disputes that do exist in the areas of healthcare and social care. It is also important to be clear that these rivalries have a conceptual origin, and are not simply a reflection of petty personal jealousies. In this section, we identify some of the sociological literature on the professions that helps to explain some of the elements of this.

Hudson (2002) has observed that a range of issues around professions and professionalism forms a key part of the extensive 'pessimistic' literature on the subject; he has further argued that pessimistic commentary outweighs optimistic (Hudson, 2007). In general terms, Hudson (2007) balances the focus on distinctiveness and differentiation that characterise pessimistic approaches with the commonality and compatibility that are emphasised in more optimistic accounts. He also proposes that there is a normative dimension of partnership working that should be acknowledged: simply put, closer working relationships between professionals are, both in and of themselves, a good thing for service users, even if they do not have a direct impact on the outcomes of care support. However, Hudson (2002) also notes the strength of the pessimistic tradition, pointing out the significance of the following dimensions in this:

- Relative status and power of professions
- Professional identity and territory
- Different patterns of discretion and accountability between professions.

The first two points are particularly significant in the development of professions at the general level: it is to a consideration of some of the literature around this that the chapter now turns.

Much early literature on professions focused on the benefits they could bring to society, and the presumed characteristics of those occupations that could be identified as professions (see Wilding, 1982). It was argued that a clear distinction could be drawn between those occupations that could be granted professional status – typically accountancy, law and medicine were held to be exemplars of these – and other occupations deemed not to be characterised by the same range of characteristics, which were consequently categorised as 'semi-professions' (Etzioni, 1969). In the context of this chapter, such occupations were usually held to include nursing – among other professions related to medicine – and social work.

From the 1970s onwards, a number of theorists advanced more critical positions on the nature of professions. For example, Johnson (1972) discussed professions in relation to the power they could exercise within society; he argued that it was vital to explore the ways in which various professional groups had managed to secure a degree of control over their occupations. In his view, what distinguished social work from more established occupations was little to do with its supposed 'traits' and more connected to its relative lack of power when related to more established occupations – particularly medicine. Johnson (1972) argued that social work in Britain was a 'state-mediated' profession and its primary location as part of the apparatus of local government served to deny it a full measure of control over the terms through which it carried out its tasks.

A number of other theorists subsequently modified and extended the critical thinking of Johnson in the direction of what Evetts (2006a) has termed a 'market closure' approach to professionalisation. For example, Larson (1977) – strongly influenced by the work of Freidson (1970) – discussed the extent to which professions have been able to organise a market for their services and thereby enhance their collective status and prestige. She termed this process of professionalisation the 'professional project', which she held to be characteristic of the way in which all professions operate. In a related argument, Abbott (1988) suggested that a core characteristic of professions is their ability to delineate a clear sphere of activity over which they can exercise control. He argued that medicine had achieved this in numerous areas of activity. A corollary of this is the understanding that social work's relative lack of power has tended to confirm its subordinate status – particularly in relation to medicine. Indeed, in a notorious critique of social work, Brewer and Lait (1980: 204) suggested that social workers should submit themselves willingly to the 'rule of medicine'. However, as Huntington (1986: 1152) has noted:

> The problem for social work in health settings from its inception … is that doctors have frequently denied or rejected the diagnostic and therapeutic contribution of social workers.

An acceptance of the 'rule of medicine' would be deeply problematic under such circumstances. Following Abbott's line of argument, it could be suggested that the failure of social work as a discipline to become accepted within such settings is as much a consequence of the way in which historically more dominant professions have restricted its opportunities as it is a statement of social work's inherent limitations. There are obvious critical implications for interprofessional working that follow such an analysis; certainly, it tends to argue that the parity of esteem and respect that are vital to successful inter-professional working would structurally be impossible to achieve.

Contemporary sociological thinking (see, for example, Evetts, 2006b) is potentially much more optimistic, both in its general implications and in relation to the establishment of effective interprofessional practice. Evetts has suggested that a more nuanced view of professions should accommodate positive as well as negative elements, and that there should be a consideration of the benefits that can derive from professional work (see also Foster and Wilding, 2000). The later writing of Freidson (2001) has been influential in this respect, significantly amending the perspectives that underpinned much of his earlier work. While Freidson's (1970) initial writing was influential on theorists of 'market closure', his later work (Freidson, 2001) focused on the extent to which professionalism could be regarded as a viable and potentially important way of organising work, particularly in relation to the dominant alternative visions of the market and bureaucracy. Central to his argument is the conception of 'trust' – the extent to which professionals can be relied on to carry out their work to the benefit of those who need services; this is a critical notion for social work specifically, and has relevance to the effectiveness of interprofessional work more generally. Indeed, it has been suggested that the numerous attempts to make professionals more accountable to the public have served to increase levels of mistrust of professional intentions and actions (O'Neill, 2002). In reality, there is a much stronger focus on accountability than trust in the public sector (Smith, 2001); this has consequences for the development of effective practice in an occupation such as social work where the creation and maintenance of trust is such a vital element.

While recognising the force of much 'pessimistic' literature (Hudson, 2002), we do believe that it is possible to be more optimistic about the potential of interprofessional activity. For example, we would suggest that effective cooperation between different professional groups is possible, provided that the differences between them – their professional goals, the nature and pace of their work, their essential orientations – are acknowledged and accepted.

For social workers, this implies not only clarity about the contribution of their own professional voice, but also an awareness of the specific knowledge and expertise that can be brought by others. The logic of this argument would see us being in favour of interprofessional arrangements that recognised, validated and worked with difference, rather than seeking to develop new breeds of workers who supposedly integrate the characteristics of different professional groupings. As such, we argue that there is considerable value in the specific contribution of social workers alongside other professional groups. We also accept, however, that the very creation of interprofessional teams will have an impact on the professional allegiances of staff when confronted with the realities of shared practice (Wenger, 1998). Regular team meetings can therefore serve as a forum for sharing and an opportunity to understand the precise contributions of others; it will be important for members to share their perspectives regularly with colleagues, developing deeper understandings of their distinctive contributions along the way. Through this process, a genuine sense of being engaged on a joint enterprise can be developed. In turn, this can lead to a working atmosphere marked by the informed and constructive criticism that characterises the most effective forms of joint working, avoiding the harsh, destructive patterns of interaction that could emerge. Mutual respect is a prerequisite of such interaction; it is precisely this absence that has bedevilled interprofessional developments in the past.

As Hudson (2002) has recognised, it is difficult to construct viable patterns of partnership working on uneven and unequal foundations; certainly, the structural inequalities of which we have written are not a fruitful starting point for interprofessional collaboration. However, he also suggests that it is important to find ways of developing such working; other writers (see, for example, Wenger, 1998) have suggested various ways in which this goal can be achieved. In particular, the creation of formal interprofessional, multidisciplinary teams could be a fruitful step in this direction. According to Molyneux (2001), there are several key factors that enable such teams to work effectively, including good quality communication within the team and the opportunity to develop creative working methods. She also emphasises the personal qualities and commitment of staff, which are particularly important factors for social workers. The following section discusses the ways in which social work practitioners can contribute to the effective working of such teams.

Making it work: social work practice in the interprofessional setting

It has been asserted that social work should be seen as 'the joined-up profession' (Frost et al., 2005: 195), providing a necessary link between different occupations within the system of welfare and between these professions and service users. However, unless accompanied by effective action on the part of social workers, this could become little other than empty rhetoric. This section, therefore, will seek first to identify what we consider to be the unique characteristics of social work, before examining a number of specific issues that relate to the attributes that social workers will need in order to play an effective role in the interprofessional environment.

We suggest that the uniqueness of a social worker's contribution to interprofessional activity rests on a combination of its knowledge, skills and values, leading to a holistic form of practice. In isolation, there is little in any of these separate areas where social workers can claim a privileged status. For example, a social worker's knowledge – drawing as it does on different elements of numerous academic disciplines – is not unique to the social work profession. Similarly, the skills that a social worker is required to demonstrate are common across numerous similar occupations. While it could be suggested that social work's values are of a distinctive nature (Thompson, 2006), it would be arrogant for a social worker to claim that aspects of this value base are not common across other professions within healthcare and social care.

However, in the above combination, one distinctive feature is also present: a social worker ought to possess an orientation that places the service user at the centre of their practice. In this way, Hugman (1998) argues that the social worker places their knowledge, skills and values at the service of the user. In his view, the conception of 'service' should ensure that social work does not become an elitist profession, more concerned with the promotion of its own interests rather than those of service users – a core element, as we have seen, in the criticisms of professions mounted from the 1970s onwards. In this way, arguably it is possible for social work to construct a new form of professionalism, based on a clear orientation to practice (Lymbery, 2001; Healy and Meagher, 2004).

This is particularly significant in the absence of detail in the definition of social work's roles and tasks. Indeed, this gap is particularly significant; the generality of social work's roles and tasks, and the functions that social workers are expected to play within society are critical, and contrast markedly with the more specific skills that are required of, for example, doctors, nurses, physiotherapists and occupational therapists. Apparently, even at government level, there is little clarity about the specific role of social work. For example, the document *Social Work at its Best* (GSCC, 2008) seeks to define the roles and tasks of social work within the context of the 'personalisation' agenda (Leadbeater, 2004) and the internationally agreed definition of social work (IFSW, 2000). Its conception of social work is perhaps more notable for its vagueness than it is for any detailed insight about the uniqueness of what social work actually does contribute. For example, it seeks to distinguish between the 'roles' of social work – in relation to its broad purposes and the outcomes that it seeks to enable people to achieve – and the 'tasks' that facilitate social workers to deliver the purposes and outcomes. However, the document states that the defined roles may only 'tend to be particular to social work' and that the resulting tasks may be carried out either by qualified social workers or unqualified social care workers, and may be, in any case, 'similar to tasks other disciplines undertake in performing their roles' (GSCC, 2008: 10). It would seem, therefore, that it has not proved possible to define precisely how a social worker is different from any other professional or indeed from an unqualified social care worker, in relation to 'roles' and 'tasks'.

The following statement confirms this impression:

> In recent years there has been a trend, reinforced by government policy, towards blurring role differences and loosening boundaries between professional systems. Unduly rigid boundaries are thought to cause problems to people trying to find their way round the system, and to make for inefficiency in the use of professional resources. Social work roles tend to be more elastic than those of many other disciplines. (GSCC, 2008: 10)

Two messages are conveyed in this short extract. The first is that the blurring of role boundaries between professions is a good thing. As we have previously noted, this does not represent our position. The second relates to this, in that the very 'elasticity' of social work roles arguably ensures that its boundaries are more capable of being blurred. All this contributes to a key point of this chapter – the fact that it is difficult to identify the specific contribution of social work within partnership working.

If one accepts our contention that it is the combination of knowledge, skills and values combined with a practitioner's orientation to their practice that can be considered to be characteristic of social work, the way in which these manifest themselves in practice becomes critical. The mere possession of a full repertoire of social work's best qualities does not necessarily lead to success in the interprofessional environment. From our experience, we suggest that there are several qualities that a social worker needs in order to promote successful partnership working. Without such attributes, it will be particularly difficult for a social worker to be effective, irrespective of their skills. Before turning our attention to these individual qualities, we first explore some characteristics of the work environment that can aid the development of successful partnerships. It is useful to reflect that there is a detailed literature on which to draw that discusses the various factors enabling effective joint working (Cameron and Lart, 2003).

Indeed, it is particularly important to pay attention to this aspect of partnership working when at the start of any new interprofessional development. While there has been a long history of interprofessional working in some areas of activity – integrated teams are common in the fields of youth offending, mental health and learning disability, for example – in other areas of practice, they are less customary. This is potentially significant as 'success breeds success': the more positive the experiences of interprofessional working, the more likely it is that similar ventures will succeed. If we reflect on our own experience, the success of the location of social workers within primary healthcare (Lymbery and Millward, 2000) led to an openness towards the idea that community nurses may be able to carry out an equally positive role within social services teams (Lymbery, 2005).

Another important consideration is the specific role and function that a social worker will play in that environment. In the history of social work's relationship with healthcare, for example, the broader contribution of social workers was often limited by the desire of doctors for social workers' primary role to be the provision of ready access to care resources (Lymbery, 2006). While this will remain a critical part of a social worker's role, we believe it should not be limited to this; indeed, if a social worker is enabled to work more broadly, this can create added value for the team and a more satisfying role for the practitioner (Lymbery and Millward, 2000). This latter point must not be forgotten: we suggest that social workers currently have to operate under three related forms of 'tyranny' – the caseload, intrusive and unnecessary managerial scrutiny, and performance indicators. None is conducive to good practice, with anxiety and a desire for self-protection dominating practitioner responses (Lymbery, 2007).

The practical implications of these 'tyrannies' can be illustrated with a simple example. It is customary for all social workers with older people to work with extremely high caseloads, the extent of which often compromises the quality of work they can accomplish. The managerial scrutiny that is applied in such circumstances is often focused on the need to reach rapid conclusions, as timescales are a key aspect of performance measurement. This may, in many cases, be inimical to good quality social work, and also profoundly demoralising to those practitioners who recognise the compromises into which they are forced.

We believe that any social worker engaged in meaningful interprofessional work must have the capacity to work independently. In many ways, this represents one of the major problems for the organisations that employ social workers, which have become accustomed – over many years (see Howe, 1992) – to act in ways that control and constrain practitioners, rather than trusting them to develop flexible and creative responses to need. As Smith (2001) has it, the policies of successive governments have replaced a focus on trust with a set of requirements that are presumed to increase public confidence in the work of practitioners. While the impact of this has arguably been sharpest in relation to adult social care (Dustin, 2008), numerous papers have highlighted a similar trend in relation to childcare (see, for example, Huntington, 1999).

We accept, therefore, that to argue for social workers to be given the opportunity to exercise a higher level of autonomy may conflict with the overall direction of policy, a problem felt internationally beyond the confines of British practice (Burton and van den Broek, 2008). As Hudson (2002) has observed, there are clear differences in the levels of discretion and autonomy that have existed within professional groups, and it is clear that these differences can be problematic in the interprofessional setting. However, from our research and observations, the more social work practitioners have the scope to practise independently, the more confident and creative their practice is likely to be (Lymbery and Millward, 2000). In addition, we suggest that independent working does not necessarily conflict with the desire for strong levels of accountability, as Eadie and Canton (2002) have argued in relation to youth justice.

This has further implications: the more an individual is confident in their own capabilities, the more they are able to have a significant impact on the workplace (Lymbery and Millward, 2000). Indeed, this learning is equally applicable to other disciplines as well as social workers (Lymbery, 2005). A closely related attribute is a level of clarity about what it is that one specific professional group can contribute to the interprofessional setting. In relation to services for older people, for example, it is apparent that social workers and district nurses will contribute to the assessment of need; however, each professional group will have a different perspective on the assessment, which can potentially benefit its overall quality (Worth, 2001; Torkington et al., 2004). This implies a level of clarity about one's own professional role and that of others, which has been argued as a prerequisite of interprofessional collaboration (Dombeck, 1997). Ultimately, this clarity would ensure that professional self-confidence would be earned. In addition, it should enable a social worker to be assertive about their contribution and open and accepting of the involvement of others. It could also enable a social worker to develop broader engagements with social issues and more purposeful interactions with service users, both activities that have been sacrificed to the requirements of bureaucratised practice (Beresford, 2008). Success in these issues can also help to enhance an individual's self-confidence, another key attribute of successful interprofessional working.

Perhaps the most critical attribute for a social worker in an interprofessional setting is the need to develop alliances with others, particularly those professions that occupy a similar structural position in relation to medicine. As we have noted, the points about social workers not having parity of esteem with doctors can also apply in relation to a number of other professions – nurses, health visitors, occupational therapists and so on. Although disciplinary differences between such professions may still exist, they are significantly less likely to be exacerbated by the impact of unequal power dynamics. Similarly, if a social worker is able to influence the practice of other professionals, the more it is likely that they can collectively present alternative strategies for responding to individual needs. In addition, the more social workers are able to create productive working relationships, the better it is for the formation of effective interprofessional collaboration and its maintenance (Freeth, 2001). While the personal enthusiasm and commitment of all team members is a critical feature of this (Molyneux, 2001), we suggest that social workers may have a particular role to play. This derives from the points we made at the start of this section concerning the particular contributions of social work to an interprofessional environment. Specifically, we believe that the orientation of a social worker is likely to be different from that of other professionals; we believe that this is certainly true in relation to work with older people (Lymbery, 2006), but also suggest that it holds more widely (Payne, 2006). Because of this difference, social workers arguably have more of an educative role than other professionals.

Conclusion

We do believe that it is possible to develop effective partnership working in health and social care; indeed, the evidence of our own experience provides a clear message that interprofessional work is simultaneously necessary and possible (Lymbery and Millward, 2000). However, we do not underestimate the difficulties that can obstruct such practice. For example, in this chapter, we have discussed the political obstacles to successful collaborative activity – particularly between healthcare and social care – and the professional dimensions that have been cited as critical problems.

Ultimately, however, we suggest that there is a normative dimension that needs to be considered: once we recognise the complexity of human needs, and the reality that numerous different organisations and professional groups have particular expertise that can assist an individual, the case for effective interprofessional activity becomes unarguable (see Hudson, 2002). If we are to provide a good quality service to people, we must find ways to operate in interprofessional environments. The purpose of this chapter is to provide an opportunity to consider the attributes a social worker requires to make this a reality.

For further discussion of the changing nature of the private and voluntary sector, see Adams et al., 2009a, Chapter 24.

www.caipe.org.uk/ CAIPE (Centre for the Advancement of Interprofessional Education) is an independent charity, founded in 1987. It is a national and international resource for interprofessional education in universities and the workplace across health and social care. CAIPE promotes and develops interprofessional education as a way of improving collaboration between practitioners and organisations in statutory and non-statutory public services.

Barrett, G., Sellman, D. and Thomas, J. (eds) (2005) *Interprofessional Working in Health and Social Care*, Basingstoke, Palgrave Macmillan. Practical and accessible resource suitable for a range of professional groups.

Bridgen, P. and Lewis, J. (1999) *Elderly People and the Boundary between Health and Social Care 1946–1991*, London, The Nuffield Trust. Outlines the central theme of this chapter in more detail, with specific reference to older people.

Hudson, B. (2002) 'Interprofessionality in health and social care: the Achilles' heel of partnership,' *Journal of Interprofessional Care*, **16**(1): 7–17. Vital for an understanding of some of the problems and limitations that can obstruct inter-professional working.

Leathard, A. (ed.) (2003) *Interprofessional Collaboration: From Policy to Practice in Health and Social Care*, Hove, Brunner-Routledge. Contains a number of detailed analyses of policy and practice in relation to interprofessional collabo-ration and is therefore essential reading.

Whittington, C., Weinstein, J. and Leiba, T. (eds) (2003) *Collaboration in Social Work Practice*, London, Jessica Kingsley. This useful book focuses particularly on the various dimensions to be considered when establishing collaborative practice in a range of settings.

Strategic planning and leadership

14

Chapter overview

Strategic management seeks to incorporate long-term aims into immediate management decisions. Personal leadership characteristics, management interaction and vision in organisations are strengthened by a strategic understanding of strands of continuity and change. Strategic planning activities can help practice and management.

This chapter considers strategic management as an activity of people at the more senior levels of an organization. It therefore makes sense to look at this alongside issues surrounding leadership.

What is strategy?

Strategy is a military analogy first applied to business planning in the late nineteenth century (Burnes, 2004). It implies a focus on an overall aim as a way of deciding on a programme of actions to achieve it. People apply this to business and public services because it is a useful way of deciding between alternative actions that seem equivalent at present, but carry implications for the future. In a complex environment that involves many different people, often you cannot achieve something immediately by just deciding to do it and putting resources into it; usually you have to take a series of steps towards it, to create a programme of action that will achieve your aim. Deciding on an ultimate aim and a programme to achieve it helps in three ways:

- It allows you to plan *resource allocation* (time, effort, money) to the steps along the way in advance, shifting resources once one step is achieved to the next step.
- It maintains *motivation and direction* by keeping the eventual aim in mind, as you deal with the tribulations involved in achieving the interim steps, and also by identifying and consolidating achievements in the major steps along the way.
- It generates *support and accountability* by enabling supporters and funders to understand progress towards a distant goal.

Although strategy is a higher level management technique, it is also a useful social work approach. Another important aspect of work on strategy is that it also involves critical thinking, because it requires examining the aims and implications of what you are doing.

There are three types of strategic activity:

- *Strategic thinking* – thinking about your work in a way that includes long-term implications as well as immediate concerns
- *Strategic planning* – actively planning what you do to include long-term aims
- *Strategic management* – managing or leading a group, team or organisation to achieve strategic objectives.

EXAMPLE

Public opinion has become concerned about an increasing number of young people who are carrying knives when they go out to clubs and pubs in the evening. Possible ways of dealing with this, all of which have been considered and used to some extent, are as follows:

- we could increase police action to search young people entering town centres or entertainment venues
- organise knife amnesties so that people can hand in knives without questions being asked about previous behaviour
- reduce drinking
- provide education about the danger of horrific injuries
- the arrest and conviction of gang leaders who create an environment of fear for young people
- keep young people at home in the evening
- provide greater police presence to prevent disorderly conduct.

Thinking strategically, first we ask about our overall aim: is it to stop fights breaking out, or is to prevent knife injuries, accepting that fights will happen, or is it to enable young people to be safe, either in general or at entertainment venues? Second, we have to be critical about what is driving the concern. Is it police concern about their budgets in managing all this, the sort of practical pressure that often sets off action to 'do something'? Or is it a more thoughtful concern about the brutalisation of a generation of young people in run-down, inner-city housing estates? This might lead us to think more widely about opportunities for young people or violence on television. Third, we have to work out a programme. It may be that more attractive youth facilities would be a good long-term aim, but how do we stop the town centre fights now: tighter liquor laws or stronger policing?

Exactly the same kinds of considerations affect social work practice. Many social workers deal with complex family situations, where it is impossible to resolve everything at once.

◇◇◇◇ CaSE EXaMPLE ◇◇◇◇◇◇◇◇◇◇◇◇◇◇◇◇◇◇◇◇◇◇◇◇◇◇◇◇◇◇◇◇◇◇◇◇◇◇

Jasmin Kuracha, aged 24, has three children from relationships with different men, poor standards of practical care, severe financial poverty and a poor environment for the children to grow up in. The school and nursery, which the children attend intermittently, are concerned about the children's progress. Her new relationship is with an older man, who has a job, provides some financial stability for the family and seems genuinely caring and supportive, but has convictions for violence and sexual assault. He says all that is in his past, and it is true that there are no recent convictions. What should her social worker do? The immediate reaction might be to say that she is a high priority for the local family support centre, which should help the children to make better progress, improve her childcare skills and allow her and the children to be monitored for signs of abuse. But if there is an immediate risk, should the children be more actively protected? If they were looked after by the local authority, would this break up perhaps her only chance of a happy future with a supportive relationship? Thinking strategically, the law tells us that the main consideration should be the welfare of the children. But what is in their best interests? The chance of an improving family life with a loving mother and supportive stepfather, the safety but perhaps poor outcomes of being looked after, the opportunities and risks of the family centre option? Thinking critically, although the children's development is the most important consideration, it is not the only one: what about Jasmin's safety and happiness and that of her new partner? The obviousness of the family centre option is partly driven by its availability, the ease of getting the family in, as they are a high priority, and the fact that it will tick several of the boxes. But will it be a wasted resource because it is not enough at an early stage of intervention? Thinking about a programme, a simple referral to the family centre may give the case a lower priority until a crisis arises. Would other involvements be needed to support the work in the centre and secure other advances in their situation?

To summarise the points made in this section, strategy is:

- a focus on an overall aim
- critical thinking about the factors that affect achieving that aim
- planning a programme of actions that will contribute to achieving the aim.

Ideas about strategy

There are four different approaches to strategy, which Whittington (2001) summarises as:

- *Classical* – this assumes that you can identify a clear aim and plan rationally to achieve it.
- *Evolutionary* – this market approach assumes that rational planning is not possible, or perhaps desirable, and that market pressures will force managers into making sensible decisions. While public and voluntary sector services do not have markets in the same way as commercial or manufacturing organisations, this approach is helpful because it identifies the importance of many different factors in the environment that influence our planning for the future.
- *Processual* – this approach assumes that you cannot take into account for rational planning all the possible factors that will affect you. Therefore you should identify the main factors that will affect your plans and set up systems to consult stakeholders so that you can gather appropriate information and take good decisions that reflect the capabilities and limitations of your organisation as you go along. This approach helpfully emphasises the value of participation and involvement in future planning.
- *Systemic* – this approach aims at rational planning, but takes account of the culture and social expectations within which an organisation or individual is embedded.

Most people and organisations would not follow just one of these theoretical types, but listing them suggests the kinds of factors that might be important in strategic thinking:

- *Aims* – the overall aim and lower level aims that might contribute to achieving it; does it all fit together logically?
- *External pressures* – examples might be the demands of service users and carers, availability of staff, provider organisations and financial resources and regulatory or legal requirements; does your plan manage all of them?
- *Involving interests and stakeholders* – this might include different professionals, different organisations, people with particular expertise, users and carers; are the right people involved enough?
- *Information and expectations* – how much you know or can find out about demand, service provision, policy, others professions' roles; should you find out more?
- *Capabilities and limitations* – of the numbers, types and quality of staff, the organisation, its partnerships, liaison and contacts and its structure, and other services; do you have or can you find the right skills or contributions?
- *Cultural and social expectations* in the environment – of service users, families and communities served and the organisation and organisations around it; does your plan fit people's important values?

In various ways, these are the sorts of issue that texts on strategic management (for example Johnson et al., 2005) cover.

What is leadership?

Leadership and developing leadership skills have been part of human civilisation from ancient times (Avery, 2004). Many people have a concept of leadership, such as the football team manager, who has an understanding of the opposition and how to organise the players on the field to win, even though he is not playing himself. Alternatively, we can think of a film director, with an idea of the overall result, directing actors and technical staff in using their special skills, which the director may not have. General ideas about leadership, therefore, involve a strong personality, an ability to have an overall conception of objectives, and to achieve compliance with their direction from people with a wide range of skills that the leader does not necessarily share. You can see, then, how leadership is linked to strategy, because an important component of leadership is the capacity to imagine and consistently pursue an overall aim.

Disentangling these ideas, writers on leadership have identified a number of facets of leadership, which are closely connected with the capacity to achieve strategic thinking and management. This account is based on the analyses of Avery (2004) and Northouse (2007).

The traditional approach has been to focus on the characteristics of the leader. These include traits or characteristics, skills deriving from these characteristics, the style of management that emerges from traits and skills, and the ability to shift that style according to the situation the leader faces. Five sets of traits are most important:

- neuroticism, a tendency to be vulnerable and hostile
- extraversion, a tendency to be sociable, assertive and energetic
- openness, a tendency to be creative, insightful and curious
- agreeable, accepting, trusting and nurturing
- conscientious, thorough, organised, decisive and dependable.

Skills, deriving from these traits, connect up knowledge about the situation, derived from training or analysis of the situation that the leader is facing, with generic skills in problem-solving and social judgement. Leadership style balances concern for people with concern for the tasks to be achieved. Situational and contingency ideas focus on how leaders change their approach between delegating, supporting, coaching and directing others. They shift their behaviour to define goals, clarify the path to the goals, and remove obstacles.

Transactional approaches to leadership focus on the interaction between leaders and followers, suggesting that the characteristics and situation of both are important. The aim is to develop a partnership between leaders and followers, defining roles, influencing each other's judgements by constant interaction and identifying people with an interest in aims and building relationships with them.

Visionary or transformational leadership involves setting a strong role model of competence in the technical tasks, articulating goals and influencing others to follow them, clear communication about expectations and a strong demand for achievement.

This enables followers to depend on and accept the objectives expressed in the modelling of the leader.

Organic views of leadership are a more recent development, and they recognise that within small-scale and expert organisations or teams, it may be more important for people working together to explore and seek to make sense of the complex environments in which they work. Leadership may change for different tasks, or may emerge from the working process, rather than coming from formal appointment. The process of leadership is about establishing shared values and agreeing appropriate processes to achieve the agreed goals.

One of the important issues for leaders is the authority and power they exercise, where it comes from and how it fits with the work being undertaken. In organic situations, for example, leadership will often come from expertise in the issue a team or organisation is dealing with. In a continuing public service, complying with legal and regulatory requirements, formal authority in a line management system and the confidence of senior managers may be more important than specific expertise in the work being done.

Leaders may focus on internal management or the staff and services they are responsible for or seek also to extend their involvement into the wider organisation or community and policy networks. Middleton (2007), an experienced voluntary sector manager, argues in her book – based on interviews with a wide range of public, private and voluntary sector managers – that it is easy and feels safe for managers to limit themselves to the areas within the organisation where they have authority. However, to achieve leadership in change, managers need to extend their activities into the wider organisation or community, where they have less authority, but may be able to achieve relationships that will make wider change possible. This analysis suggests that wider involvements and consultations are important in achieving change and development in a creative and forward-looking way. Also, a focus on the present staff and activities may not be a good preparation for strategic management in a situation where change and development is required.

Continuity and change

Much strategic thinking focuses on change and development in organisations, but it is equally possible to be strategic about managing continuity. However, focusing a strategy on continuity is potentially easier than change because you can see and analyse the present situation, while change requires a more conceptual grasp of something you cannot see and so contains more uncertainties. In any case, choosing between change and continuity is often not a possibility; instead you may be able to retain some aspects of an organisation or a practice, and will have to change others. A focus on continuity would emphasise a quality management agenda, doing the job better every day, achieving quality targets and constant steps in improvement, rather than restructuring the organisation or identifying and planning for different aims.

In a research review on improving social and healthcare services, Fauth and Mahdon (2007) suggest that there are three elements to taking action to change:

- leadership that reviews the present situation, compares it with policies and organisational aims and then can articulate and motivate people to make the necessary changes or improve the present approach
- employee participation in planning the change
- stakeholder participation.

Areas of strategic thinking

There are several areas that strategic thinking can usefully focus on:

- the processes within an organisation or a particular piece of work or project, in particular the professional and practice techniques, the flow of work, for example between general or intake teams and more specialist staff, or between teams with different functions, communication and decision-making
- the resources of staff and money and the facilities to carry out the work
- the boundaries between the different parts of the organisation or between the organisation and other organisations or teams
- organisational design, for example whether it needs to be centralised or localised, whether or not to attempt multiprofessional practice, whether or not the work is on several different sites.

Some techniques

There are some widely used practical techniques for getting involved in strategy that leaders and practitioners might use.

Creating mission and vision statements helps to clarify aims. A vision states what the world would look like if you are successful, while a mission expresses precisely what you are going to do to achieve it. A useful guide is 5WH: why, who, what, where, when and how you are going to achieve this outcome. Both positives and negatives may help you to set boundaries, for example not only who is going to be involved, but who is not needed.

A SWOT (strengths, weaknesses, opportunities, threats) analysis involves looking at the internal and external factors that affect a team or organisation. It is usually done by a group of workers making notes about their personal analysis, then coming together to build a complete picture. Figure 14.1 outlines the process. The group examines the internal strengths and weaknesses that the organisation may have in achieving the goal. What are they good at? Are they able to recruit staff with the right training and experience? Then the group examines the opportunities that the organisation might be able to achieve, and the threats, such as a lack of resources or criticism of the failure to achieve results. It can be helpful if work on internal factors includes analysis of any distinctive features of the workforce, leadership styles and actual past performance.

Similarly, it helps if the external factors examined focus particularly on uncertainties and resource availability (Buchanan and Huczynski, 2004: 538).

	Positive factors	Negative factors
Internal factors	STRENGTHS	WEAKNESSES
External factors	OPPORTUNITIES	THREATS

Figure 14.1 A SWOT analysis

A forcefield analysis (Figure 14.2) enables you to look at factors that will help and hinder you in achieving a change. You list factors that are positive, which are pushing you towards your aim, and restraining factors that get in the way. Then you give each a weight; 5 where it is very positive or restraining, 1 where it is a minor factor. You can do very little about some of these factors, even some of the big ones, but with others you can make a difference. Perhaps one major restraining factor is immovable, but you might find other less important factors that you can change, so that a combination of small-scale positive forces can overcome the main obstruction. This technique works well to clarify what to do in projects or developments in a team or agency and in working with service users and families.

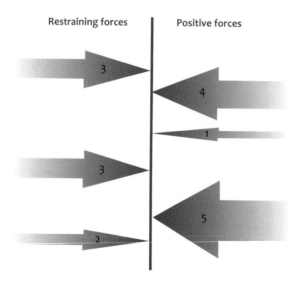

Restraining forces · Positive forces

3 · 4 · 1 · 3 · 5 · 2

Figure 14.2 A forcefield analysis

Prioritising is another important possibility, identified in Chapter 12 on managing a workload. This involves listing everything that you want to achieve and putting them in order of importance. You could also put objectives into separate lists of achievability: quick, medium and long term.

Conclusion

Strategy is about identifying and maintaining long-term aims within everyday management and practice. Strategic management and thinking are an important function of senior management staff in agencies, but the approaches can be adapted to thinking strategically about practice and teamwork as well. Leadership is crucial to strategic thinking and management, because in many situations, someone must take responsibility for maintaining understanding of and motivation towards wider objectives. However, participation in identifying and committing everyone involved to those objectives is also needed. Strategic leadership involves thinking about organisation, task and people and their contribution to an overall objective. However, leadership is not only a set of traits or characteristics contained in a visionary person, but also a responsiveness to the environment, culture and relationships needed to achieve the objectives of an organisation.

For further discussion of organisational aspects, see Chapter 19.

Avery, G. (2004) *Understanding Leadership: Paradigms and Cases*, London, Sage. Concise, practical and widely used book on leadership ideas, with case examples of how they were put into practice from different cultures.

Bruce, A. and Langdon, K. (2000) *Strategic Thinking*, London, Dorling Kindersley. Although a business text, it is engaging, heavily illustrated and offers good ideas that you can apply to thinking strategically in partnership with a team or with service users and their families.

Fauth, R. and Mahdon, M. (2007) *Improving Social and Health Care Services*, London, SCIE. Good summary of relevant research on strategies that might help in improving social care services.

Johnson, G., Scholes, K. and Whittington, R. (2005) *Exploring Corporate Strategy*, 7th edn, Harlow, Prentice Hall. Extensive text on strategic planning.

Whittington, R. (2001) *What is Strategy – and Does it Matter?*, 2nd edn, London, Thomson. Good brief introduction to strategic planning by an important management writer – focuses on business management, but many of the ideas can be adapted.

15 Supervision and being supervised

Chapter overview

This chapter asks why, when so much of social work is being questioned, rethought and restructured, the ideas and practice of social work supervision remain remarkably consistent. The chapter looks at whether or not this consistency is helpful to developing critical practice.

Contemporary social work has been described as contested, compromised and challenged (Healy, 2000) and many believe that the social work profession, like others, is in crisis (Rossiter, 1996). The reasons for this buffeting are numerous and include the changing design and delivery of social work and an increasing dominance of managerialism, and the impact of imperatives of challenge and auditing embedded in Best Value and evidence-based practice, as well as the destabilising that postmodernism has prompted (Leonard, 1997). Service users too continue to question social work practices and theories (Wilson and Beresford, 2000). Together, these challenges have unsettled social work's identity, purpose and processes.

Yet social work supervision, a fundamental plank in ensuring social work's focus and effectiveness (Brown and Bourne, 1996), appears to be largely untouched by these seismic upheavals. The steady flow of books and articles on supervision largely refine and develop it rather than question it fundamentally (for example Knapman and Morrison, 1998; Hawkins and Shohet, 2000). Is this because all is well with supervision or might its very continuity be hindering the profession's ability to respond critically to the changes and develop critical social work practices that emphasise an emancipatory social change orientation (Healy, 2000: 3)? Might it be enhanced by being challenged itself? A preliminary excursion into reconsidering social work supervision is the focus of this chapter. It uses a questioning process that critical practice also requires and begins to consider supervision's potential to facilitate critical social work.

Uprooting the roots of supervision

Brockbank and McGill (1998) suggest three roots to contemporary supervision:

1 *Industry*, with its perceived need to oversee employees and their work.
2 *Therapy*, where counsellors and therapists are regularly supervised to ensure the cognitive and emotional 'fitness' of the therapist and therefore the safety of the client.
3 *Academia*, where learners are attached to a 'master' (p. 232).

Each root emphasises different aspects of the functions of supervision: the control of the behaviour and output of the worker, support and 'fitness for purpose', and learning and development. The three roots find their way not only into conceptions of supervision's functions (for example Kadushin, 1976; Richards and Payne, 1990) but also into many agency supervision policy documents and Diploma in Social Work handbooks. Together they are regarded as a key to ensuring social work's purpose and efficacy. Thus Brown and Bourne (1996: 9) argue that:

Supervision is the primary means by which an agency-designated supervisor enables staff, individually and collectively, and ensures standards of practice. The aim is to enable the supervisee(s) to carry out their work ... as effectively as possible.

The ultimate aim is 'the provision of the best possible service to service users' (Brown and Bourne, 1996: 10).

It is usually suggested that the effective implementation of the functions is ensured through mechanics such as recording proforma (which are often shaped by the functions), contracting and having a regular time, space and place for supervision. The role of authority and the supervisor's expertise in practice, management and in supervision itself are also requisites for effectiveness. This depiction of supervision is of a formalised, regulated and largely private process into which supervisors are trained, but where supervisees are infrequently offered parallel training in being a supervisee.

This portrait of supervision's purpose, functions and implementation, as already suggested, appears remarkably consistent in literature and policies, while other realities are largely ignored. For example, workers and students also depend on 'on the hoof' supervision in the corridor or office, while supervision of large groups of workers at infrequent intervals, such as in domiciliary care, is rarely acknowledged or considered in detail. The latter is largely by and with women about an area of practice seen as relatively unskilled, although much appreciated by service users. What might these omissions suggest about the orthodoxies of supervision?

There is some acknowledgement in the supervision literature of difficulties with the formalised model. For example, Brown and Bourne (1996) point up the danger of assuming that supervision is a convenient hybrid of three different kinds of meetings, each with their allotted time on the supervision agenda. This 'runs the risk of reducing supervision to a rote practice capable of maintaining only minimum standards' (1996: 61). Hughes and Pengelly (1997) depict the functions as a triangle and thereby reveal a problem they describe as ' three into one won't go', where there is a danger of over- or

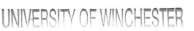

underemphasising one of the corners/functions at the expense of the other two. The functions are not themselves queried.

Power dynamics and aspects of identity are also increasingly acknowledged as an important issue in supervision. Concerns about the potential for the abuse of power embedded in the typically hierarchical structure of student and staff supervision are raised (for example Evans, 1999; Hawkins and Shohet, 2000).

In this author's experience, much practice teacher training rightly emphasises this potential and the need to be vigilant against it. However, this orthodoxy too may be problematic in practice, for Brown and Bourne (1996: 33) also suggest that social work supervisors are not comfortable with their authority and power and seek to sidestep it, thus confusing the supervisee. Maybe the models of power and empowerment espoused in the supervision literature and training also need to be questioned. Perhaps they do not adequately reflect the complexity and impact of identity aspects such as race, gender, disability and sexuality, as explored by Carroll and Holloway (1999). For example, Lee Nelson and Holloway's (1999: 30) review of gender relations in supervision shows complex and changing power dynamics over time that are affected by the gender alignments of supervisee and supervisor:

> Only dyads with male supervisees followed the path of becoming more collegial over time, while dyads with women supervisees over time, tended to reflect a greater imbalance of power.

Lee Nelson and Holloway (1999: 31) quote Jordan's study, which contended that power in supervision cannot be considered without also considering affiliation and women's need for a sense of mutuality and to 'participate with others in a mutual give and take of empathy and understanding'. While the study concerns counselling, it raises questions for student and staff supervision. Studies on the impact of sexual orientation, 'race' and disability in the same volume confirm the need to see power relations as complex, dynamic and affected not only by the structure of supervision but also by wider societal structures and ideologies such as the medical and social models of disability (see also Thomas, 1999). Like Healy's contention that critical social work has developed its own orthodoxy in seeing worker power as essentially oppressive, maybe supervision also needs further work on exploring the positive dimensions of power imbalances, how power relationships change over time, as well as different sorts of authority models such as proposed by Jones (1993).

So while there are some ripples of disturbance in the conventions of writing and thinking about supervision, what of the experience of supervision?

Experiencing supervision

Information from social work students, practitioners and managers suggests that while there are great expectations of supervision and some good quality supervision is experienced, many people are disappointed by either what they can offer or receive. Some examples suggest differing components to the dissatisfaction.

◇◇◇ Case Examples

> It's quantity supervision, it's like a game of tag where you touch base and then shoot off again. (Williams, 2000, personal communication)

As the previous month's supervision had been cancelled, there were now 17 'cases' for update as well as other agenda items. Mrs J was one of them. She'd been in hospital for three months and was desperate to go home. The discussion was brief and focused on finding and contracting with care providers. The other 'cases' were also skimmed through; mutual support was offered about the workload pressures both worker and supervisor were experiencing; some agenda items were postponed. It was all that was possible in the hour and a half. Later, when the delay continued, the supervisor realised that no contingency plans had been discussed, neither had the worker's feelings, and as for research into the impact of delayed discharge on older women ...

The female senior manager described how when she went into supervision, she seemed to spend a lot of time listening to her supervisor's problems with his senior management colleagues; till at last, fed up, she went outside the division for support and advice (Phillipson and Riley, 1991).

◇◇◇◇

It was a tense moment in what had seemed, initially, a positive supervision session. They'd exchanged news about their respective weekends and agreed the agenda and note-taking. Their shared discussion about theory teaching at college was lively. But then the practice teacher's verbal feedback on the student's written work was met with rebuttal. He'd commented gently on the way she sometimes seemed dismissive of her practice skills by writing statements such as 'I just let her talk'; his attempts to encourage her to inquire further about her thinking, feeling and responses to the family were countered, laughingly, by 'you make it too complicated, you're too analytic.'

These examples highlight the difficulties of 'overseeing' the sheer volume of work; relationships that may be both enabling and oppressive, tensions between aspects such as speed and depth, support and challenge, thinking and feelings. For students, there may be a tension between proving competence and acknowledging difficulties. The tensions experienced in supervision are not surprising, as 'tensions and contradictions lie at the heart of much social work' (Lawson, 1998: 248). Social work practices include fleeting encounters as well as sustained relationships, they are about power and control as well as empowerment, they necessitate the often simultaneous performance of activities, some of which require considerable skills and others which do not. Both social change and conformity are demanded of social work. Social work supervision is likely to mirror these tensions and paradoxes (Mattinson, 1975). Supervision policies and rituals seem designed to contain and shrink these complexities and tensions, and maybe this too mirrors social work, with its concern to 'manage risk' (Parton, 1998).

Using provocations to question how supervision might be different

Healy (2000), as part of her critique of past attempts at critical social work, uses the postmodernist tools of querying, dismantling the orthodoxies and destabilising the ideas and practices of critical social work to move it forward. Being contextually sensitive and self-reflective are two key tools. Applying this latter approach to my own work as a supervisor and supervisee, I sought to disturb my own orthodoxies about supervision by questioning my own practice and reading accounts that provoked and helped me to do this. Three are offered below, not as essential reading but as exemplars of the process. A novel by A.S. Byatt (2000), research by Jan Fook (2000) and writing by Celia Davies on nursing (1995) all provided fertile provocation.

Davies' study *Gender and the Professional Predicament in Nursing* highlights the way in which the parallel developments of organisational and professional development have been essentially a process of masculinisation. Her analysis leads her to point up the way gender is not only 'on the surface', in terms of aspects such as speech, dress, presentation and ways of interacting, but also a constitutive element in organisational structure and logic. The notion of a 'job', the concept of 'career', the supremacy of hierarchical organisational structures, the assignation of tasks and thereby status to different ranks are all gendered. This gendered organisational logic affects other aspects such as the expression and suppression of emotions, sexuality and even what counts as legitimate knowledge. This analysis provokes consideration of the way in which the conception and practice of supervision might itself be gendered, for example in its own predominately hierarchical model, the content, focus and processes. Might this explain the lack of attention paid to 'on the hoof' supervision and group supervision for predominantly women workers? How might gendered organisational logic and expression impact on my experience as a woman supervisor and supervisee? And how might this link to the development and promotion of critical social work, which espouses the importance of the wider structural context, change and standing alongside oppressed and marginalised peoples?

Fook's (2000) research into the development of social work expertise also uses postmodernist critiques and tools. Like Davies, she sets this within a feminist framework that attempts to characterise social work expertise in ways that are more representative of the experience of social workers and service users, many of whom are women. Her study showed that

> rather than entering situations with superior and fixed notions of desirable outcomes, derived from the legitimacy of professional knowledge, practitioners often engage in a mutual process of discovery with service users (Fook, 2000: 114)

and they were context sensitive and used uncertainty and playing it 'by ear'. This echoes Parton and O'Byrne's (2000: 3) description of practices they call 'constructive social work', where 'an ability to work with ambiguity and uncertainty in terms of process and outcome is key'. Such social work suggests a richness of practice that emphasises a 'plurality of knowledge and voice, the use of paradox, myth, enigma and narrative'.

Neither Fook nor Parton and O'Byrne discuss the implications of their research and practice accounts for supervision models and processes. But their work prompts the possibility of valuing and surfacing uncertainty, ambiguity, plurality and narrative in supervision as well as in practice. This may be 'counterculture' in organisations where 'getting the work done' is essential and where, like the White Queen in *Alice Through the Looking Glass*, people often feel that they have to undertake 'six impossible things before breakfast' and supervision (of any sort) is just one of these.

The third provocation is *The Biographer's Tale* by A.S. Byatt (2000). The novel begins with her hero Phineas G. abandoning the 'stultifying' criticism and tortuous deconstructions of postmodernism that he has been studying:

> It was a sunny day and the windows were very dirty. I was looking at the windows and I thought I am not going on with this any longer … I need a life full of things, full of facts. (Byatt, 2000: 3–4)

Instead, he decides to become a biographer in search of uncontestable facts. The novel is redolent of the tension between facts and assumptions, the search for certainty and the discomfort of questioning. I recognise the temptations of looking for and assuming the solidity of facts, of leaving critical self-reflection and the uncertain 'swampy lowlands' described by Schön (1991) behind. Supervision is not exempt from such yearning or a pressure to deal in 'facts'.

Regrowing supervision for critical social work

These provocations encourage a reconsideration of how supervision might be used to develop and sustain critical social work in an era of challenge and contestation, and how supervision itself might model this approach.

If practice is to be flexible, pragmatic and non-dogmatic, supervision could model this in terms of its 'when', 'where' and 'how' without abandoning the more formal expectations and opportunities. Practitioners and managers reveal that much significant 'supervision' takes place spontaneously, often among peers, yet this is rarely formally acknowledged, recorded or used to expand the notions of supervision. Domiciliary care workers in particular are often dependent on a quick phone call to a supervisor for advice, support, workload management and even quality assurance. Supervision in its formalised, one-at-a-time version is likely to be unavailable or infrequent for such workers – new supervision models are needed that respect and problematise their work. Surely critical social work cannot be the prerogative only of social workers? New technology also offers the possibility of new models of supervision.

Fook's (2000) research suggests that there is a challenge to develop a new discourse of expertise derived from practitioner experience. The discourse of critical practice might include the contradictions and uncertainties of what it constitutes as well as developing some 'facts' about it. Emancipatory practice might well take place in the everyday activities of social work practices as well as the more usually assumed wider political spheres or indeed in both. How, for example, are practitioners engaged in identifying and recording the 'unmet need' of both service users and carers? How might they tackle people's unmet needs and at the same time promote social change? This is a practice, management and political issue, yet personal experience of supervision notes rarely show this being debated or recorded. What might it be like to have 'emancipatory practice' as an agenda item? The example of the supervision session in which Mrs J was briefly discussed might have thought about her not only in terms of 'setting up a package of care', but also in terms of how information about the shortfall of care might be collected, made known and acted on individually and collectively. The possible impact of aspects such as ageism, sexism and racism and medical models of care might also be crucial. In this way, the focus of the supervision 'lens' might itself be open to debate, such as: 'Why are we discussing this aspect?' 'What are we not looking at and why?' 'How are we talking about it?'

Critical social work requires an ability to be both self- and politically reflective. If supervision's aim is to ensure the delivery of the 'best possible' service, then 'best possible' could also be contested in supervision in terms of beliefs, policy and practices. Johns' (2000) suggestion that a key aspect of reflection is to expose and understand the contradictions between what is desirable and actual practice could form part not only of the destabilising and contesting but also the construction of knowledge through telling the practice stories in supervision.

Conclusion

It has been suggested that the theory and policies of supervision have remained largely untouched by the debates about social work. This is perhaps not surprising, given its origins in the largely hierarchical organisational settings in which it is still mainly implemented, where questioning, contesting and political challenging are constrained. By using questioning and self-reflection, other possibilities for supervision have been suggested. And yet maybe this discourse of questioning is itself a new orthodoxy. Maybe supervision remains undisturbed because the definitions of its purpose, the analysis and implementation of its functions are apt and appropriate? The need for regular space and time for review, reflection, action planning and quality control continue to be what people say they want and hope for. Perhaps the roots should be cherished and nurtured, not questioned. But I am not convinced that this is enough for the development and enhancement of critical social work.

For further discussion of preparing for practice learning, see Adams et al., 2009a, Chapter 25.

Bond, M. and Holland, S. (1998) *Skills of Clinical Supervision for Nurses*, Buckingham, Open University Press. Detailed look at supervision as a 'working alliance' that offers a multitude of practical ideas as well as being thought-provoking.

Brown, A. and Bourne, I. (1996) *The Social Work Supervisor*, Buckingham, Open University Press. Social work text focused on supervision, with useful chapters on the necessary value base and the impact of difference for supervision.

Hawkins, P. and Shohet, R. (2000) *Supervision in the Helping Professions*, 2nd edn, Buckingham, Open University Press. Key book for understanding processes in individual and group supervision, revised to include more debate on working with difference.

Healy, K. (2000) *Social Work Practices*, London, Sage. Challenges some of the orthodoxies of critical social work, highlights the importance of everyday practice and questions itself.

Lahad, M. (2000) *Creative Supervision: The Use of Expressive Arts Methods in Supervision and Self-supervision*, London, Jessica Kingsley. A small book rich with ideas and stories of imaginative ways of working in supervision that are fun and illuminating.

16

Managing risk and decision-making

Chapter overview

This chapter examines some of the possibilities and pitfalls of refocusing risk assessment and risk management towards being an aid to professional decision-making and problem-solving in uncertain social situations.

It has been argued that governments and agencies have directed much of social work towards differentiating high-risk from low-risk situations, so that limited resources can be more effectively used to protect people from harm (see, for example, Parton et al., 1997; Parton, 1999). Houston and Griffiths (2000) claim that in terms of organisational development, risk assessment and risk management have become bureaucratic procedures overconcerned with prediction, control and culpability. In his study of 'risk paradigms' used by health and social care staff, Taylor (2006: 1424) concluded that 'decision making seemed to be more about what was defensible than what was right'.

◇◇◇◇ CASE EXAMPLE ◇◇◇◇◇◇◇◇◇◇◇◇◇◇◇◇◇◇◇◇◇◇◇◇◇◇◇◇◇◇◇◇◇◇◇◇◇◇

Nazeen is an experienced social worker who has been involved in a review of whether or not Zena, a young person on a care order, should return home. Zena is 10 years old and has made remarkable progress since coming into care 18 months ago. A court made Zena the subject of a care order after years of emotional abuse by her mother, who has mental health difficulties and struggles to cope with the care of her daughter. Zena's mother wants her daughter home and the care order discharged. The independent review officer and Nazeen's line manager believe that Zena's needs would be better met at home, and if this is not feasible, her care plan changed to working towards adoption. Nazeen is concerned that if Zena was returned home, she would again suffer from emotional abuse and re-enter care, triggering her into a downward spiral. Zena does not want to be adopted and is not sure about returning home as she feels secure where she is for the first time in her life. The review decided against the option of applying for a discharge of the care order and the independent review officer requested a risk assessment of Zena being placed with her mother. Nazeen is sceptical of the vogue currently sweeping her agency for risk assessment as the answer to everything and is wary of placing too much confidence in the human ability to predict the future with certainty (Dingwell, 1989). Nevertheless, she is in favour of having a reasoned basis for making decisions, and sets about endeavouring to undertake a critical risk assessment.

Nazeen's starting point is that people need to feel empowered to make their own decisions about their future but the nature of decision-making in social work means there are different levels of client involvement (O'Sullivan, 1999). Zena's situation is typical of many in social work in which the right to take risks is not straightforward. Adult clients may be considered to have the right to take risks with their own bodies, if they have the mental capacity to make that decision, but not the right to harm others (Cupitt, 1997). So Zena's mother's wish to have her daughter home is important from a number of points of view, but she is not considered to have the right to expose Zena to harm. In deciding between the different courses of action, there are tensions between Zena's and her mother's right to live their lives free from interference and Nazeen's duty to protect Zena from self-harm and harm from others. Nazeen wants to promote the conditions of open discussion with Zena, her carers, her mother, the line manager and the independent review officer, so that reflexive communicative reason, rather than control-oriented instrumental reason, can form the basis of decisions (Blaug, 1995).

Nazeen poses herself four questions to be asked by critical practitioners involved in making decisions in uncertain situations:

- What is meant by 'risk'?
- What are the societal contexts of the concern with 'risk'?
- How are risks to be assessed?
- What approach to risk management is to be taken?

What is meant by risk?

One of the pitfalls for Nazeen and her colleagues is regarding 'risk' as an unproblematic and taken-for-granted concept. Stalker (2003: 216) states that:

> The theories [of risk suggest] that social work theorists and practitioners should adopt a critical approach to their understanding of and response to risk.

One of the first steps in taking a critical stance towards risk is to appreciate that the word 'risk' represents a contested concept that is embedded in a number of different discourses. There are a number of conflicting discourses of risk (Kemshall, 2002a), two of which will be identified here. The first, currently dominant in social work, concerns danger, safety, caution and avoiding blame, and relates risk to the chance of bad outcomes occurring. Douglas (1992, cited in Parton, 2001: 62) argues that 'the word risk now means danger', and Alaszewski and Alaszewski (1998: 109) found that the professionals they interviewed defined 'risk' in terms of danger. The second, which has a longer history, sees risk as being an unavoidable aspect of life, which involves risk-taking and decision-making resulting in actions taken to achieve benefits that may result in a loss. Rather than risks being avoided, they are managed in a critical way.

Nazeen is tempted to take the advice of Dowie (1999) and abandon the term 'risk' as redundant and substitute it for the concept of 'uncertainty' as suggested by Parton (2001: 69). She settles on endeavouring to use the word in a more sparing, precise and careful way. Within a professional decision-making framework, there needs to be clear conceptualisation that includes a differentiation of the concept of 'risk' from the related ideas of hazard, strength, danger and benefit. Zena's situation is typical of those found in social work where all options involve possible dangers and benefits, and there are complex balances between situational hazards and strengths. There are uncertainties about the outcomes of staying in care, returning home or being adopted. All three courses of action could possibly led to a good outcome; however, they all involve the possibility of sustaining a loss. The questions are: Which option gives the best chance of a good outcome? Are there other factors, other than likely outcomes, that need to be taken into account, for example issues of autonomy and social justice?

What are the societal contexts of the concern with 'risk'?

Nazeen lives in a global society that has been characterised by sociologists and anthropologists by its concern with risk (for example Beck, 1998; Douglas, 1992; Giddens, 1998). There are a number of important connections between the debate on a societal/global level and the work of Nazeen. At the core of the risk society are uncertainty and unpredictability (Ungar, 2001), features that have always been present in social work in the sense that the outcomes of care plans cannot be predicted with certainty. Nevertheless, the hidden catastrophic dangers of global warming, nuclear accident and mass contamination of food generate different social anxieties from the negative impacts of being brought up in care. The observers of social anxieties would be forgiven for believing that the world has become more hazardous but, as Giddens (1998) has pointed out, they reflect a society increasingly preoccupied with the future and safety, rather than the world being a more dangerous place. Douglas (1992) argues that all societies, past and present, have systems of blame for misfortunes and that risk has taken on this function in modern society. In a blame culture, there are pressures to proceduralise how uncertainty is dealt with, to ensure that there is always something or someone to blame when things go wrong. Workers can be blamed for not following the procedures correctly, or, if the procedures were followed, the procedures can be blamed for not being adequate. In such a safety climate (Furedi, 2002), critical social work becomes a challenge, as Parton et al. (1997: 240) state:

> Once concerns about risk become all pervasive, the requirement to develop and follow organisational procedures becomes dominant and the room for professional manoeuvre and creativity is severely limited.

Dangers are always in the background, in everyday social work and everyday life. For all these dangers to become the subject of decision-making would disrupt one's own life and the lives of others. How some dangers come to the foreground of concern is related to, among other things, risk perception or, more accurately, danger perception. Nazeen is concerned about fears engendered by panics generated from time to time through the mass media (Jenkins, 1992; Thompson, 1998) and how these can impact on professional perceptions of danger. During periods of heightened sensitivity following the discovery or rediscovery of a social problem, there is a danger of excessive caution. The independent review officer's concerns about Zena remaining in care can be cast as being partly shaped by the latest agency panic engendered by the government's concern about the negative outcomes of care. Panic and deliberative decision-making do not go well together, and an unintended consequence of legitimate government concern can be the generation of anxieties that translate into panicked agency responses. Many children are harmed by the experience of being in care, but this is different from saying that all children who are in care are inevitably harmed by the experience. The independent review officer and the line manager had accused Nazeen of not taking seriously enough the reality of being in care but this was to misunderstand her position. She, as an experienced social worker, knows better than most what the dangers are of remaining in care (Owen, 1997). She did not question the reality of children being harmed, but argued that it is the particularities of each situation that are important.

How are risks to be assessed?

There is a range of potential approaches to the assessment of risk. Sinclair et al. (1995) state that assessment is a basis of decision-making and different types of assessment can be distinguished by their purpose. Risk assessment tends to come into play when there is uncertainty and concern that a person may be exposed to harm. In its current dominant forms, 'risk assessment' tends to be limited to dangers and hazards and focuses on just one option. Some 'risk assessments' might go further and estimate how likely the dangers are to occur and the likely extent of harm if they do occur. The result is a particular representation of reality, which raises at least two issues: Is the narrow focus on the negative side of risk justified? Does the method of risk assessment give a distorted and unbalanced representation? No course of action is inherently a risk in itself but equally anything can be a risk (Ewald, 1991). This means that any situation can be considered in terms of risk or alternatively seen through some other lens. An issue for Nazeen is whether the focus on the possible negative outcomes becomes isolated from other concerns. She believes that risk assessment needs to be an integrated part of a full assessment of Zena's situation, including her wishes and feelings, her progress in care, her needs and her mother's caring capacity and resources. Milner and O'Byrne (2002) have recognised that the development of an overarching framework for assessment in social work has been hindered by differing emphases on risk, needs and resources and there is a need to see risk as one side of a triangle that has needs and resources forming the other two sides.

The use of risk assessment instruments

One potential distorting effect is through the use of risk assessment schedules, which form part of what Webb (2006: 151) refers to as the 'technologies of care'. Nazeen has witnessed a trend for all assessments to become more routine and more structured, sometimes being reduced to checklists and tick boxes of risk indicators. Her agency has just introduced a risk factor checklist for children subject to care orders returning home. Risk assessment instruments attempt to reduce difficult and complex decisions to a limited number of questions. In the past, risk assessment checklists have been taken seriously (for example Greenland, 1987), only to have their predictive validity subsequently questioned (Parton, 1991). Even the most carefully researched predictive instruments are regarded as having too high an error rate to be relied on exclusively (Sargent, 1999; Munro, 2002). Nazeen and her colleagues have an ambivalent attitude towards the agency risk assessment schedule. On one hand it gives a degree of protection to workers and can take much of the anxiety away from making difficult decisions. On the other hand they question the face validity of some of the risk indicators, particularly when the prediction of harm occurring is reduced to the presence or absence of a limited number of factors. Using checklists can undermine professional wisdom and the sensitivity to context and creative thinking needed to deal with the complexity and uncertainty of social situations. There is a danger that Nazeen uses the agency checklist in a mechanical, routine and non-reflexive way to give herself and her agency some protection from criticisms if things go wrong (Wald and Woolverton, 1990). Even when checklists are used to guide and focus professional judgement, the predictive validity of the featured factors needs to be critically examined.

Is a critical risk assessment possible?

There is no consensus as to what form critical risk assessment would take and indeed whether such a thing is possible. A starting point would be that such an assessment would need to be carried out in a reflexive manner and involve what Parton (1998: 23) refers to as 'situated judgements' rather than checklists. The assessment would be the product of open dialogue between the participants and would place strengths alongside hazards and include the benefits of taking the course of action alongside the dangers. A further step would be to compare all identified courses of action in terms of their possible outcomes, whereas often only the one perceived to pose risks receives attention. The aim would be to assess the balance between the options, in terms of the chances of a good outcome occurring. The process would need to be carried out with reflexivity, as regards the judgements and interpretations made and the knowledge used. In sum, this would amount to placing 'risk assessment' explicitly within a participatory reflexive decision-making framework. There would need to be critical recognition that a risk assessment carried out in the above manner would be located within what Clark (2000: 72) refers to as 'consequentialist ethics' and that other ethical theories may also be relevant.

Decisions such as Zena's future care plan need to involve deliberative processes, part of which is structuring or framing the decision situation (O'Sullivan, 1999). Dialogue needs to take place between Zena, her mother and Nazeen to discuss the uncertainty of what the future holds and what the possible consequences of each option are and their situational strengths and hazards. The quality of Nazeen's practice and thinking is crucially important in producing a well-reasoned frame of the decision situation that is based on carefully gathered and sifted information. The particular balance of hazards and strengths in Zena's and her mother's present situation will influence the chances of a good outcome occurring. One of the issues of carrying out such an analysis is the basis on which predictive factors and possible consequences are identified. There are a number of potential sources of distortion, including confirmation bias (Sheppard, 1995a), the use of stereotypes (Milner and O'Byrne, 2002), taking a deficits approach and the 'rule of optimism' (Dingwall et al., 1983).

Limitations of evidence-based practice

Nazeen claims to be using her professional wisdom (Scott, 1990; Sheppard, 1995b; O'Sullivan, 2005) accumulated through her own experience and knowledge gained from reading and studying. However, she works in a context of mounting pressure to base decisions exclusively on research evidence but is aware of serious flaws in this approach (Webb, 2001). She takes a pragmatic approach to evidence-based practice, seeing the findings of empirical research as potentially useful to practitioners to inform rather than dictate their practice. She is worried about 'the rhetorical force of the word evidence' (Trinder, 2000: 158) and its potential negative impact on practice. She is aware of research that has been carried out in relation to returning home (Biehal, 2007), adoption (Quinton et al., 1998) and young people being brought up in care (Cashmore and Paxman, 2006). She welcomes the light studies shed on the factors that may be involved in certain outcomes occurring, but the uncritical use of research findings poses a number of dangers. One is regarding such research as providing the whole answer or a definite conclusive answer. Another is when research findings are misinterpreted due to a failure to appreciate the difference between co-relational and causal relationships, hence confusing the descriptive with the explanatory (Biehal, 2007).

Research studies need to have a supportive rather than determining role in relation to decision-making, with a critical approach taken to methods, findings and interpretations. When making decisions in uncertain situations, there are serious flaws in relying solely on the number of research-based factors present (Howe, 1998; Cooper and Kapur, 2004). A mechanical, narrow and exclusive focus on the presence or absence of factors is not warranted or likely to be advocated by researchers. The construction of research-based predictive factors is made possible by the application of computer technology to produce, from the deconstructed details of individual situations, 'statistical correlations of heterogeneous elements' resulting in 'a combination of factors liable to produce risk' (Castel, 1991: 288). The identified factors may give pointers to what may be influential in a majority of situations, but not what will be influential in a particular situation. Users of checklists need to critically appreciate the need for interpretation and the issue of the reductionism that involves focusing on a limited number of factors to the exclusion of other, more specific situational factors. Nazeen, alongside Zena and her mother, can critically assess the applicability of the factors on the agency checklist to their particular situation, so that they can add the presence or absence of relevant factors to their own strengths/hazards analysis.

What approach to risk management is to be taken?

Risk management can generally be thought of as minimising bad outcomes; however, three approaches to risk management can be identified: defensive caution, informed risk-taking, and excessive risk-taking. In terms of decision-making, the approach adopted to managing risk will influence the choice of option. Nazeen is aware of how the future plans for Zena will be affected by the independent review officer's approach to risk management, particularly the prevailing attitude to risk-taking. Within defensive caution, concerns with safety predominate, with the option perceived to be the safest being followed, even when a more critical assessment would have shown how unintended harm could be caused. Fears about things going wrong, and not being blamed if they do, become more important than the negative consequences for service users. There is a danger that in the current cultural climate, the independent review officer would take a safety first approach and uncritically perceive Zena returning home as being the safest option.

Excessive risk-taking is when, either through overconfidence or the need to avoid a loss framed as 'certain' (Whyte, 1998; Kelly, 2000; Milner and O'Byrne, 2002), decision makers take unjustified risks that can lead to disastrous outcomes. In the specific circumstances of Zena's age and her not wanting to be adopted, the 'being adopted option' could be categorised as excessive risk-taking. The independent review officer can be cast as framing both Zena remaining in care and being placed at home as 'certain' losses, and would rather Zena had a chance to avoid these by risking the even greater loss involved in her experiencing an adoption placement breakdown. Nazeen was advocating an informed risk-taking approach to decision-making and risk management that involves careful analysis of the situation as a whole and a preparedness to take risks in order to have the chance of achieving benefits (Carson, 1996). Nazeen was aware of the dangers of Zena remaining in care but considered these were, in her situation, outweighed by the chances of benefits. From the relative security of care, Zena has been able to develop her relationship with her mother in a way that is likely to extend well into adulthood. An issue for Nazeen is how to take practical steps to reduce the chances of the dangers of being in care occurring, while not significantly reducing the chances of achieving the benefits sought. Within the 'remaining in care option', she plans to take an active approach and do everything she can to reduce the hazards and build on the strengths, for example by providing supportive relationships and monitoring Zena's progress. One pitfall is that such actions can become overly intrusive and inadvertently bring about the feared dangers.

Conclusion

The review finally accepted Nazeen's argument that remaining in care was the best option for Zena. Although pleased to have convinced the review, Nazeen was acutely aware that she had gone against current thinking and in doing so had exposed herself to future criticism if the situation develops in an unfavourable way for Zena. Despite a decision being carefully thought through, with a wide variety of factors and views taken into account, negative outcomes can still occur. A colleague responds to Nazeen's anxiety about being blamed if things go wrong by reminding her that a desired future cannot be brought about in some definite way, but rather carefully judged, nurtured and promoted in the face of complexity and uncertainty.

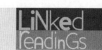

For further discussion of tackling oppression in practice, see Adams et al., 2009b, Chapter 19.

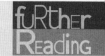

Carson, D. and Bain, A. (2008) *Professional Risk and Working with People: Decision Making in Health, Social Care and Criminal Justice*, London, Jessica Kingsley. Takes a balanced approach to risk, Chapters 4 and 5 focusing on 'risk assessment' and 'risk management' respectively.

Denney, D. (2005) *Risk and Society*, London, Sage. Chapter 7 considers the dominance of the notion of risk within state social care.

Munro, E. (2002) *Effective Child Protection*, London, Sage. Chapter 6 gives an account of some of the issues in carrying out risk assessments.

Stalker, K. (2003) 'Managing risk and uncertainty in social work', *Journal of Social Work*, 3(2): 211–33. Reviews the social work literature on managing risk and uncertainty.

Webb, S.A. (2006) *Social Work in a Risk Society*, Basingstoke, Palgrave Macmillan. Chapter 5 critically examines the technologies of care, including risk assessment.

17 Managing finances

Chapter overview

How can social workers reconcile a desire to advocate for the poor and disadvantaged while rationing services and being responsible for means testing care? This chapter explores these dual pressures, setting them in the context of the personalisation of care.

The UK social work profession has generally sought, unlike many other countries, to separate itself from income maintenance systems. It looks increasingly likely, however, that it will have to engage more with finances when working with individuals within social work agencies, and in work with partnership organisations. Financial literacy is now a professional imperative.

In the UK, the twin services arising from the postwar welfare initiatives located welfare, and some health services, within local authorities and this confirmed central government's control of most income-related systems such as national insurance, general taxation and national assistance. Exceptions existed and continue to do so. Growing numbers of central government initiatives aim to reduce social exclusion, with initiatives to develop skills, enhance motivation and offer practical assistance and encouragement to those out of the labour market. Such initiatives compel a personalised approach and blur the boundaries of government departments, the third sector and private companies.

This chapter asks a number of questions about the role of social workers in managing finances, noting that few texts and guides tackle this subject, particularly at the level of social work practice, but also at the level of social services' overall financial resources. Significant exceptions include Glennerster's (2003) comprehensive outline of government welfare funding and Glasby and Glasby's (2002) more practical guide.

Poor clients

Curiously, for a profession that evolved out of critical responses to the Poor Law (the system for the provision of basic social security in operation in England and Wales from the sixteenth century until the establishment of the welfare state in the twentieth century) in the UK, social work has an ambivalent relationship with poverty. Many of its origins stem from attempts to ameliorate the problems of the urban poor and were a combination of acts of practical philanthropy and community development. Although closely associated with the Poor Law systems, early social workers argued that poor families could be assisted by better housing, employment and cash provision. Many recognised that social change would be necessary to break cycles of deprivation and entrenched inequality.

Although the slums of Victorian Britain were the crucible of social work, the paradox of professional social work is its increasing distance from the issues and experiences of poverty. This paradox arises despite considerable evidence that:

- poverty 'creates' social work clients
- the most common characteristic among social work clients or users of social care services is their poverty.

Despite social workers' daily encounters with poverty and its effects, the responses remain similar to those of earlier decades. Becker (1997) was highly critical of social work's attempts to 'manage the poor'. He described a collection of individualised social work responses to requests for help on the discovery of poverty among service users:

- advice on benefits
- referral to other sources for advice
- assistance, if criteria are met
- reliance on a good interpersonal working relationships between social workers and the Department of Work and Pensions.

These responses have their failings. Many social workers are not trained and not interested in benefits (Glasby, 2001), often to the detriment of services users. To take one example, Nosowska (2004) reported that despite the high levels of contact between older people dying from cancer in a hospice and professionals such as social workers, many were badly informed about their eligibility for financial assistance. Overall, social workers have long been judged as often ill-equipped to offer advice and few social workers have the confidence and experience to advocate for users in potentially complex administrative and legal arenas of welfare. Concern about this in the 1980s led to the development of welfare rights specialisms, often located within local authority social services departments, where 'poverty problems' could be separated off from matters of psychosocial functioning. As Hill (2000) outlined, such developments may combine advice to clients and their social workers, and a typical social services authority will offer an information service and training for frontline staff with specialist referral points. For social workers, four main dimensions arise for practice:

- the model officially embraced by their employing agency
- linkages with social security and advice agencies

- the culture of the office or team
- their personal inclinations, knowledge of and empathy with service users and carers.

These four elements draw on the discretion still open to social workers in determining the boundaries of their work. Thus, one practitioner may conceive their role as close to advocacy, while another may be quick to refer problems on in order to concentrate on the 'underlying pathology'.

The matter of referral can be seen as one way of 'managing the poor', in Becker's terms. Charities and self-help groups continue to receive supplicants for assistance, prompted and supported by their social workers. Although social workers have generally been adverse to involvement in establishing the priorities of the Social Fund (grants and loans for necessities and in times of crisis), they have been less reluctant to push the merits of their clients for charitable relief. In practice, this can involve dilemmas for social workers in heightening the claims of some individuals by portraying them as part of the 'deserving poor'. Key aspects of such a label may include:

- the person was 'not to blame' for their predicament – by implication, unlike others
- the person is 'worthy' of one-off assistance – to get back on their feet
- the person 'acknowledges' their position with due deference
- a sense of gratitude and/or apology.

In practice, few social workers would represent this process so starkly, but many feel forced to collude in respect of their client's best or immediate interests. There is cold comfort, for example, in being without basic essentials but keeping one's dignity. Recent developments in social work education offer suggestions for social workers in working more collaboratively with people using services who are living in deprived circumstances (SCIE, 2008).

Social workers' management of the poor may also extend to other referrals, such as to welfare rights specialists, debt advice agencies or community legal services. In practice, the ever-changing and complex world of benefits, tax, court summonses, unpaid bills and income maintenance can defeat even those practitioners who wish to maintain expertise in the field. For some, the personal solution, or a strategy agreed with colleagues, may be to develop:

- a particular expertise or specialism, for example in fostering allowances, the Social Fund, child support
- systematic screening for opportunities to provide initial advice on benefit claims
- regular audits of service users' circumstances
- proactive information in conjunction with other agencies
- sound and appropriate referral routes to other agencies.

In such ways, individual practitioners counter Hill's painful allegation that they 'very often turn a deaf ear to material needs' (2000: 132).

Turning the screw

Although social workers generally have a high awareness of service users' poverty, recent years have witnessed three countervailing approaches:

1   Social workers have increasingly become the agents of local authorities in means testing or seeking information about service users' financial circumstances in order to see if they will be asked to pay for social care services. This has often led to a neglect of people who have resources and become 'lost to the system' – known as self-funders (see Henwood and Hudson, 2008).

2   They act within local authorities, many of which, simultaneously, have placed the reduction of poverty on their corporate agenda. Such a position creates a series of multiple dilemmas but also opportunities.

3   Social workers are at the vanguard of the personalisation agenda (HM Government, 2007), enabling people to arrange their own care and support, through direct payments and personal budgets.

There have, of course, been selective consumer charges for social care over many years. Although central government has encouraged and enabled local authorities to charge, it permitted them to operate a discretionary system. For people using social care services, charging systems can be confusing, contradictory and complex.

At the practice level, there are a number of dilemmas. These appear to account for the ambivalence of many social workers towards operating means-tested systems. In research exploring financial assessment for the costs of residential care, Bradley et al. (2000) found that care managers:

■   felt caught up in conflicts of interest between older people, their relatives and the local authority

■   were uncomfortable in giving information or advice and varied considerably in the extent they did so

■   worried about distinctions between avoidance and evasion of charges

■   felt unsupported by managers and politicians when they had suspicions of financial abuse or deception.

Half the care managers interviewed considered themselves inadequately trained but, for many, further training would appear more beneficial if it addressed ethical decision-making rather than knowledge-based skills. As they observed, people undergoing financial assessments may be unwell, confused or extremely anxious. Social work skills may be helpful in building relationships and presenting a holistic picture of people's needs and resources. For this reason, we consider that financial assessment, in whatever form it is likely to take for social care in the short term, is best undertaken by care managers or social workers rather than by a separate workforce. The systems of direct payments and personal budgets, where people eligible for services may receive cash instead of care, remain means-tested.

Within social services, as noted above, a new interest in poverty, and a recasting of it as social exclusion, emerged following the 1960s. Such thinking informed the Children Act 1989, which stated that if a child does not have the opportunity or is unable to achieve or maintain a 'reasonable standard of health or development', the child is to be regarded as being 'in need', which in turn means they are eligible for support services. According to section 17 of the Children Act 1989, a child is considered to be in need if:

> he is unlikely to achieve or maintain, or to have the opportunity of achieving or maintaining, a reasonable standard of health or development without the provision for him of services by a local authority ... [or if his] health or development is likely to be significantly impaired, or further impaired, without the provision for him of such services.

As the Social Care Institute for Excellence (SCIE, 2005) noted, this might, for example, include children living in substandard or unfit accommodation. This perspective places individual casework in the context of local anti-poverty or community regeneration strategies. For social workers in adult services, at an individual level, the growing ability to respond to need with cash, not care, enables people to be in greater control of their own support. This may apply particularly to people who may have found existing systems do not meet their needs:

> In one London borough that has been more successful in promoting direct payments among ethnic minorities, care managers found that the payments were helpful for engaging people who had previously been reluctant to accept support. Key to this was an outreach approach whereby workers from independent organisations, such as Age Concern which employed someone to liaise with the Bangladeshi community, could be involved in the initial assessment, alongside social services. Service users there were particularly appreciative of this advocacy role. (Swift, 2007)

More than a sticking plaster

Although much of social work's origins lay in local responses to poverty, the development of anti-poverty work in the 1990s broadened to include areas outside the inner cities and draw on a wider range of partners – both horizontally with partnerships of local agencies and vertically with links to government strategy – for social renewal, full(ish) employment, regeneration and inclusion. Social work's focus on individuals rather than groups and on client status rather than locality has created some difficulty in aligning social work priorities with broader anti-poverty moves. The emphasis on risk and danger, which developed during the 1990s as a rationale for social work's focus on certain targeted groups, has also contributed to a reactive rather than preventive model of practice. In the world of social inclusion initiatives, social services departments have become part of locality based initiatives, such as Sure Start programmes, that emphasise the value of multi-agency approaches and regeneration schemes, generally taking a steer from the corporate local authority. In most parts of England, the division of social services departments into adult services and children's departments has enabled new .

links with professionals who see individuals and families in the context of preventive work, rather than at times of crisis.

For social workers, anti-poverty strategies have been one way of combating poverty and promoting social justice beyond casework (Craig, 2002). Craig (2000) has identified several ways in which social workers can support such strategies, including:

- monitoring of service use to identify take-up or withdrawal by those living in poverty
- assessing the impact of policies in terms of reducing poverty through 'poverty proofing'
- pooling data with other agencies to monitor poverty levels locally
- listening to the voices of those 'on the sharp end of poverty' to hear their views of new approaches.

Developing skills

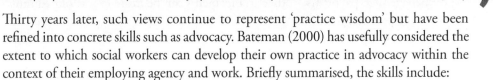

Social workers ... have to engage with poverty in two ways. One involves a general response to its impact on their clients, with an obligation to describe and discuss for a wider audience whose concerns can be mobilised. The other ... requires the social workers to consider the most effective ways of helping the individual in poverty who is a unique person in unique difficulty. (Stevenson, quoted in Hardiker and Barker, 1988)

Thirty years later, such views continue to represent 'practice wisdom' but have been refined into concrete skills such as advocacy. Bateman (2000) has usefully considered the extent to which social workers can develop their own practice in advocacy within the context of their employing agency and work. Briefly summarised, the skills include:

- understanding the 'best interests' principle – now encapsulated in the Mental Capacity Act 2005
- purposeful and in-depth interviewing
- research skills
- organisational skills
- assertive, negotiating skills
- knowing when to act and when to refer.

These can be incorporated into placement opportunities or within social work curricula at pre- or post-qualifying levels.

Cash not care?

Increasingly central to the work of adult social services has been the provision of support to disabled people. The Community Care (Direct Payments) Act 1996 gave local authorities powers to make cash payments to service users to purchase their own assistance. Such schemes are popular and successful among many disabled people. Users have valued the greater independence, choice and control underpinned by the ability to organise their own support and have argued that the staff they employ are more reliable, more flexible and personally suitable. As such, this form of cash assistance is empowering.

Early research, however, pointed to the difficulties of translating the ideals of such schemes into practice. Leece's (2000) study of the early days of direct payments found that social workers did not always appear confident in the schemes or were reluctant to communicate information to potential participants. Dawson (2000) argued that social services departments needed to change attitudes to risk management and learn to compromise in order to enhance the independence of service users. Rummery (2003) suggested that debates about citizenship would need to build on early work on welfare rights.

Other research has pointed to practitioners' dilemmas in encouraging choice and user control while protecting disabled people from exploitation or neglect (see Manthorpe et al., 2008). These risks are not new. Ryan (1999), for example, developed frameworks to help practitioners to manage their own reservations about direct payments that remain highly relevant. These include:

- accepting that service users can receive direct payments and assistance from other people – the two are not exclusive
- distinguishing between the 'willingness' to take on direct payments and the ability to manage such payments – other arrangements can be made to sort out administrative or practical matters
- maximising opportunities to learn about the scheme and respecting that people may lack initial confidence
- considering the use of independent living trusts and supported decision-making systems
- establishing a range of safeguards to assess and manage risks.

Such points may provide social workers with greater confidence in the system of direct payments and new personal budgets. Evidence from direct payments and the 'in Control' organisation is that such schemes potentially offer people opportunities to arrange support that:

- is flexible in timing and extent
- is individually tailored
- promotes a sense of control.

Trusting poor people with cash has for many years been a difficult matter for state agencies, as the existence of subsidies or benefits in kind, for example free school meals and milk tokens, demonstrates. It will be a key part of social workers' roles to enable people to develop skills and experience in this, and to recognise if or when they need outside support.

Cash and capacity

This section moves to discuss social workers' roles in enabling individuals to maintain control over their own financial resources in the face of attempts to remove such abilities on the grounds of ageism or disablism. For people whose mental capacity is becoming significantly impaired, social workers may play a key role in advising them about possible measures that can be taken and plans that can be made. Individuals who have learned that they have early dementia, for example, may be usefully supported by social workers in making legal arrangements for lasting powers of attorney under the Mental Capacity Act 2005 (England and Wales) and thinking about advance decisions. For those without such arrangements, social workers may be involved in liaison with the Department of Work and Pensions or the Office of the Public Guardian.

Evidence for the need to be alert to the possibility of financial abuse has come from a variety of accounts about the harm that may be caused by such betrayals of trust or deprivation of quality of life. The national prevalence study of elder abuse (O'Keefe et al., 2007) found that financial abuse was the second most common form of mistreatment and neglect reported. Pritchard (2000) has suggested that the distress of financial abuse in later life among older women may be compounded by the lack of adequate response or support they receive should they disclose their predicament. Feelings of self-blame and helplessness were common among the women she interviewed.

While deprivation of cash or possessions may be an important indicator that a person is being mistreated or abused, social work values and the Human Rights Act underline people's right to self-determination in all but the most extreme circumstances, generally if severe harm would be caused to themselves or others. At times, social workers will find themselves respecting the rights of people to be 'foolish' or eccentric and this may cause conflict with relatives or others in the social network. Similarly, disabled people who are vulnerable to becoming involved in debt (Grant, 2000) may benefit from sustained support rather than crisis intervention. Such support is, of course, difficult when social care policy focuses on people in most need and may exclude those whose disabilities are classified as 'moderate'. The building up of relationships between service users and individual practitioners, which might promote trusting communication, is often reported to have declined as practitioners' focus more on assessment rather than ongoing support.

Conclusion

In this chapter, we have seen how social workers' ambivalence to working with finances reflects a desire to avoid crossing the boundary into territory of income and expenditure. New models of social care support combined with growing means testing mean that, like it or not, finance is central to the helping and empowering relationship. Similarly, the role of social workers in managing budgets and contracts with service providers means that ignorance of finance is untenable and unprofessional.

However, technical, financial skills are not sufficient, because, as we have shown, money, or the lack of it, is central to the lives of people using services. An understanding of the impact of poverty or financial abuse may contribute to a broader understanding of why individuals may react to their situation in certain ways, what factors enhance coping or resilience, and what might prompt change. Listening to the experiences of people who are poor needs to be part of a continual process of reflection for practitioners, in respect of their work with individuals and families and with regard to the policies and resource allocations of the broader agency. And whatever new organisational structures arise for social work, managing to champion the interests of the most disadvantaged may be the one distinctive and enduring contribution of social work.

For further discussion of the implications for policy and practice of research into poverty, see Adams et al., 2009a, Chapter 7.

Davey, V., Fernandez, JL., Knapp, M. et al. (2007) *Direct Payments: A National Survey of Direct Payments, Policy and Practice*, London, TSO. First major study pulling together information about the use of direct payments.

Glasby, J. and Littlechild, R. (2009) *Direct Payments and Personal Budgets*, Bristol, Policy Press. Early look at the meaning of personalisation when applied to social care provision.

Glendinning, C., Challis, D., Fernandez, J. et al. (2008) *The Evaluation of the Individual Budget Pilots: Final Report*, Social Policy Research Unit, University of York, php.york.ac.uk/inst/spru/pubs/1119/. Research study that looked at the implementation of individual budgets in 13 pilot local authorities in England.

Social Care Institute for Excellence (SCIE) (2008) *Personalisation: A Rough Guide*, SCIE, www.scie.org.uk. Clear, if uncritical, outline of government policy, with practice points.

Quality assurance   18

Chapter overview

This chapter deals with the different mechanisms by which central and local government bodies assure the quality of social work services. I look critically at four main perspectives on quality assurance, located in the wider context of public services.

Quality is a matter of debate and controversy

The question of assuring the quality of public services as a whole, and social work services in particular, is somewhat controversial. There is general agreement that it is a good thing but methods of doing it remain debatable. This is for three main reasons:

1 It is by no means agreed how the quality of public services should be judged.
2 A succession of scandals in the delivery of social services to children and disabled people, and in hospital and community health and social services to people with mental health problems, to which the mass media often draw attention (Franklin and Parton, 1991), has shaken public faith in the authority of professionals.
3 The fact that the funding of public services comes from the public purse tends to give the politicians, central government agencies and local authority managers first claim on how their quality should be judged, yet service users are increasingly vocal in claiming they should have a say in judging the quality of services.

Policy and legal context

The history of external scrutiny of the quality of public services is somewhat chequered. Systems for regulating and inspecting the quality of public services have been introduced on a piecemeal basis since the 1830s; but they only began to develop into coherent national or UK-wide systems of quality assurance from the 1980s onwards. The Audit Commission – an independent public body – was set up in 1983 to monitor the extent to which public money was being spent efficiently and economically. Since then, its initial responsibilities as a financial auditor have shifted somewhat to monitoring services (Cope and Goodship, 2002). The scandals referred to above have spurred governments to set up heavily centralised systems for quality assurance in the health and social services.

At times, policy and practice may seem to be driven by the concerns of the general public. However, public bodies are not primarily accountable to the public but to their local and central government treasuries for the money they spend, and public expenditure in services delivered through local authorities and their independent (voluntary and private) agency partners has increased by 40 per cent between 1998/99 and 2003/04, while capital expenditure has more than doubled. The quality of local authority managed and commissioned public services remains one of the priority areas to be tackled under the Labour government's twenty-first century plans for the modernisation of public services.

The Local Government Act 1999 increased the inspectorial powers of the Audit Commission over local councils and required these and national park authorities, fire and rescue authorities and some parish councils to set up systems for continuous improvement known as Best Value. Inspections by the Audit Commission began in 2000/2001, but there was clearly a need for a more coherent approach than hitherto, reflected by the somewhat uncoordinated system of audits and inspections. By 2001/2002, these audits and inspections were combined and in 2002 a system of comprehensive performance assessment (CPA) was set up, comprising a four-part assessment:

1   a three-year cycle of corporate assessment of every council was carried out – 150 single tier and county councils and 238 district councils were inspected and reports published by December 2004
2   annual service assessments
3   annual resources assessments
4   a direction of travel assessment, intended to judge the likelihood of the council's future performance improving.

Similar arrangements for audit that were broadly harmonised were made in the other three devolved countries of the UK:

- The Accounts Commission for Scotland was set up in 1975, independent of central and local government, to oversee public spending, and under the Local Government in Scotland Act 2003, Audit Scotland works on behalf of the commission to monitor public services.
- The Northern Ireland Audit Office was set up under the Audit (Northern Ireland) Order 1987.
- The Public Audit (Wales) Act 2004 instituted similar arrangements.

From April 2009, a new inspection framework – the comprehensive area assessment (CAA) – was introduced for local authorities, intended to replace annual performance assessments and joint area reviews (JARs) of children's services. The intention of the CAA was to reduce the total burden of inspection on authorities and to focus on the outcomes

achieved by local authorities, either working alone or in partnership with other authorities and organisations, including those in the voluntary and private sector.

Until 2005, annual service assessments of services for children and young people
and adult social care were carried out by different inspectorates. Since 2005, JARs of
children's services have been carried out by Ofsted and the Commission for Social Care
Inspection (CSCI). National performance indicators (PIs) are used as the basis for these
inspections. The CPA framework draws on a variety of sources of information – PIs,
audit reports, inspection reports, assessments of corporate capacity and the views of
stakeholders, including service users, or experts through experience, and carers.

The Care Standards Act 2000 set up the National Care Standards Commission
(NCSC), responsible for regulating the quality of a wide range of services, from fostering and adoption, through domiciliary care, hospitals to care homes for older people
and residential childcare. The quality of services has to be registered under section 48(1)
of the NHS and Community Care Act (NHSCCA) 1990 and inspected under Part II
of the Care Standards Act 2000. The inspection of services and premises falls under
section 31(2) of the Care Standards Act 2000 and is the responsibility of the Care
Quality Commission (CQC) created under the Health and Social Care Act 2008.

Until 2008, the Commission of Healthcare, Audit and Inspection (generally called
the Healthcare Commission) and the CSCI were responsible for regulating health and
adult social care services. The Mental Health Act Commission monitored and regulated
mental health services under the Mental Health Act 1983. The Health and Social Care
Act 2008 replaced this system and these bodies from April 2009 with a single integrated
body – the CQC – with responsibility for regulating health and adult social care,
including mental health services. The Act also put in place a coordinated and managed
system for inspecting these services and a system of registration of services to cover
essential standards of safety and quality, to operate from 2010.

Arguments for these new arrangements include support for integration and the view
that they will be simpler to administer and less onerous for local public services, being
regulated through local authorities, voluntary and private agencies and organisations.

Critics of the reformed arrangements argue that:

- there are no structural safeguards to ensure that care issues are not overlooked
- there are no bodies catering for the needs of people who are excluded or seldom
  heard
- the former duties of the CSCI to review particular services (such as led to the report
  on home care; CSCI, 2006) are downgraded from a duty to a power of the CQC.

Similar concerns about the quality of services have been voiced by an independent
working group, which commented on the plans to expand significantly the involvement
of the independent and voluntary sector in the delivery of health services (Timmins,
2006). The working group recommended that the patient representative element was
removed from foundation trusts and transferred to primary care trusts (PCTs), which
would have membership councils so that the voices of patients could be heard, accompanied by the expanded principle of patient choice (Timmins, 2006: 35). This is

consistent with a pattern across health, social care and social work to involve patients and people who use services in the inspections of services. A Commission for Patient and Public Involvement in Health was established in 2003 and was replaced under the Local Government and Public Involvement in Health Act 2007 by Local Involvement Networks (LINks) to enable independent individuals and groups to have a stronger say in how their health and social care/social work services are delivered. The extent to which inspection and LINks arrangements are real rather than tokenistic depends on the commitment of public bodies and the assertiveness and criticality of the people who become involved. Given the intrinsic power of entrenched managers and professionals and the structural and dispersed (geographically and socially isolated) situations of many patients and service users, such arrangements need to be worked at and will not automatically be effective.

A wider range of legislation has a bearing on quality assurance and adds to the complexity of the field. Some legislation creates, or reflects, this pressure more than others. Two examples are health and safety and anti-discriminatory legislation.

Health and safety cover a wide range of aspects of the quality of people's working and living environments, so are relevant to sustaining the quality of all health, welfare, social work and social care settings. The Health and Safety at Work etc. Act 1974 was a consolidating law, which brought together a huge mass of previous legislation and required employers to provide a healthy and safe workplace and required employees to take responsibility for their own safety and that of other people with whom they worked. A great quantity of regulations, or secondary legislation, normally in the form of Statutory Instruments, was introduced following this Act, covering many aspects of work with people, such as lifting and handling regulations, which affect the work of professionals in many aspects such as disability, geriatric and palliative care. Health and safety are regulated by an increasing number of directives from the European Union, which are binding on member countries including those of the UK. Health and safety in social work and social care establishments and services in different countries of the UK are governed by a memorandum of understanding between the Health and Safety Commission and the Health and Safety Executive, set up in 1999 and responsible for the regulation of social care in England, Scotland and Wales.

Campaigns for equality and anti-discrimination have been promoted since the 1970s by professionals, pressure groups, the general public, ethnic minority groups and, more recently, the disability movement. The Equality Act 2006 represents the high point of these equality- and rights-based movements. It replaces existing commissions (Commission for Racial Equality, Disability Rights Commission and Equal Opportunities Commission) with the Commission for Equality and Human Rights, which has the aim of eliminating all forms of prejudice based on age, gender, ethnicity, 'race' or disability. The single equality scheme was developed in the NHS (DH, 2007) to ensure compliance with legal duties regarding gender, 'race' and disability legislation and to anticipate new duties in relation to age, religion, beliefs and sexual orientation.

Concepts of quality and quality assurance

Quality assurance as a concept has a life of its own. We shall see in the next section that it has been borrowed from other disciplines and applied in the public services sector. Hence the language it uses is somewhat strange to social workers, and, not surprisingly, the term 'quality assurance' means many different things to different people. As a lowest common denominator, we can say that quality assurance refers to

> processes, procedures and techniques aiming to guarantee that social work services to clients and carers meet their needs through their appropriateness, consistency and excellence. (Adams, 2000: 279)

We have seen from the example of equality and human rights that the operation of systems of quality assurance cannot be segregated from the general work of public service authorities. In this sense, quality assurance is part of the politics of policy and practice. It is affected by debates about why and how particular approaches to service delivery are adopted.

It follows that the concepts of 'quality' and 'quality assurance' are contested concepts whose application is as deeply enmeshed as any aspect of social work in the politics of its management. Although quality assurance procedures may seem to take place in the margins, alongside the main business which is to commission, contract and deliver services, they do not take place in a vacuum, in two main ways:

1 They are part of the politics of policy-making and service delivery. Considerations of what constitutes a good service are matters of opinion and judgement rather than fact.
2 They are locked into their time. Judgements about what is 'good' quality in services change through time. For example, the process by which the menu is arrived at and meals served, whether in a residential home for older people or through meals on wheels, is affected by national debates about fat and salt in the diet, obesity and the health of the nation. One decade's staple diet could turn out to be another decade's poison.

Quality assurance is an ambiguous concept, being both an empowering tool to improve the practice of social workers by giving clients a stronger role, and a means of regulating professionals. These functions may be compatible, but where they are not, assuring quality remains a problematic goal. The Best Value culture of quality assurance in health and social services creates its own language of regulating bodies, standards, procedures and PIs against which practice is evaluated. The critical practitioner should not be swamped by the detail of these and just follow them slavishly, without an awareness of their inbuilt assumptions and limitations.

Methods of assuring quality

The methodologies on which quality assurance in the health and social services draws originate in the disciplines of economics, politics, mathematics and management. Some examples are briefly examined below.

Welfare economics and policies into practice

Judgements concerning the achievements of organisations and professionals about delivering services to people originate in a branch of economics known as 'welfare economics'. This draws on different theories and approaches that help economists and social policy makers to decide how to make socially desirable and, one hopes, socially just decisions about how to allocate health and welfare – including social work – resources, among many other resources, of course. Welfare economists use their own complex arguments and assumptions to guide them towards these decisions. One traditional set of assumptions – known as 'Pareto efficiency or optimality' – refers to the best possible distribution of services that can be made, such that no further improvement can be made to anybody's situation without harming somebody else's situation. This reasoning does not tackle the situation many social workers face, which is that excluded or vulnerable individuals and groups may need more resources in situations where they are unequally divided in society between people who are extremely well off, and becoming better off, and people who experience persistent poverty.

Cost–benefit analysis

One of the most commonly used methods of comparatively evaluating different resources and services is cost–benefit analysis (CBA). The CBA is carried out by totalling the value of the benefits of the policy, facility or service and then subtracting its costs. This sounds simple, but in reality the tasks of apportioning a value to benefits and identifying the total costs are complex, since they are likely to include not only financial but other measures such as individual and social costs (including environmental importance) and people's perceptions and experiences. Sometimes managers will try to overcome these problems by putting a financially estimated figure on these other costs and benefits.

Quality adjusted life year

Associated with efforts to quantify both qualitative and quantitative aspects of benefits to people's lives is the notion of quality of life. Efforts to try to arrive at a commonly agreed measure of this have led, in health settings especially, to the quality adjusted life year (QALY). A QALY is a measure of people's quantity and quality of life (the extra longevity and wellbeing), which is produced by combining an estimate of life expectancy and the quality of the remaining life years. Thus, the QALY calculates a value on the time spent in a given state of health, scoring a year of perfect health as 1 and death as 0, although some states of poor health are estimated to be worse than death and are scored less than 0.

Cost–utility ratio

This brings us to the cost–utility ratio as a way of using the QALY to compare different interventions and services. The cost–utility ratio calculates the extra cost of generating a year of perfect health for a person, that is, one QALY. Different treatments and services can be measured using this as a comparative measure. Those with a relatively low cost per QALY are relatively inexpensive and those with a relatively high cost per QALY are relatively expensive. Although these calculations and comparisons are fraught with difficulties and sometimes extremely controversial, the cost–utility ratio provides evidence as a basis for choices between different groups of people receiving different services and interventions. Staff commissioning services gain an insight into the possible benefits of investment in new treatments.

Risk analysis and management

One of the most tricky aspects of comparing different treatments and services is working in uncertain conditions where people's actions and responses to circumstances are difficult to predict, that is, they represent differing degrees of risk. A major proportion of professionals' time is taken up with analysing and managing risks. Risk analysis focuses on the threats facing people and/or situations. A risk is generally defined as what people perceive as the extent of possible loss, harm or damage to a person, situation, goods or services. In material terms, it is possible to calculate a value for a risk as the likelihood of an occurrence times the cost of the occurrence.

NICE and the SMC

We can see the importance of the above concepts and methods in operation in the procedures adopted in the UK health services for approving drugs for treatment. The National Institute for Health and Clinical Excellence (NICE) was founded in 1999 as the independent body responsible for deciding which drugs and treatments the NHS in England should provide. The Scottish equivalent is the Scottish Medicines Consortium (SMC), set up in 2001. In Wales, the All Wales Medicine Strategy Group has more restricted oversight of the use of medicines and prescribing.

NICE tends to use cost-effectiveness as the main determinant for usage of a drug or treatment. It has adopted the cost-effectiveness baseline of £20–30,000 per QALY. According to Carroll (2008), this is a rule of thumb that has been adopted in the absence of an adequate empirical or theoretical evidence base (House of Commons Health Committee, 2007). The average PCT allocates between £12,000 and £19,000 per extra QALY in circulatory disease and cancer respectively (Carroll, 2008).

The decisions reached by NICE in respect of particular treatments and the length of time it takes to reach them are the subjects of fierce controversy, made more acute by the fact that the SMC – using less rigorous and time-consuming research – reaches decisions in an average of 12–16 weeks compared with 62 weeks by NICE (Carroll, 2008). Some critics allege that the cost of about £80,000 per appraisal by NICE is not 'value for money' – another commonly used measure of quality of services.

Best Value

The Local Government Act 1999 imposed the duty on local authorities in England and Wales to achieve Best Value, that is, continuous improvement in carrying out their functions with regard to the economy, efficiency and effectiveness of service delivery. In Scotland, the Scottish Local Authorities (Tendering) Act 2001 marked the shift from the system of compulsory competitive tendering to the Best Value approach. In Northern Ireland, this was achieved under the Local Government (Best Value) Act (Northern Ireland) 2002. A Best Value Authority is one which complies with the requirements of best value, in working towards meeting local and national targets and reporting on past, current and future performance. There is evidence that Best Value has had a positive effect on the quality and accountability of local authority services, but little effect on the costs of services (Boyne et al., 2001).

We have surveyed some of the main concepts and methods involved in quality assurance and now need to change focus, in recognition that perspectives on assuring quality in social work differ in major ways.

Four main approaches to quality assurance

It will help us to clarify the priorities for critical practitioners wishing to draw on ideas and practices concerning quality assurance if we simplify the different perspectives, methods and techniques and relate these to assumptions and views about quality in public services. Adams (1998b: 28) identifies four main perspectives on quality assurance:

1 rectification of errors and shortcomings in quality
2 maintenance through standard-setting and inspection
3 quality enhancement through audits and evaluation
4 quality maximisation.

These are somewhat idealised and artificially distinguished from each other, whereas in practice the territories they occupy often run into one another. It is likely that different approaches can exist side by side in the same setting, in response to different policy initiatives, for example (see Table 18.1).

Let us examine these in turn, bearing in mind that only some of them are visible in the public services at any one time, but setting them out in this way helps to clarify what is going on.

Table 18.1 Four approaches to quality

Approach to quality assurance	Dominant process	Person holding power	Dominant management style
1 Rectification	Control	Manager	Commercial managerialist
2 Maintenance	Regulation	Expert	Scientific management
3 Enhancement	Consumer satisfaction	Professional	Consumerist managerialist
4 Maximisation	Empowerment; learning culture in the organisation	Service user, worker, manager and politician	Democratic

Source: Adapted from Philips et al., 1994; Coote, 1994

Rectification of errors and shortcomings in quality

The rectification culture is managerialist, dominated by the efforts of managers to retain control in a time of crisis, that is, there are errors or shortcomings in services that must be remedied. To the extent that there is scope for individual enterprise and creativity on the part of practitioners, or for service users, it is within the framework of initiatives led by managers. So, the decisions of professionals such as social workers are underwritten by management, that is, they are primarily shaped and rationed by costs and only secondarily by service users' priorities.

The history of the emphasis in social services on remedying shortcomings is unfortunate but some would say inevitable, given the poor quality of work in some areas. Critical commentators draw attention to the

> climate of negativity whereby few have a good word to say publicly [about social work and the] 'deficit' culture which positions social work as fair game for persistent criticism, not only from politicians, the media and inquiries into apparent 'failures' to protect children and adults but also from some social work organisations themselves and from some academics and social work literature. (Jones et al, 2008: 1)

A so-called 'blame culture' may result from efforts by managers to identify blameworthy individuals. Failures are given a high profile in the mass media and the responsibility often focuses on faulty practice by individuals, including social workers. This has the effect of reinforcing an ideology that punishes individual weakness and rewards individual enterprise, responsibility and competition. Workplaces beset by scandals and subsequent investigations are understandably not happy places. Staff and clients, some of whom may have suffered from the effects of the original incidents, are likely to feel the depressing and stress-provoking impact of their aftermath.

So, we have evidence to support the view that the rectification culture predominates in social work, in that the most widely publicised approaches to quality assurance in the public services in general and social work services in particular are those arising from the mistakes, problems and shortcomings of services. Since the early 1970s, there has been a long succession of inquiries into disasters and scandals in Britain in childcare and mental health, in particular. The mass media tend to nurture the sparks of public interest in incidents and ensure that many of the small fires of concern become major conflagrations. In their turn, the authorities often rely on inquiries and investigations as their main means of translating remedies into practice.

The following case example highlights the operation of this first approach to quality assurance.

CaSE EXaMPLE

Eleanor is a social worker, whose client, lone-parent Mary, takes her youngest child Stephanie to a nursery school within walking distance of her home. The nursery school has a new head, Gail, and is staffed by nursery nurses and teachers. Mary's widowed mother, who has had a stroke, has been admitted to a local, privately run residential nursing home for older people.

There has been a complaint about conditions in the residential home. An inspector from outside the local authority comes to interview Mary and visits Eleanor. Mary's mother has become seriously ill with food poisoning. The inspector wants to know whether Mary mentioned her worries about the physical deterioration in her mother since admission to the home. Eleanor admits that she didn't follow this up, or visit Mary's mother and check out the quality of care in the home. The inspector comments in passing that the most cursory visit to the toilets in the home would have revealed serious shortcomings in hygiene, which would have been clues to other possible problems in the home.

Maintenance through standard-setting and inspection

The maintenance culture is that of scientific management, which works on the mechanistic assumption that members of the workforce function as the equivalent of cogs in the machine. The dominance of scientific principles over the regulation of the workplace is maintained by experts – not professional social workers or service users. They are located towards the bottom of the hierarchy. The overriding priorities are to maintain the system, the structure of power, as it is and not to disturb the status quo in any way. To this end, there is an emphasis on working to set minimum standards and laid down procedures. Procedures very much dominate professional practice as well. In some scientific management cultures, even professional social workers may become virtual slaves to proformas, which must be completed in the face of unmet requirements, wishes and needs of people who use services.

A particular concern in the UK in the twenty-first century is whether the inspection regime is rigorous and robust enough to expose weaknesses and abuses in the private and voluntary sectors, given that the local authority commissioners of such services have a shared interest with providers in maintaining, for example, a particular residential home, even though deficits in service are exposed. There is bound to be a temptation to collude rather than a ruthless culling of inferior providers.

In the maintenance organisational culture, the emphasis is on squeezing the most work out of staff for the least expenditure. There may be pressure on the warden of a privately run sheltered housing complex to cut costs, with the aim of maximising profits rather than the quality of life of residents. There may be little or no investment in staff. At worst, they are simply exploited. Rhetoric about standard-setting and quality indicators masks the cutting of resources, so that fewer staff work harder, experiencing greater stress, to sustain a growing range and depth of services, with evermore risk that mistakes will occur and vulnerable people will suffer. The number of full-time staff in the core workforce declines and services are sustained by an increasing number of part-time, sessional staff. Meeting budgetary targets dominates the agenda. The pressure is on staff to accept working conditions. The implicit message, discouraging staff from looking critically at working practices in the organisation, is: 'If you don't like the job, leave and we'll find somebody else to do it.' In such circumstances, ironically, quality may actually decline.

CaSE EXaMPLE (cont'd)

Ofsted inspectors have reported on the nursery. The new head of the nursery has come from a teaching background. She has decided to respond proactively to the report's observation that the first half-hour of each day is not spent productively enough, and introduces a formal period of teaching for the first half-hour of every day.

However, Mary's daughter Stephanie is causing problems. Parents used to stay with their children, but Mary now delivers Stephanie at nine o'clock and leaves immediately because she feels in the way of the teaching. Stephanie has been extremely distressed every morning for two weeks. The work of seven other children in her group has been interrupted by her prolonged crying. Stephanie's key worker nursery nurse asks the head if Stephanie can come half an hour later. The head refuses, on the grounds that parents sign up for the entire curriculum or withdraw their children. There are not the resources to give Stephanie individual attention first thing in the morning. Stephanie must be unsuitable for nursery education, she comments.

Mary confides in Eleanor her distress at what is happening to Stephanie. Eleanor backs away from challenging the inspectors' recommendations, now implemented, that is, the emphasis on schooling in the nursery, at the expense of care tailored to the individual needs of the children.

Our example raises a number of critical questions about the limitations of such quality assurance procedures. How far, for example, can such measures recommend the resourcing of new and additional services where there is unmet need? How can they judge whether services are being delivered at prices that existing and potential clients can afford? How can the multiplicity of different standards for service provision in authorities throughout the UK be reconciled with the principle that all clients should have equal access to services of an equivalent quality that meet their needs? Where there is discretion, the variations in services offered will not always be ideal.

For a number of reasons, largely due to human rather than technical factors inherent in the principle – it is a good one – of inspection itself, procedures for inspection as a means of imposing standards of service cannot of themselves assure quality. There is much that is good about setting standards and attempting to measure performance by monitoring and inspecting, using them as benchmarks. The appearance of objectivity in published standards may offer a false reassurance of quality being delivered.

Quality enhancement

The quality enhancement culture allows professionals some scope to influence decisions about the management and delivery of quality services. Staff still are required to work to laid down standards, but there is more scope for individual initiative and less absolute reliance on procedures and checklists. Managerialism still dominates, but promotes consumer choice from within an array of existing options defined by politicians and managers. Among the positives, in this case, are approaches to quality assurance that in some ways move beyond maintaining existing levels of service, to enhancing them. Also, some inspection systems have the brief of enhancement, whereas others are still concerned to regulate the status quo. The greater involvement of professionals, including social workers, enables more of the wishes of service users to be heard and, hopefully, acted on.

Quality maximisation

Many different labels approximating to this broad perspective have been developed, such as total quality or total quality management, which in business usually refers to an organisation-wide approach to producing the best quality product or service at the lowest possible price.

There is a huge literature about organisational leadership and management describing the profile of the organisation where quality is maximised:

- the organisation is change oriented
- staff are encouraged to take calculated risks in innovating
- there is no blame culture if things go wrong
- professionals, for example social work practitioners, receive encouragement, resources and the authority to develop creative and critical, rather than merely competent, practice.

People receiving services need to be empowered so that they can exercise a signifi-cant say in the quality of services they receive. The democratic nature of the culture in the organisation frees politicians, managers, professionals and service users to negotiate a variety of different ways of working together. They are partnerships. Some of them are traditional, in that the managers and professionals still lead. However, the tendency towards extending the provision of services into the voluntary and private sector creates opportunities for service users and, in some circumstances, carers to take the lead.

Measures to enable people to respond to the suspicion of abuse or neglect include support for whistle-blowing – the act of bringing hitherto hidden shortcomings to public notice. People can make complaints about the quality of services or that they have not been assessed as needing a service, under the Local Authority Social Services Act 1970 and the NHSCCA Act 1990. Under section 50 of this Act, local authorities must draw up and widely advertise a complaints procedure, in respect of their services, including social work and social care services. Practitioners across the health and welfare sector may feel an ethical duty to expose shortcomings and malpractice in their organ-isation (Hunt, 1995, 1998a), but in practice in social work, their situation vis-à-vis their relationship with employers tends to be precarious, as Hunt demonstrates (1998b).

◇◇◇◇ CASE EXAMPLE (cont'd) ◇◇◇◇◇◇◇◇◇◇◇◇◇◇◇◇◇◇◇◇◇◇◇◇◇◇◇◇◇◇◇◇◇◇◇

Eleanor is in a quandary. She knows she isn't helping Mary, Mary's mother or Mary's children. She is confused about what to do. She feels guilt at not picking up what was happening in the nursing home. Should she intervene proactively in the nursery school? A tutor on a quality assurance course she attended talked about quality maximisation, but she finds the implications of this – empower-ing practice with Mary and her family members – somewhat challenging and difficult to envisage in practice. Eleanor is not going to be popular with the head of the nursery if she insists on a meeting to examine the extent to which the needs of Stephanie are being met.

Eleanor reconsiders her situation. She looks critically at her practice in this case so far, and is aware that she has not been assertive enough on behalf of her clients. She decides to insist on the meeting, as her overriding priority is to achieve the highest possible quality of service for her client. She takes Mary into her confidence regarding her doubts, as part of her preparation for the next stage. She wants Mary to be as empowered as possible. She cannot predict what will happen.

Repeated evidence shows that clients' perceptions and views too often are ignored. Over decades, children, young people and adults have protested against the conditions in which they are incarcerated, schooled and 'cared for'. An examination of the strong tradition of protests by pupils (Adams, 1991) indicates that while those receiving services may protest, invariably their protests are not attended to. Their views should be taken seriously and not ignored or responded to punitively.

Empowerment can be too politically, financially and managerially dangerous. It is easier for the powerful to continue to manage the powerless in society. Empowerment could be about offering people informed choice, and thereby enabling exclusion to be challenged at the personal level. At the collective level, empowered people could tackle the political, social and economic causes of their and others' exclusion (Adams, 1998c). This is superior to top-down approaches where projects and programmes are designed without involving clients at all. In childcare, for example, children could be offered greater control, choice and independence over when and what happens, at the expense, perhaps, of some protection. Immediate intervention may be traded off against providing the child with more support and scope to explore, with key adults including professionals, alternative strategies for addressing problems that may be improved despite being complex and deep-rooted.

Quality maximisation requires staff to turn repeatedly to carers, parents of children being looked after by the social services, and others receiving services, and ask them for their perceptions of those services.

Implications for critical practice

Four general implications for critical practitioners can be drawn from this brief discussion of the four main approaches to quality assurance:

- We cannot maximise quality through quality assurance alone, or through approaches based on imposing regulation and standardisation, or one based largely on problem rectification. It is difficult to envisage how regulating a system that is not working will improve it significantly. Such a system needs reforms outside the quality assurance process and, probably, more resources.
- There should be no upper limit set on the level of expertise that it is possible to achieve. Expertise is linked with excellence, rather than with the pursuit of minimum standards of achievement (Adams, 1998b).
- We cannot maximise quality without empowering clients and workers, including managers as well as professionals. A deskilled, demotivated, stressed and overworked workforce is not well placed to help other people.
- Professionals and managers will continue to have an uneasy, and potentially bumpy, relationship. The way to address potential conflicts between professional and managerial interests is for managers constantly to check out with social workers any implications for them of proposed new approaches to quality assurance. Likewise, practitioners have a responsibility to go beyond maintaining handed down standards and to criticise approaches to quality.

Conclusion

Despite the tendency towards quality assurance to be driven by central government and applied through local authorities throughout the UK, the fact that health and social services increasingly are delivered by a growing number and variety of voluntary and private providers makes the task immensely more complicated. Behind the actual mechanisms for assuring quality, there is much scope for critical debate about the different perspectives on quality and the methods associated with each of these. One particular area of controversy is the role of the service user in assuring their quality, and what weight to give this voice alongside the views of managers, professionals and the public who pay for these services.

Approaches to quality assurance based on rectifying shortcomings and maintaining present standards have little to offer in the rapidly changing circumstances facing our complex probation and social services organisations, in contrast with approaches based on enhancing professional practice and maximising quality through empowering all stakeholders in services. Equality-based and self-critical organisational cultures with an open, democratic style of working are more likely to lead to service user satisfaction than those dominated by managers and professionals (Adams, 2000: 280). Such organisational cultures cannot automatically resolve conflicts of perspective and preference between adults and adults, and adults and children. The task of managing these falls, among others, to critical social workers. This entails moving beyond the procedurally driven analyses of shortcomings in quality and the crisis-inspired responses to them.

For further discussion of empowering organisations, see Adams et al., 2009b, Chapter 16.

Adams, R. (1998) *Quality Social Work*, Basingstoke, Macmillan – now Palgrave Macmillan. Critical examination of the four main approaches to quality assurance.

Adams, R. (2000) 'Quality assurance', in M. Davies (ed.) *The Blackwell Encyclopaedia of Social Work*, Oxford, Blackwell. A summary of the main elements of quality assurance of relevance to social work.

Evers, A., Haverinen, R., Leichsenring, K. and Wistow, G. (eds) (1997) *Developing Quality in Personal Social Services: Concepts, Cases and Comments*, Aldershot, Ashgate. Series of studies of quality assurance in a European context.

Kelly, D. and Warr, B. (eds) (1992) *Quality Counts*, London, Whiting & Birch/Social Care Association. Good spread of critical chapters on different aspects of quality in the social care field.

Kirkpatrick, I. and Miguel, A.L. (eds) (1995) *The Politics of Quality in the Public Sector*, London, Routledge. Diverse collection of studies providing a context for quality assurance in practice.

19 Change and continuity in social work organisations

Chapter overview

This chapter examines the major factors affecting both continuities and aspects of change in social work organisations and deals with some of the main consequences of these for people in management roles.

Introduction: social work in the context of change

The international definition of social work (IFSW, 2000) remains fundamental to any social care organisation and to social workers:

> The social work profession promotes social change, problem solving in human relations and the empowerment and liberation of people to enhance wellbeing

within a framework of human rights and social justice. This firmly locates social work in the context of social change, which is nowhere more visible than in the changing organisational environment in which social work is managed, administered and practised. This chapter deals with the following aspects of organisational change, which particularly affect the practice of social work:

- change in the UK context, arguing that change in social care services and social work has been constant throughout the history of the welfare state
- constancy through change, arguing that an important role of social work practice is to create certainty and security for service users
- organisational links, exploring the importance of communication and links within social care organisations and across their boundaries
- organisational stresses, exploring the interacting stresses that affect practitioners, middle managers and people in leadership roles.

The chapter concludes with a brief note on challenges for the future.

Change in the UK context

At the beginning of the twenty-first century, the organisations that employ social workers experience regular changes from their own internal improvements and stresses, and are subject to changes from wider society, which sometimes have powerful and unexpected impacts on the organisation. This is particularly the case in the UK as social work has a policy framework within the public sector: *Putting People First* (HM Government, 2007) and *The Children's Plan* (DCSF, 2007) create the current framework, and are examples of the way in which government policy directions are developed into comprehensive statements designed to influence organisational policy and through this professional practice. Social workers are also nationally registered professionals and as such are expected to work within practice guidelines and follow a code of conduct established by the care council for the relevant UK nation; many other countries have similar provisions. Social work in the UK is seen as an important element within a welfare state, in which the state takes responsibility for important aspects of citizens' wellbeing, through providing professional services, including social work, developing a partnership between state welfare policy development, service delivery organisations, professional practice and service users and their families and communities. Social work is therefore subject to political changes in public policy – in this way it is no different from practice in any other public state agency. The changes to the organisational framework are felt as keenly by colleagues in the main universal services of health, education and the criminal justice sectors. Changes in related sectors are significant for social workers, in that these will have a knock-on effect on social care services. Consequently, the social worker needs to be aware of the impact of changes in public policy and the impact of this on related services. For example, the introduction of antisocial behaviour orders (ASBOs) impacted on the criminal justice system, as well as social care children's services. Change is therefore a constant factor in the political environment and in public services in the UK.

The money that funds the organisations that employ social workers in the UK is, on the whole, from the public purse, and consequently social work organisations are publicly accountable bodies. Statutory agencies such as adult social care departments within a local authority (LA) receive their funds directly from taxation, while agencies providing a statutory service, such as a contracted adoption agency, or a voluntary sector agency that contracts to provide services as part of a partnership with LAs, such as the national Children's Society or the Alzheimer's Society, receive their funding indirectly from central and local government bodies. Private care providers, such as those in the residential and daycare arena, are also substantially funded from the public purse. Public accountability has to be demonstrated and there is a network of devices to measure and judge value for money and fitness for purpose in all organisations that provide a public service.

The current picture of organisations providing social work and social care is very different from the starting point of the welfare state in the 1940s, when social workers were seen as workers who could operate within the new state structures of children's departments, welfare departments and the health and criminal justice services. Change within the organisations of state welfare has therefore been a constant feature of organ-isations employing social workers and providing care services as they have made adaptations to policy and social circumstances, and this will inevitably continue, as organisations try to develop and improve their services, making them responsive to current needs. The picture at any one time is only a snapshot; to practise effectively, students and practitioners need to be constantly updating themselves as change affects their own organisation and those in their partner services.

Constancy throughout change

What has not been subject to change are the core values and approaches to people taken by social workers in their work. It is these values that have enabled social work to survive and adapt to changes. These have been reinforced by the introduction of the UK codes of practice for employers and social care workers (GSCC, 2004) and the statements in *Social Work at its Best* (GSCC, 2008). The form of the statements is periodically reviewed and may change, but the values they represent remain unchanging. This means that as the codes are extended to cover more groups of workers within social care, social work values will come to influence social care practice more widely.

It is often forgotten how unique the values held in social care are. The values are deceptive, in that they underpin most twenty-first century, democratic Western socie-ties. Applying them within social work practice is, however, challenging and needs the mandate of the state and social care organisations in supporting the social care worker:

> Social work embodies a set of core values and principles. It is committed to the rights of the child; respects the equality, worth and human rights of all people and their individu-ality, privacy and dignity; and challenges discrimination and prejudice. (GSCC, 2008: 4)

Practising according to such values has proved to be particularly challenging, especially when confronted with the might of powerful care and treatment institutions, such as the long-stay hospitals, care homes and prisons. To respect and support the individual who wants a different life challenges the rationale of group living situations. This same challenge is also fundamental in protecting and supporting minority groups, since working with diverse cultural and ethnic groups and promoting equal opportunities mean acknowledging the right of the minority to be different from the assumptions of a powerful majority. Social work is therefore particularly valuable 'in situations where there are high levels of complexity, uncertainty, stress, conflicts of interest and risk' – especially among children and vulnerable adults (GSCC, 2008: 4). What has changed in public policy is some of the emphasis given to the practice of these values. For example, the work of the organisation 'in Control' in leading the introduction of direct payments and independent budgeting requires social workers to enable users to be self-directing in choosing help that will best meet their own conception of their needs, rather than the worker creating a package of care that reflects the assumptions of need determined by the agency. The role of the social worker shifts from care management towards guiding, advising, informing and facilitating the means to achieve this.

The uniqueness of the social work profession lies in the fact that these values drive the whole approach, style, decisions and actions that social workers take. This can lead to a lonely and conflictual path when the social worker acts as an advocate for a client and voices opinions not seen as popular or acceptable to colleagues in other professions, or to managers with a budget to maintain. By taking a position alongside and with the service user, the social worker is often able to present a different set of options that are particularly valuable when working in a multidisciplinary team. The value base and the style of social work have correctly been seen as being particularly valuable in reaching out and engaging with many individuals who often are and feel alienated from others in society who set the assumptions about what is 'appropriate'.

The nature of the organisations employing social workers has not always been able to provide a supportive structure for this diverse and often challenging focus of social work. Organisations, particularly large organisations, are often more rigid and less flexible than individual workers. This has led to a wide diversity of organisations in social care and a network of voluntary sector organisations, whose role is to challenge and provide alternatives. While this may be uncomfortable to the individual practitioner caught up in a dispute on behalf of a service user or their family or community, the support of the codes of practice is a useful counterbalance to the organisational power that often seems to be an insurmountable barrier to enabling users to achieve their preferred choices. Careful study and discussion within teams of practitioners and social care organisations of what each item in the codes means to daily practice can be a useful support to practitioners in carrying out their challenging task.

To conclude, we can see that change does affect practice but the core of practice values remains constant and it is this that has enabled social workers to adapt to a changing environment.

Organisational links

The leadership of organisations has to ensure that the organisation is fit for purpose. To do this, it must demonstrate that it can deliver public policy to a budget, help meet individual users' needs, and ensure that the workers can operate appropriately and safely. There is often an inevitable tension between different workers in the organisation, in particular frontline staff and their middle managers and agency leaders. Social workers and other frontline staff are dealing with the immediate pressures presented to them from users and the community. They are often dealing with situations in which there is no easy answer and which are unique to the individual user. Social workers require an organisational response that is flexible so that it responds to individuals' needs, is speedy and accepts the uncertainty that comes from the social pressures affecting the user, their family and their community. The resources and organisational light-footedness necessary for this are not easy to achieve and are not always available; also, competing pressures have to be balanced.

Middle managers deal with the consequences of a volume of requests within organisational constraints and work closely with the leadership to ensure a flow of information up and down the organisation. Middle managers have a crucial role in balancing often competing tensions between the different workers in the organisation.

The leadership of the social care organisation is involved with the overall direction of travel in the agency. This strategic view is long term, as changes in the organisation have a long timescale and involve the agreement of many different players. Therefore, a communications and consultation strategy that engages with the perceived issues in the front line as well as strategic imperatives is an important means for all parties to manage their responses to the complexities of the environment that frontline practitioners and managers at every level work within. This needs to involve a range of stakeholders including local committees, trade unions, staff groups, service users' interests and the media. In addition, existing budgets will have to be reconfigured and staff may have to be retrained. Services may have to be closed in one form and reopened in another form. A three-year perspective is common in changes that affect the whole organisation. This needs to be planned and moved forward at a steady pace (see Chapter 14 on strategic leadership and planning). In addition, it has become increasingly common for pilot projects to be established as forerunners of a larger change. This can be seen locally in the introduction of Sure Start programmes, or in the implementation of direct payments. The core purpose of the leadership is to ensure that the framework of the organisation operates good organisational practices and is fit for purpose now and in the future, so that practitioners can carry out their work effectively and flexibly.

Figure 19.1 sets out the impact of these stresses coming from different parts of the organisations, and interacting with each other. Practitioners and managers needs to come to a balance between them.

Organisational pressures		Social worker pressures
Budget management	⟶	Rationing
Performance standards	⟶	Recording
Service developments	⟶	Changes
Provider choices	⟶	Information
Interagency partnerships	⟶	Communications
↑		↑
Responses to need		Individual needs

Figure 19.1 Organisational stresses impacting on the social worker

These five highlighted aspects of organisational stresses are budget management, performance standards, service developments, provider choices and interagency partnerships, which are now discussed.

Budget management

This is an area of constant tension and the form it takes varies across the UK. This is because LAs have considerable discretion in how they allocate their funds within the broad parameters of public policy. This discretion enables them to reflect the differences in local needs and to implement local priorities. The unevenness of service provision from area to area makes the development of a strong and consistent lobby for improvement slow. For example, all LAs have the freedom to interpret the adult social care eligibility criteria (*Fair Access to Care Services*; DH, 2002) according to their local resources and local political priority. Gradually, over a period of years, local decisions have been taken to limit the operation of the criteria from the four areas of need – reflecting critical, substantial, moderate and low needs – down to three by dropping low needs from consideration, then two and, in some instances, to only one, the highest. As the impact of this across the country began to be realised, so lobby groups representing the interests of particular service user groups, or groups with an interest in the level of community and public services and financing more generally, began to organise and raise this issue on the national agenda. The role of the local leadership ranged, therefore, from national lobbying at the Department of Health and the Treasury on the impact of this policy, seeking to influence guidance in ways that will meet the needs of service users appropriately, through to damage limitation in the local political arena.

The impact of local financial pressures and local decision-taking in this area directly affected the practice of social workers. They had to introduce the local rationing rules to service users, and manage the complaints and distress these decisions caused. Endeavouring to be fair to and flexible with users within a framework of financial constraints can become a major driving force for an organisation's leadership and middle managers. This seems a deviation from a focus on developing and providing good services, but with financial constraints a reality, 'taking hold' of what is going on, as Chapter 11 on management and managerialism puts it, is a crucial role of management.

Performance standards

The performance of the local children and adults services is crucial to the overall performance of the LA against national standards. Performance is rated against a set of goals and targets that are rigorously monitored by national regulators. The impact of this is that agencies must be able to record and measure many areas of their activity. Therefore systems to measure the daily activity of the workforce have had to be introduced – this includes recording the volume and type of work, and the decisions made by staff, and these are measured regularly. Frontline staff therefore have routine information systems to complete. Chapter 11 discusses how, in the UK, this implements an international trend towards managerialism, that is, using numerical quality indicators as a way of responding to questions about the legitimacy of state provision as state welfare expenditure is increasingly devalued. Bell and Payne (Adams et al, 2009a, Ch. 21) describe the development of these performance management systems, recognising that they also make a contribution to an effective review of practice. For many social workers, this has changed the balance of their work to ensuring that they have time to access computers and record activities efficiently. With the increased move for many practitioners towards working from home, the administrative monitoring of activity has to be factored into work planning.

Service developments

The impact of financial pressures as demand rises of user expectations, complaints concerning services provided, plus the impact of political changes in public policy as welfare expenditure is politically questioned have a profound effect on service provision. Consequently, a number of issues have been debated, and politicians, practitioners and managers in each local area try to arrive at a resolution that is right for their locality: What services are required to support families and carers? How are these best provided? What range of services are required to best meet local needs? What services provide best value for money? The local pattern of care services has been subject to constant pressure and the most dramatic changes over the past 30 years. From a baseline of public services to provide support in people's homes to the provision of residential care alternatives, the network of provision has constantly changed as conceptions of what the overall service should achieve and the mix and range of provision that would achieve it have developed. The most fundamental change has been the shift from public sector provision to services provided by quasi-markets incorporating for-profit and not-for-profit organisations in partnership with public sector bodies. To dismantle existing public services and re-establish services in other sectors have been extremely time-consuming and difficult for the local leadership and have required planning change on a three- to five-year timescale. The value of these changes and an understanding of the benefits that differing political ideologies expect to achieve with them are difficult for frontline staff to absorb and explain to worried service users and contacts in the local community. Moreover, as they progress, it is often hard to envision and explain the expected shape and benefits of the final outcome.

The impact of this shift has also affected the roles and tasks required in the LA. The development of contracting and regulating services has become an important dimension of work, which is very different from the starting point of direct management of a complete system of provision. In addition, the relationship with the service user has changed and social care tasks increasingly involve brokerage and giving advice, information and advocacy, as service users exercise choices from a range of services available to them.

Provider choices: commissioning

The need to ensure that the range of local provision is able to meet local needs is now a critical element of leadership. This can only be done by engaging with frontline staff about what are the perceived gaps in service, understanding the issues surrounding local needs, and through consulting in public dialogue with service users and carers, while ensuring that nationally recognised best practice is adapted to local situations. This has led to the emergence of commissioning as a core organisational activity. This involves assessing local need and demands against local resources and priorities to plan the range of services to be developed.

The result of this approach, taken over many years, is that, in many areas, there is now a wide network of local provision that balances a range of services across the public, private and voluntary or third sectors. Although this may still be patchy and fragile in parts of the country, the range and balance of provision have seen a dramatic development. This has been reflected in the emergence of user empowerment; consultation and partnership are now crucial in the development of commissioning plans. In addition, the exercise of personal choice is now a major plank of public policy. The development of direct payments and self-directed independent budgets has opened up more flexible choices for many individuals of support that they find best for their own understanding of their needs and preferences.

This change in emphasis has become a preoccupation of the local leadership who have to work closely with a range of local stakeholders to make these changes. As change can often lead to conflict, this has often been time-consuming and difficult work. The social care staff need an understanding of the pressures for and ideas that lie behind the need for change, so that they can explain to users what is available and how to access this, energising them to take up their rights to an increasingly flexible self-directed response to their needs. In addition, social workers are in a crucial position to evaluate, monitor and influence the quality of the new services now being provided.

Interagency partnerships

Health services	Social care services	Quality of life service
Hospital services	Assessment	Poverty
Community health	Service providers	Housing
General practice team		Leisure
		Communication technologies
	Social work practitioner	
Individual needs		Carer needs

Figure 19.2 Interagency partnerships

Figure 19.2 sets out the role of social work practitioners in interpreting and pushing forward the needs of service users and their carers not only within their own agency, but within a wider network of agency partnerships. Social care agencies have always seen that operating with other related agencies is crucial to their ability to best meet individual needs. Referrals flow into, out from and between a network of local agencies. Negotiating and advocating across boundaries on behalf of their service users is a critical activity for social workers. Other public sector agencies have a universal service perspective in which they are working with the total population, and without the personalised approach of the social care agency, this can result in a low priority being given to social care users whose needs may be excluded from consideration by the service priorities implemented by other professionals. Social workers and their social care agency need to negotiate a framework for best practice and conflict resolution. It is important that the leadership of care agencies work with their colleagues to create an environment of common understanding across local networks of related services and to ensure that there is a degree of mutual concern for social care users.

Increasingly, interagency partnerships are being developed with common plans, shared budgets, joint services, joint training and shared information bases, and these are some of the positive moves that have helped different professional workers to develop common causes. Some of these developments have been radical, in that they can change the shape of the local organisations, and there is a move in a range of areas towards integrated teams bringing together people from different workforces.

To adapt and manage change of this kind creates constant tensions within the organisation, but has different effects on frontline workers as they relate to service users and carers, and affecting middle managers differently again, as they manage patterns of service connected to the needs of particular communities. For change to occur seamlessly, all staff need to be aware of the journey the organisation is taking as a whole, and everyone needs to understand the advantages of change, while ensuring that the process of change preferably benefits and also causes the least damage to the security of the service users, carers and communities on which their roles focus. Partnerships with service users are essential throughout change processes, and ongoing, open communication and information are therefore vital, so that middle managers and practitioners can interpret the direction of travel and intentions, while reflecting back to local leadership the hotspots of conflict and uncertainty and unfortunate side effects.

Conclusion

Challenges for the future

This chapter, examining past change and present developments, has suggested that change is inevitable, arising from the impact of political and policy developments, social change and the need to improve the quality and flexibility of practice as it responds to changing needs and policies. Change is not, therefore, to be regretted and resisted, because it will have to be embraced. However, continuity and security for both practitioners and services users emerge from the fundamental values incorporated into social care services. These derive from social work professional values, expressed currently in the codes of practice.

Social workers and their organisations will continue to move forward within the policy agenda as laid out in the goals spelt out in *Every Child Matters: Change for Children* (DfES, 2004) for children's services and *Our Health, Our Care, Our Say* (DH,

2006) for adult social care services. These have many similarities that present key challenges. The most important similarity remains to ensure the provision of the best and most appropriate care for those with the greatest needs. There is, however, a renewed focus on preventing need occurring and escalating and this is a constant pressure. Early identification of those with the greatest needs and introducing measures to prevent escalation of need remain a constant challenge but a vital responsibility to secure good access to effective services and therefore social justice for some of the most deprived and oppressed people. However, public policy has recognised that the protection and support of the most vulnerable people also have to be a wider responsibility of all partner agencies. A whole system approach is clearly described in the goals and objectives of the policy as described in *Every Child Matters* and *Our Health, Our Care, Our Say*:

- *For children:* to enable them to be healthy, to stay safe, to enjoy and achieve, to make a positive contribution and to have economic wellbeing.
- *For adults:* to enable health and wellbeing, to access high-quality services, to support those in greatest need and to offer appropriate care close to home.

These goals can only be achieved if organisations work together. For all the related agencies, the challenge is to identify those at risk early, involve other relevant agencies quickly, determine the assessment of risk and take the most appropriate and relevant actions to provide help. However, the free flow of accurate and worthwhile information across agency and professional boundaries is deeply flawed and needs renewed attention, recognising increasing concerns in society about excessive surveillance and poor information security by public bodies. In addition, agreement on the best action to take remains restricted by scarce resources and interprofessional and interagency misunderstandings and therefore interorganisational conflict about who does what. For example, an important area affecting children and adult services remains some of the limitations in accessing the appropriate mental health resources. For social care, this is crucial. Social workers, therefore, need to work in supportive organisations, develop skills in communication. negotiation and advocacy and be able – working with their team, middle managers and the community – to obtain and use a good knowledge of available local services and their interconnections.

For further discussion of ideas about management, see Chapter 11.

www.scie-peoplemanagement.org.uk/ The SCIE people management website provides many useful resources for working on change in a social care organisation.

Aldgate, J., Healy, L., Pine, B. et al. (eds) (2008) *Enhancing Social Work Management: Theory and Best Practice from the UK and USA*, London, Jessica Kingsley. Useful collection of discussions on various issues concerned with managing social services organisations.

SCIE (Social Care Institute for Excellence) (2004) *Learning Organizations: A Self-assessment Resource Pack*, London, SCIE. Provides a practical way for teams and organisations to examine how they can respond more effectively to change.

Smale, G. (1998) *Managing Change through Innovation*, London, HMSO. Thoughtful introduction to change in social work organisations, highly regarded by practitioners and managers.

Sullivan, H. and Skelcher, C. (2002) *Working across Boundaries: Collaboration in Public Services*, Basingstoke, Palgrave Macmillan. Useful review of a wide range of policy and practice issues around developing coordination in public services; its perspective covering all public services is particularly useful in reducing the insularity that sometimes affects people working within one particular service.

Part 3

RESEARCHING SOCIAL WORK

Practitioners are required to develop their research awareness as part of their developing expertise in evidence-based practice. It is understandably difficult, however, for many beginning practitioners to balance the requirements of research-mindedness against the demands of practice. We set out in the final part of this book to provide basic guidance on what is entailed in developing research as a practitioner.

At the outset, it is necessary to couch research requirements in terms of ethical requirements, while recognising the inherently problematic nature of the research task (Chapter 20). The research process begins with a period of clarification and 'ground clearing', during which goals are established (Chapter 21). It is necessary early on to visit the relevant literature and locate the research in terms of what other similar work has been carried out (Chapter 22). The research project should generate excitement in the practitioner, tempered by realism brought about by critical awareness of what it is like to undertake research (Chapter 23).

Practice research can offer much to the prospective researcher – more pragmatically and practically through evaluating practice (Chapter 24), through delivering critical commentary on practice (Chapter 25) and through offering the prospect of the wider development of the research agenda (Chapter 26).

Social work research: contested knowledge for practice

20

Social work research is contested territory, with stakeholders arguing about what counts as research, who should do it and how. Service user demands for a say in research can be met by engaging a diversity of voices in research design, data collection, analysis and dissemination. This can raise the status of research by drawing on both empirical and experiential evidence.

Chapter overview

Research has gained a new prominence in British social work. This development has been driven by:

■ managers and policy makers promoting evidence-based practice and evaluations of practitioners' performance and responses to new policy initiatives
■ practitioners undertaking their own research, known as practitioner research
■ service users' demands for a say in the research used to determine the services they could access
■ academics being assessed on their research activities for funding purposes in ongoing research assessment exercises (RAEs).

The concern to be a research-led discipline predates these emphases. Research-based social work was endorsed by the 'founding mothers' of the profession who believed that its status would be enhanced if it included research and PhD students. Eileen Younghusband's (1959, 1960) reports on social work education in the UK and Hong Kong argued strongly for a research-led profession, as had Jane Addams earlier in the US (Elshtain, 2002). Extracting funding for their aspirations proved a major barrier to the realisation of their vision and until recently more effort was expended on education and training (Lyons, 2004). Encouraging qualifying students to undertake small-scale research is crucial in building future capacity for social work research and can be supported by specific units covering research methods and a history of the struggle to validate the importance of social work research. This last part of the book aims to assist that process.

In Britain, research has not been given a high profile by those bodies responsible for social work education, despite notable exceptions such as Whittaker and Archer's (1990) study on practice research. The low profile of research in social work has been exacerbated by:

- the disinterest in research shown by social work's current regulatory bodies, the General Social Care Council in England, Care Council for Wales and the Scottish Social Services Council in Scotland, which concentrate on training social workers rather than fostering research in their programmes of study
- the absence of social work as a named discipline in the deliberations of the Economic and Social Research Council (ESRC) until 2007
- the Department of Health's support for applied research linked largely to concerns in child protection and welfare.

Additionally, the Department of Health's focus on applied research or research concerned mainly with what happens on the ground has been replicated in the research endeavours of other bodies with an interest in social work research, namely the Social Services Research Group, the Association of Directors of Adult Social Services, the Association of Directors of Children's Services, and voluntary organisations undertaking research such as the National Society for the Prevention of Cruelty to Children, National Children's Homes and Barnardo's. This applied focus neglects conceptual or basic research.

This position is being altered somewhat by the Social Care Institute for Excellence (SCIE), which has been charged with improving practice by using research, especially that linked to 'what works', to do this. Much of its research tends to downplay the distinction between social work and social care, and has a narrow, evaluative focus that is unlikely to produce a substantive foundation for the theoretical and methodological innovations that social work needs (Dominelli, 2004). At the same time, SCIE has supported social work research by producing guides that students can use in their research projects and has supported other research initiatives, including the group of nine universities comprising the Making Research Count network that was formed in 2005, and Research in Practice for Adults under the auspices of the Dartington Hall Trust. It has endorsed the initiatives of the Joint Universities Council Social Work Education Committee (JUC SWEC) to raise the profile and status of social work research. Other recent initiatives that have made up for these weaknesses cover naming social work as a discipline on funding forms for the ESRC in 2007, and the wider research agenda being promoted by the Department for Children, Schools and Families.

Basic research focuses on the fundamentals of knowledge – its conceptual building blocks – rather than how knowledge is used, which is considered the province of applied research. Basic research enables us to ask fundamental questions about social work – what it is, how it works, how to gather data about it, how to make predictions about practice and how to test theories. Basic research aims to improve human wellbeing and ask questions that might otherwise be ignored. As basic research is led by experts in their field, it can be used to discredit the contributions to knowledge made by those holding what Foucault (1980) termed 'subjugated knowledges', that is, knowledge that comes from the experience of being a service user. It is difficult to find words that accurately describe people who access services. I use the terms 'service user' and 'client' inter-changeably, while acknowledging that each is problematic and socially constructed. The privileging of expert knowledge, particularly those forms that adopt the supremacy of natural science paradigms, can carry intellectual arrogance as a by-product. This approach holds sway in the social sciences and disinherits social work research with service users from a valued place in the academy. Basic research has also been critiqued by the Service User Research Enterprise (SURE) at King's College, London for being unable to deal helpfully with the messiness of issues explored in the social sciences (SURE, www.iop.kcl.ac.uk/iopweb/departments). Endeavours aimed at building theory from practice have featured in the pages of *Qualitative Social Work*, a relatively new journal promoting qualitative social work research.

In the absence of an assertive promotion of social work research by the profession itself, other social science disciplines, especially psychology, sociology and social policy, have appropriated much of the research agenda in social work and made its research issues their own. In the process, social work research and what it had to say about itself as a research-based discipline and its input to other disciplines have been marginalised, a condition that is unlikely to shift easily in the current configuration of research. Social work managers, practitioners and educators have the responsibility of reclaiming these knowledge domains and taking an active role in (re)defining and (re)affirming their own contributions to general social sciences research.

In 2006, concerns about the low status of social work research, the lack of research capacity in the discipline, the low levels of funding for social work research and the lack of recognition of the governance structures in social work research led the research subcommittee of the JUC SWEC to form a research strategy working group to develop and begin to implement a 20-year strategy for social work research to address these issues and develop endeavours aimed at enhancing both applied and basic research. Working under the aegis of JUC SWEC, the British social work academics involved have attempted to claw back and/or identify this terrain by arguing for recognition of the distinctiveness of social work research. Ron Amann, head of the ESRC in the mid-1990s, challenged social work educators to make the intellectual case for the recognition of social work as a discipline in its own right when replying to a letter I wrote to him asking for this in May 1996. The social work educators' response to his challenge ulti-mately yielded collaborative endeavours under the auspices of JUC SWEC, which led to the formation of the Theorising Social Work Research (TSWR) seminar series, funded by the ESRC for three years in 2000, the current strategy implementation group, and several capacity-building proposals under the ESRC's ongoing Researcher Development Initiative. The TSWR produced publications that explored a range of important research issues and began to advance social work as a research-led discipline (see www.scie-socialcareonline.org.uk).

The TSWR raised a number of issues for discussion and debate that continue to be addressed by the JUC SWEC research subcommittee. These include the updating of a code of ethics for social work research and a place for social work in the ESRC's decision-making bodies. The latter began with success in gaining a place for social work on the

ESRC's Training and Development Board. This gain raised the educational status of social work and enabled Joan Orme, social work's first main representative, to use this position to leverage movement on the provision of doctoral studies and studentships, a crucial element in developing a research culture and contributing to the RAE. Ian Diamond, the current head of the ESRC, has consolidated these gains by recognising social work as a named discipline with regards to doctoral studentships in 2005 and as a discipline for research grant purposes in 2007. These developments should be welcomed as opportunities for building capacity in social work research for the future. In addition, the ESRC has encouraged practitioner involvement in research-based studies through the development of collaborative (CASE) studentships that involve partnerships between academic and practice-based institutions. As CASE funding involves a substantive contribution from an individual agency or employer, these are difficult to establish in significant numbers in a given locality, and so the number of PhD students doing social work research remains low. Another reason for this is that some students doing social work research are registered in other disciplines, for example sociology and social policy, and so the total figure remains unknown (Lyons, 1999).

The ESRC's endeavours have been paralleled by initiatives from other regulatory bodies. For example, after publication of the 2001 RAE results, the Higher Education Funding Council for England (HEFCE) agreed to fund a capability fund to improve social work's research base. The HEFCE accepted the arguments that having a practitioner base disadvantaged social work research and consequently provided extra funding to those getting 3 (national rating) in the 2001 RAE to raise their outputs to an international level (5 or 5*). The 2008 RAE assessed the impact of this particular approach to the issue. The lack of research capability in social work in the US shows that this is a concern elsewhere (Gillespie and Glisson, 1992).

In this chapter, I argue that social work has to strengthen its research standing vis-à-vis other disciplines, while ensuring that more research is undertaken by social work academics, practitioners, service users and students. I suggest that those engaged in the profession should become more research literate, that is, be familiar with a wide range of research methods, and understand what research is, how it can be conducted as an ethical endeavour, what it has to offer practice and how social work educators, practitioners and service users can play a greater role in its development. Responding to this agenda requires social work academics, practitioners and managers to ask more searching questions about their contribution to social work research and problematise social work research in ways that enable it to engage meaningfully with the contested nature of knowledge and include service users more effectively in knowledge creation, validation and distribution.

What is social research?

The British TSWR group considered the question 'What is social work research?' without reaching a conclusion, except to say that social work research was not unique as it drew on the same methodologies as other disciplines in the social sciences. However, it was deemed distinctive, in that it had to address the implications of research for practice rather than undertake research purely for its own sake.

As a member of the TSWR group, I agreed with these conclusions, which have been further examined. What constitutes research is a contentious issue, as Jackie Powell also suggests in Chapter 26. Traditional empiricist approaches to research, as propagated through positivist methodologies, assume that knowledge is acquired through observation and experimentation. This way of proceeding has been termed the Enlightenment approach to knowledge creation (Crotty, 1998). It has been critiqued by feminists (Stanley and Wise, 1997), postmodernists, poststructuralists and constructionists (Crotty, 1998). Their work emphasises how researchers examine the relationship between human thought and social existence when creating knowledge (Usher, 1997) to suggest that there is no 'truth' as such, but a description of things as we interpret them (Crotty, 1998). Thus, knowledge does not portray universal truths, but is situational and context specific (Gibbs, 2001b).

The controversial nature of research becomes even more evident in social work research because it straddles the academy's concerns for rigorous methodologies while engaging with the realities of practice and everyday life and developing critical reflexive practitioners, difficult as this may be, as Sewpaul and Raniga (2005) demonstrated. Social work researchers have to explore further important research issues. These include having to:

- Rethink what kind of research carries credibility and validity
- Question what counts as legitimate knowledge
- Deprivilege clinical knowledge and its claims to hold higher status because it defines itself as being more 'scientific' than other approaches
- Articulate alternative voices including those of service users and practitioners in discourses about research
- Reverse the undervaluing of the applied research undertaken in social work.

Sherman and Reid (1994: 1) define social work research by dividing it into qualitative research 'that produces descriptive data, spoken or written words and observable behaviour' and quantitative research, which is concerned primarily with 'numerically measuring the degree to which some feature is present'. This distinction is blurred by the achievement of qualitative researchers in developing systematic ways of picking up and enumerating or counting data. These definitions are helpful in highlighting important differences in what can be achieved by either approach. Both have their different uses and validity. There is a richness in small-scale qualitative research that is absent from quantitative studies, while the latter gives indications of frequency that are absent from the former. The simple division of research endeavours into these two mutually exclusive categories is not always constructive. There are areas of overlap between them, particularly in their search for authenticity and attempt to clarify the nature of knowledge and 'truths' about the world. Research is a complex undertaking that involves people forming research relationships that (re)configure knowledge and the status held by those who create it.

By understanding what is meant by social work research, social work educators can defend their distinctive stance to research and problematise dominant paradigms. Additionally, I think that social work research, which I define as a field of systematic investigation that examines human interactions around human wellbeing (or its lack), has to encompass more than a general concern with practice. Social work research involves researchers and those participating as the subjects of research in building egalitarian relationships around a study and its outcomes. The creation of such relationships enables the findings to shape the subsequent actions for both and thereby carry implications for both their lives. Otherwise, research has the potential to become a site of exclusion. Thus, social work researchers should give thought to the consequences of their research (Dominelli, 2005). Power relations are at play within the dynamics of inclusion and exclusion, even in research. Not least among these is that of who forms part of the research community that decides what counts as research. Research is an expression of power relations, with a direct bearing on the products of the research or knowledge-building enterprise. Social work research focuses on marginalised groups or people who hold limited social power. It seeks to bring about social change that enhances human wellbeing. So, social work research enacts a moral and political standpoint rather than being indifferent to the purposes for which research is used, as is suggested in positivist approaches to empirical work.

Research serves several purposes in social work. It can be used to:

■ Enhance the status of the profession in both the field and the academy
■ Improve services by finding out what service users think about those that have been delivered to them
■ Evaluate the extent of their use and who utilises them
■ Highlight issues of concern
■ Elucidate depth and complexities in practice
■ Explore problems
■ Raise additional questions
■ Enhance critical reflection.

Responding to service user agendas and shifting the lack of high regard for social work research in academia highlight a need for research materials that can be used to (re)theorise social work practice and guide it in new directions. This can draw upon applied and basic research and opens new arenas for social work researchers, including students.

Service user researchers are a recent phenomenon. Their demand for full participation in research has arisen from several insights. One is that some, for example those in the new social movements such as the disability movement, have demanded this as a right and have introduced a new paradigm to convey their thoughts – 'emancipatory research' (Barnes and Mercer, 1997). As experts on living in a disabling society, disabled people argue that they have valid information to impart to others who are not. They see controlling what happens in research as a right of citizenship, while creating knowledge and having it recognised is an entitlement they intend to have. Their demands also aim to bring 'subjugated knowledges' from the margins to the centre, and in the process require expert researchers to reflect critically on the nature of their enterprise and seek to transform it in more empowering directions.

Service users who indicate an interest in research are ordinary members of the public who are involved in a research process in which they are interested, for example to see an improvement in services, or if they have been asked to participate in it by someone outside or within their own community. They may have to acquire formal research skills through training either before engaging in the research or alongside it. This will require the researcher working with them to demystify the research processes and expertise associated with these, shift the researcher–researched power dynamic in more egalitarian directions, and embed the research in a holistic environment.

Researchers with an interest in social work, for example Barnes and his colleagues (Barnes and Mercer, 1997; Barnes et al., 1999), have challenged the idea that only experts can undertake research and argued for it to involve experts, practitioners and service users, or a combination of these. Experts in research are usually called 'researchers'. They hold a privileged status in knowledge creation by virtue of having specific skills in research methodologies and being paid for doing research by an organisation charged with the task of crafting knowledge. The expert approach to research tends to favour those who maintain a distance between the researcher and those on whom they do research. By framing their efforts as 'doing' research, they establish 'power over' relations in which the researcher is the subject who controls the process and research respondents become the objects of their expert ministrations. This sets up an unequal researcher–researched dynamic and a hierarchy of valuing what the researcher rather than the respondent says (Dominelli, 2005).

The research expert may be a consultant who claims a capacity to do research and undertakes a given piece of research through a specific contract. Many of these may be freelance operators rather than employees in a research-oriented organisation such as a university or research institute. Unless these experts in research also happen to have expertise in social work education and/or practice, they will not bring specific understandings of social work to bear upon their studies, a point discussed at length by Beth Humphries in Chapter 25.

Practitioner researchers are likely to have been or remain involved in practice and bring a greater awareness of the field and research that carries significance or relevance for practice. They may find it easier to access service users and be strongly motivated to form research partnerships involving practitioners, academics and service users. This approach can be problematic, with examples of it being discussed in all the chapters in this part of the book. If practitioner researchers remain committed to the field, they may find time for research squeezed against the demands of the vocational parts of the job and lack of immediate access to library facilities, computer-based technologies and statistical information. Students experience this pressure when doing research for their dissertations while on placement. Practitioners may risk promotion if their findings reveal material that is negatively perceived by employers. These difficulties identify significant dimensions in the 'politics of research', an issue that is explored throughout this part of the book.

Practitioners and students as stakeholders in the social work enterprise are doing research all the time. Research skills such as collecting information, evaluating it, theorising from it and acting on it constitute activities that mimic research expertise in the daily routines of practice. These actions are usually taken for granted and not considered research. They can cover data collected during everyday investigations into people's problems, including life histories and analyses of hidden social issues. This information is seen by other practitioners, managers and magistrates who would not consider this research per se. Yet, a systematic analysis of these documents could produce invaluable insights into retheorising social problems and finding new solutions, alongside showing how individual problems are rooted in social conditions. Ethical approval for using this information for these purposes would have to be obtained. Ethical issues in research merit further investigation not possible here (see Dominelli and Holloway, 2008).

The distinctiveness of social work research

Social work researchers determine whose story counts as worthy of being told and decide which group of people will be subjected to the research gaze. In deciding who to include in a research project, they should not limit their investigations to excluded groups and forego studies of power elites. In a traditional researcher–researched relationship, this gaze favours the ruling elite who can find out what they want to know about subjugated peoples without exposing their own positions because there is no accountability back to the research subjects. This relation can be reversed through social work research that poses questions about dominant elites that are articulated by marginalised groups, including those who access services. Students are well placed to support service user research agendas.

Research may carry an emotional content that has to be taken into account. Social work researchers have to address the emotional investment that each group of participants has in a research project, giving it a holistic dimension often absent in research in other disciplines. Funders, researchers and the subjects of research will each have specific views about research and its end products. The commitment to enhancing wellbeing is a contentious position and not accepted by power holders who fear losing their privileges if the research gaze focuses on their comings, goings and doings. This problem is evidenced in Sewpaul and Raniga's (2005) research. It shows how in controversial situations, regional and local authorities play safe by going along with the dominant discourses and following central government research agendas rather than setting their own. These trends may impact on student research and they may need to be supported through difficult questions of access, endorsing service user agendas and political and economic exigencies.

Social work research is a creative process requiring knowledge of a range of methodologies and research methods and involving hard work and a coordination of activities between researchers and the subjects of research. Researchers have to care for and about those with whom they are doing research. Power relations between researchers and the subjects of research pose ethical dilemmas to be taken into account:

- permission to do the research
- obtaining informed consent
- making arrangements for its smooth conduct
- disseminating the findings.

The research subject is respected and treated as a person with agency, that is, an active contributor to the research, not a passive object waiting for researchers to ask questions and evaluate their answers. Agency raises significant ethical points for social work researchers to consider systematically and explicitly, including in research conducted by students. Another difficulty in developing a distinctive approach to the holistic agenda of social work research is that the Department of Health, a key funder of this research, applies narrow, positivist models of NHS research and governance structures to social care, in which it includes social work (see www.dh.gov.uk/policyandguidance/research-anddevelopmentAZ/researchgovernance/fs/en).

If social work researchers are to identify those features that distinguish them from others doing research in similar areas and using similar methodologies, they should also develop:

- A change orientation
- A more egalitarian relationship between themselves and the subjects of research
- Accountability to clients/service users for the products of their work
- A holistic engagement with the different aspects of the problem(s) or people they are researching with.

Social work researchers can engage with practice to transform it, alongside raising questions about what it is and what it can(not) do. They should identify:

- The arguments for transformative change
- The basis on which such change is to be conducted
- The opportunities for different actors to participate in these changes
- How to evaluate existing endeavours
- The potential for future developments.

Involving service users in research design, delivery and dissemination can be used to hold practitioners and academics accountable to those who are affected by their work and question the privileging of their research. In Chapter 25, Beth Humphries argues that engaging in holistic research is empowering.

There are other researchers for whom the first two requirements apply. For example, feminist researchers examining domestic violence without a social work dimension would want:

- change that eliminates it
- to create a relationship with the women they interview for the study
- to make arrangements to provide services for those who might be emotionally distressed by the research process (Stanley and Wise, 1997).

In this sense, they are involved in caring about others. However, they would not be held accountable for changing social work practice with the victims/survivors of domestic violence, nor do they have to confront the ethical challenge of reporting potential risks to others, especially children, arising from knowledge gained during the research.

Social work researchers have to consider not only what happens to the women victims/survivors and men perpetrating these assaults, but also to children living with them. This consideration becomes part of the 'holistic' dimension of social work research. Some of these concerns are explored by Sewpaul and Raniga (2005) in their research on HIV/AIDS. Social work research may have to meet the practice aspirations of an entire community, not just the agencies or individuals directly involved in the research. Social work students may find such expectations onerous and require additional support from tutors.

Social work researchers are distinctive in ensuring that their research integrates theory with practice. But this is precisely where social work research is weak. As Gillespie and Glisson (1992) contend, social work research is inadequately theorised and has failed to spell out a research practice and methodology that it can call its own. Their position is contested. Some argue that social work research draws on skills that are evident in practice. Sherman and Reid (1994) suggest that Mary Richmond's (1917) classic, *Social Diagnosis*, is a form of qualitative social work research that covers questions of judgement, choice, interpretation and situations that social workers investigate. Patton (1980) contends that a case study is a well-known form of in-depth social work research.

Gilgun (1994) suggests that grounded theory, proposed by Glaser and Strauss (1967), is a social work research method because it replicates skills that social workers draw on and are familiar with from practice. These include the concern to maintain confidentiality, interviewing and communication skills, analytical skills involved in rigorously examining the data collected and dissemination of findings. Its rigorous approach to coding and theorisation from the data is a skill to be learned. Gilgun (1994) also claims that grounded theory gives voice to service users and enables their words to become the basis for theorising their experiences. Reissman (2002) and Fraser (2004) make similar points about narrative analyses. Those advocating these positions make crucial points, yet none considers the actual involvement of clients or service users in the evolving research process.

Involving service users in research is not straightforward. The terms on which they are integrated are important. Researchers' assumptions about knowledge and truth underpin the relationship between them (Usher, 1997). Unless researchers value their participation, research will be conducted without their input except as objects of the research. Elsewhere (Dominelli, 2005), I examine the weaknesses of grounded theory in this regard. The contractual conditions of research, ownership of findings, institutional privileging of those labelled 'researchers' and the failure to benefit service users are not addressed in grounded theory, so new forms of social exclusion can be created in the process of involving service users and validating their knowledges (Dominelli, 2005). I also suggest that maintaining service user agency in research is a constant factor in research relationships. It is not a one-off event that can be forgotten once service users are included. Engaging service users as full partners in research is an essential aspect of every component of the social work research process, a point emphasised by those in the disability movement. It remains an issue for further work. Sarah Banks and Di Barnes demonstrate in Chapter 21 that social work research involves an iterative process that engages the researcher and subject of the research.

Beth Humphries' contribution in Chapter 25 identifies difficulties in using research to empower service users. Researchers have been employed to do research because they are skilled in this work. Training service users in these skills occurs under tight schedules and conditions that limit the amount of knowledge and skills that can be passed on. It assumes that existing research skills are those that clients should adopt. This ignores the issue of engaging service users in developing new methodologies and techniques that are rooted in their ways of knowing about and experiencing the world. The wonder is that several researchers have claimed considerable success in sharing research skills without devaluing service users' involvement in knowledge creation processes while not producing innovative research methodologies (www.iop.kcl.ac.uk/iopweb/departments).

Empowering clients in the research process involves several moves (Dominelli, 2005), including tackling language and power relations inherent within it. Referring to those involved as 'subjects of research' or even 'owners of research' conveys different meanings from that of research 'interviewees'. Differentiated power relations are evident in getting research funders to pay for time spent on training research subjects. Making a case requires effort, but the request may not be accepted. Funders have to be convinced that the approach 'adds value' to support it financially. The organisational culture has to be changed to value the newly acquired research skills of the subjects of research if the label of 'researcher' is associated with someone from a university. Also, there is an issue of whether research questions should be asked differently to ensure that those who are not directly employed in research can engage effectively in knowledge creation processes. An example is not referring to 'evaluation' if people perceive it as an incomprehensible procedure and are put off, but asking instead a straightforward question that has the same effect, such as: 'How do you know what does or does not work?' These questions are considered by Carol Lewis in Chapter 23.

Becoming more research literate and responding to controversies in social work research

In the past, British social work students and practitioners have given research a miss whenever given a choice, as research methods courses were considered an optional extra. Students' eyes tended to glaze over when listening to lectures about research methods and practitioners were happy for someone else to engage in this activity. Even research-led teaching took a back seat on too many courses and requiring students to read social statistics engendered a fear that prompted most of them to avoid the subject wherever possible. As a result, the current social work labour force lacks the requisite research knowledge and skills and is poorly equipped either to undertake or use research in a critical reflexive manner. This reality constitutes a compelling reason for encouraging social work educators, practitioners and students to take an active role in promoting and engaging in social work research and giving space for research-mindedness to be given a high profile on courses. The JUC SWEC has embarked on a process of capacity-building and raising the level of funding in social work research and has developed a 20-year research strategy to achieve these goals.

Many changes in practice are making research important for practitioners. In Britain, a movement towards evidence-based practice (EBP) (Sheldon, 2000) and government determination to have practice demonstrate effectiveness – the penchant for 'what works' – have rekindled interest in social work research and required practitioners to become more research aware. Becoming research literate is critical in forming views about research, given the contested nature of what counts as evidence and who decides what or whose knowledge counts. Social work managers and practitioners commission research to improve practice. Gaps in knowledge about social work will be filled, but not necessarily by those who best understand the profession, if social work educators do not promote research and socialise researchers to do this work in future. Producing critical, reflexive researchers and practitioners with an interest in undertaking social work research is to be encouraged.

Linking research accountability to 'what works' approaches to research is problematic because questions are framed in terms of effectiveness and assume that there are fixed answers that are right or wrong. But practice is full of uncertainties and ambiguities and there may be more than one way of responding to a given situation (Parton, 1998), none of which can guarantee a particular outcome. Practice also tends to be messy and indeterminate (Parton, 2000). Grappling with these realities makes finding new ways of doing and theorising social work research an urgent matter. I am not convinced that approaches rooted in EBP as defined by Sheldon (2000) will provide the way forward. These focus on a narrow view of research that emphasises quantitative methods over qualitative ones and randomised controlled trials as the way of verifying research results. This formulation sets up an unnecessary division between the two methodologies, which, as Sherman and Reid (1994) and Kirk and Reid (2002) argue, have a lot in common, including issues of judgement, choice and interpretation, activities involved in designing and executing both types of research. This view of EBP also foregoes rich insights gained from qualitative methodologies and ignores its positivist base in the systematic collection of anecdotal evidence (Dominelli, 2004).

EBP conceptualises data as unitary and knowable rather than disputed and disordered. Researchers' knowledge is privileged over respondents' knowledge, although the entire research enterprise rests on their contribution to data collected, that is, the respondent is the data. Their interdependence can be ignored because respondents in these studies are treated as objects of research and denied subjectivity. Consequently, the order imposed on the information collected by the researcher through the processes of analysing the material collected and finding meaning in or interpreting data is presumed, while that provided by the research subject or 'knower' is deemed irrelevant. Treating knowledge as fixed encourages students and practitioners to look for a 'toolkit' that equips them with answers and a checklist that can provide them with the correct response to a complex situation. The search for certainty ill-prepares practitioners to deal with the uncertainties, ambiguities and complications of practice (Parton, 1998). It permits social workers to ignore processes and power relations in specific interactions including those evident within research relationships.

Power and subjectivity in the processes of social work research

The neglect of process raises the issue of bypassing voice, that is, who is creating the statements and making sense of them to produce what counts as knowledge or is accepted as such? The processes of EBP research exclude people who are positioned at the margins of society except to treat them as 'objects' of study able to give statements that are ordered by an allegedly impartial and disinterested researcher in ways consistent with hegemonic expectations about knowledge (Belenky et al., 1997). Feminists like Harding (1991) have argued that people's 'standpoint' or location in a society influences their views of what constitutes knowledge and understanding. EBP has a bias towards quantitative research and privileges experts' assertions regarding what is valued. It belongs to a tradition of research that privileges men's expertise and ways of knowing above those of women and marginalised others and divides the world into mutually exclusive, hierarchical and dichotomous categories (Harding, 1991; Belenky et al., 1997; Usher, 1997; Dominelli, 2004).

EBP has not made explicit its ontological or epistemological underpinnings and is oblivious of its emphasis on social science research that privileges ways of working that are consistent with natural science approaches to knowledge. This treats research respondents as passive objects whose essence is there to be discovered by those doing the research. Social work research that emphasises the connections between people and acknowledges service users as co-creators of knowledge or key players along with researchers in the knowledge creation process cannot get away with doing this. To gain research literacy that can handle these complexities, social work researchers treat research as an interaction that involves researchers and subjects of research as participants in mutual knowledge-creating activities (Dominelli, 2005). Beth Humphries highlights the significance of this way of proceeding in Chapter 25. Those advocating a narrative-based approach to practice (Hall, 1997) make similar claims: both practitioner and client are creating the intervention that makes sense in their jointly agreed version of events. They construct the story and each other in the process of articulating what occurred.

To effectively commission research, practitioners and managers require knowledge sufficient for evaluating competing claims to the knowledge creation process and must choose wisely from a vast array of research designs and methods. They will have to acquire skills that enable them to draw meaningful conclusions from the products of research. They may weigh up insights gained through an impressionistic study in which informed hunches are followed through to their logical end against a more systematic formal approach. What is done by those involved in impressionistic inquiry still constitutes research. It creates data that are collected by listening carefully to anecdotal evidence and systematically trying to make sense of what is being said. Its findings may be as valid as those emanating from a sophisticated, systematic and well-tested method that has utilised quantitative or qualitative methodologies or triangulated them (Belenky et al., 1997), but they will be less robust and less generalisable. Managers and practitioners have to know what counts as evidence in research and who determines what counts and why, and hold the skills for evaluating experimental forms of research, experiential expertise and more exploratory, unfocused studies that seek to break new frontiers. They may have to explain to sceptical others why scarce funds should be expended on research rather than much-needed services. In Henkel's (1995) words, they have to act as 'reflective participants in, rather than privileged observers of, particular phenomena and situations'.

Changes in contemporary practice supplement pressures from academia to actively and simultaneously encourage practitioners to do research as part of lifelong learning and career progression, including at PhD level. Social work students are increasingly engaging with small pieces of research as part of their studies in writing dissertations for qualifying programmes and more courses are offering research methods or research-mindedness units in preparation for this. These developments have to be nurtured. Sizable student stipends can enable those with domestic duties to participate in research.

Involving service users more completely in research begs questions about the links between research and practice. These have to be better understood than is currently the case. Their potential to contribute fully to the research design, implementation and dissemination processes remains underdeveloped. It will be a while before they are integrated as equal and active subjects in research. There are a number of barriers to their inclusion. Lacking skills in formal research methods is a key one. Funders are reluctant to pay the additional costs associated with their involvement, although some, like the Joseph Rowntree Foundation, pay small honoraria for the time that service users spend on research projects. Differential pay privileges researchers who receive an agreed salary and makes the statement that a researcher's time is more valuable than that of the research subjects (Dominelli, 2005).

Current funding schemes do not cover the initial stages of developing proposals and service users tend to be excluded at this point. Decisions about research design, methodologies to be used and processes for delivering a project have been made before they become involved, and so the role of service users in deciding the research question, how the research is to be conducted and who is to do it is diminished. Once funding is secured, it is usually easier to bring them on board and involve them in dissemination to ensure that findings influence policy and practice.

Given the critique of traditional or positivist approaches to research, there are three possibilities for future development in social work research:

1   To find ways of including service users more fully in the research process so that they can influence it from the beginning as well as engage in endeavours aimed at changing policy and practice at the end.
2   Creating the theories, knowledge and skills that will enable social work researchers to

engage in research endeavours that link to practice and claim validity beyond the local-ity in which the research was conducted to address the question of generalisability.

3   To ensure that the personal elements in research are connected to their structural and contextual components. If it can achieve these, social work research will differ from psychological studies and sociological research as traditionally conducted and will be forging new paths for researchers not just in social work, but in the social sciences more broadly.

Conclusion

Social work research has to meet new challenges and engage with those that bedevil research more generally. Crucial to this are:

- Emphasising the role of research subjects in the research process and ensuring that they are engaged as full participants in research
- Finding new methodologies that will meet the specific concerns of practice, namely discovering ways of dealing with uncertainty and ambiguities
- Inventing approaches that will enhance service user wellbeing
- Retheorising social work research
- Working out how practice-based research can involve practitioners without jeopardising their career prospects when they uncover material that portrays their employers in a negative light
- Involving service users as full partners in research.

Responding to these concerns may precipitate more controversies in social work research, but facing these cannot be avoided if social work researchers are to articulate distinctive approaches to this enterprise.

In the process, researchers who engage in participative research fully with service users and practitioners have to deal with pitfalls and take advantage of the opportunities offered by moving further in this direction. As they do so, social work researchers have better possibilities of responding to service user agendas while advancing and protecting the place of social work research in academia. They can work towards ensuring that social work becomes a social science disci-pline that does not authorise becoming caught up in replicating models of research popular in the natural sciences, as these treat people as the objects of their ministrations. These paradigms do not meet the needs of people interacting in a research relationship. Consequently, social work researchers have to work together with service users, practitioners and managers to develop new and different methodologies and insights for social work research.

For further discussion of ethical aspects, see Adams et al., 2009b, Chapter 4.

Becker, S. and Bryman, A. (2004) *Understanding Research for Social Policy and Practice: Themes, Methods and Approaches*, Bristol, Policy Press. Comprehensive book of particular interest to social work students because it focuses on the importance of research for policy and practice.

Cree, V. and Davis, A. (2007) *Social Work: Voices from the Inside*, London, Routledge. Illustrates how research can be used to highlighted marginalised voices and bring them into the mainstream.

Nutley, S.M., Walter, I. and Davies, H.T. (2007) *Using Evidence: How Research Can Inform Public Services*, Bristol, Policy Press. Useful in exploring how evidence of various kinds can be used to inform policy developments in the public services.

Royse, D.R. (2003) *Research Methods in Social Work*, Belmont, CA, Wadsworth. Summarises a range of research methods that are useful for social workers.

Planning research and evaluation projects in social work

21

This chapter examines some of the processes and issues involved in setting out to do a piece of research as a practitioner. Specifically, it covers some of the tensions, dilemmas and ethical issues that may arise when working with service users, practitioners and agencies in the course of participatory research.

Chapter overview

Although this chapter is about 'getting started' in research, it is important to anticipate and plan for as much of the research process as possible in advance, including consideration of how the research might end and the results disseminated. This enables all the research participants to have a clear idea about what is expected and allows agreements to be made with various stakeholders that are both feasible and ethically sound.

In this chapter, we assume that a research topic has been decided on, therefore we cover matters relating to:

- Deciding on an approach to the research
- Confirming values and principles
- Clarifying roles and purpose with stakeholders
- Negotiating access and anticipating and agreeing issues relating to ownership of the research, privacy, consent and anonymity.

However, it is important to emphasise that the choice of topic in itself raises ethical and political issues. If research is funded or sponsored by an agency, government department or funding council, the boundaries of what counts as a researchable topic may already have been defined, and this severely limits the extent to which research can be initiated from the 'grass roots'. Frequently the topics for which funding is available are those that match with the latest government agenda or 'moral panic', with the result that much more research is undertaken on 'problematic' issues, such as young people's involvement in crime or drugs, than on the everyday routine matters, or positive aspects of people's lives.

The nature of research and evaluation

The title of this chapter refers to 'research' and 'evaluation'. Although there is considerable overlap between what we commonly think of as research and evaluation, it is important to distinguish between the two. 'Research' is a broad term generally associated with a systematic investigation, involving a process of discovery or critical inquiry. According to Robson (2000: 9), it entails the activities of 'description, explanation and understanding'. An example of a piece of research might be a study of the levels and causes of youth crime on a particular housing estate.

'Evaluation' has a rather narrower meaning – literally 'an assessment of value'. In the field of public services, the importance of evaluation has grown rapidly alongside a growing concern with value for money and the targeting of services to meet the greatest needs. Evaluation involves making a judgement about the worth of a specific activity, project, programme or policy. An example of an evaluation might be a study of the effectiveness of a particular youth crime project in reducing reoffending on an estate. Insofar as evaluation should involve careful and systematic inquiry, then we would argue that it is a particular type of research. Sometimes the terms 'evaluation research' or 'evaluative research' are used (see, for example, Cheetham et al., 1992). It is in this sense that we are using the term 'evaluation' here.

Practitioner research

Practitioners may often find they are involved in research, whether as a researcher, commissioner, consultee, research user or a combination of these. In this chapter, we are specifically concerned with the practitioner, or student practitioner, as researcher. This type of research has sometimes been termed 'practitioner research' (Broad and Fletcher, 1993; Fuller and Petch, 1995). The term is used rather loosely, but tends to denote the fact that the person doing the research is a practising professional in the field they are researching. Therefore they may have insider knowledge and contacts, and a direct interest in both setting the research question and the results of the research. Practitioner researchers may undertake research in the setting or agency where they work. Alternatively, the research may be undertaken in different agencies/projects or using national data sources. Sometimes the 'practitioner researcher' is distinguished from the 'academic researcher'. While this is rather a false distinction, it does highlight the fact that practitioner research is usually concerned with practical applications, whereas academic research may be concerned more with understandings or theoretical insights.

The following are questions for the intending researcher to consider:

- Do I think of myself as a practitioner researcher? For example, am I a full-time practitioner researching in my own setting, a part-time student practitioner, a full-time student with practice experience or a full-time researcher with practice experience?
- What are the advantages and disadvantages of this role?

Applied, action, participatory and emancipatory research

Categorisations such as 'applied research', 'action research', 'participatory research' and 'emancipatory research' are often used in the context of practitioner research. These types of research are not mutually exclusive. A piece of research or evaluation may fall into several categories, to varying degrees, depending on the purposes of the research and the principles by which the key stakeholders wish to operate. But the labels provide some useful headings for researchers to consider when placing themselves in relation to their research.

Applied research

The term 'applied' refers to the fact that the subject matter and findings of the research can be applied to matters of practice or policy relevance (Everitt et al., 1992). This is usually contrasted with 'pure research', where knowledge and understanding may be sought for its own sake. However, this distinction is not clear-cut, and is better thought of as a pure–applied continuum rather than mutually exclusive categories.

The following are questions for the intending researcher to consider:

- To what extent is the research in which I will be involved expected to be relevant to policy or practice?
- What does this mean about who should be involved/consulted in designing the questions and hearing the results?

Action research

This refers to research that has an explicit focus on bringing about change or improvement (Reason and Bradbury, 2005). This type of research is often undertaken by practitioners (see Hart and Bond, 1995; Winter and Munn-Giddings, 2001), but not exclusively. A classic example of action research in the UK is the Home Office-sponsored community development projects set up in 12 neighbourhoods in the late 1960s, where teams of researchers from universities worked alongside community workers, feeding in the results of their research as the projects developed, with the aim of contributing to government understanding of the causes and effective responses to poverty and to the improvement of the practice of the projects (see Green, 1992).

The following are questions for the intending researcher to consider:

- To what extent will the research focus on the aim of changing or improving policy/practice?
- Will it inform practice as it proceeds on an ongoing basis?
- How will this be achieved and what might be the barriers?

Participatory research

Participatory research involves those who might traditionally have been categorised as subjects of research, for example service users, young people or professional workers, in carrying it out, usually alongside a principal researcher/evaluator (Feuerstein, 1986). The concept of 'stakeholders' is useful in this context, referring to all those who may have a stake in a piece of research, ranging from sponsors/funders to service users. Barr and colleagues (Barr and Hashagen, 2000; Barr, 2003) have developed an increasingly popular model for evaluating community developments based on involving as many stakeholders as possible in designing the evaluation. Some people regard 'stakeholder' research/evaluation as a separate category (for example Robson, 2000), but for our purposes, we see it as encompassed within 'participatory research', although stakeholders often play more of an advisory than an active participatory role. Participation in research can cover a broad spectrum of involvement, ranging from stakeholders, in particular service users, merely being consulted about the design or findings through to them having full control over the whole research process.

The following are questions for the intending researcher to consider:

- Who are the stakeholders in the research and to what extent will they be involved at each stage of the research?
- Will some, all or none be advisers, designers, co-researchers, analysts, report writers?

Emancipatory research

Increasingly, the term 'emancipatory' is being used in relation to research that is designed to focus largely on enhancing the power of service users (Zarb, 1992; Dullea and Mullender, 1999). Some of this is located at the radical end of the participatory research spectrum (for example Whitmore, 2001). However, some commentators imply that it is a distinctive approach, involving research that clearly originates from and is conducted by service users (Evans and Fisher, 1999). This focus on emancipatory research has developed out of an increasing concern in social welfare work with the empowerment of service users and the promotion of anti-oppressive practice, along with developments in critical social research (Harvey, 1990) and feminist research (Roberts, 1981; Reinharz, 1992).

Critical research and evaluation have been put forward as a model that is particularly appropriate for social work (see Everitt and Hardiker, 1996). This is a form of participatory action research based on critical theory, which aims to work towards developing research participants' understanding of the political and policy context in which they are operating, with a view to bringing about radical change. The focus goes beyond simply developing the skills and confidence of service users by engaging them in the research process as participants, to a more radical educational process, akin to the approach promoted by Paulo Freire (1972), the Brazilian educator, where the aim is to challenge the existing power structures, with a stress on liberation and transformation. Feminist critiques of the traditional model of the researcher as a detached, objective collector of facts have also been influential in social work research and evaluation, with the emphasis on the researcher taking an explicit value position and engaging in reciprocal relationships with research participants (see Humphries, 1999).

The following are questions for the intending researcher to consider:

- To what extent can or should the research be empowering in its process (participants gain respect, confidence and skills) and/or its outcomes (it results in changing power structures)?
- Do all the stakeholders, including the commissioners of the research, share this aim?
- How can these ideals be put into practice?

Issues of philosophy and values

Traditional social science textbooks and courses on research often start with philosophical questions about ontology – the nature of the social world – and epistemology – how we come to know the world. While important, a more logical and accessible starting point might be a consideration of the issue of ethics – values and moral commitments about what makes for a good life or society and how we ought to behave towards other people.

Social work and related occupations rest clearly on a value base that entails respect for service users, promotion of their choices and rights and stresses the aim of working towards equality and social justice in society (Banks, 2006). So, in taking on a piece of research as a practitioner, we would expect these values to be paramount. Indeed, in their codes of ethics for social work, most professional associations include a section applying to practitioners undertaking research and stress that the research process should be congruent with social work values (for example BASW, 2002). Butler's (2002: 239) code of ethics for social work and social care research states that social work/social care research should, where possible, 'seek to empower service users' and researchers should 'seek to promote emancipatory research'.

Butler's code of ethics for social work research, unlike most of the ethical statements for generic social research (for example BSA, 2004), seems to commit social work practitioners to a particular type of research endeavour – 'emancipatory research'. However, it is important to bear in mind that, like many codes of ethics, this code encourages the expression of statements of universal ideals that are open to interpretation and may be impossible, or inappropriate, to achieve in particular contexts (see Banks, 2003). For example, we need to consider whether the research should aim to be emancipatory in its process and/or its outcomes. We should also be wary of imposing our values on stakeholders who may not share them and hiding behind the illusion of equality in what is still an unequal relationship, as discussed in the previous chapter (see Humphries, 1997 and Shaw, 1999 for a discussion of some of these points). There may be situations where improvement or reform is desired, rather than liberation.

Nevertheless, this code is useful in that it reminds us that we need to have the debate about what counts as 'emancipatory', whether 'emancipatory research' is what we can or should be doing, and if not, why not? It reminds us that it is important to offer an alternative to the traditional model, in a climate where much research and evaluation is commissioned and controlled by government bodies and senior agency managers, with the assumption that service users will feed into the process as passive respondents.

The practitioner researcher's own ideological and value position will inevitably make a difference to the type of research approach chosen. However, this does not preclude the use of traditional research methodologies in bringing about change, as in certain contexts it may be important that research results are regarded as credible in order to make an impact on policy makers.

In the light of this brief discussion, a crucial question for practitioners embarking on a piece of research might be: What are my personal, professional and political values and commitments? This might include considering questions such as:

- Who am I, for example what are my origins, job, gender, ethnicity?
- Where do I stand on certain issues, such as religion, politics, feminism, ecology?
- What values do I hold as an individual and a professional practitioner, for example honesty, integrity, equality?
- Do others share my values?
- What does this mean for how I/we conduct this research?

This involves being clear about which value commitments one might be prepared to negotiate on and which are non-negotiable (see Everitt et al., 1992: 137–8 for a list of values for social work research). It also involves a process of reflexivity – identifying, acknowledging and questioning what we bring with us to the research process (see White, 2001 for a useful discussion of reflexivity in research). This process should continue throughout the process of a piece of research, as practitioner researchers continually question their own role and interpretations, and stand back and see the people/policies being studied with fresh eyes in a broader social and economic context.

Although research that is participatory and empowering for service users fits well with the values of social work, this approach is fraught with challenges and can be more complex and time-consuming than more traditional models where the researcher has complete control. To illuminate our discussion about some of the practical and ethical issues to take into account in setting up a research project, we outline a research study with which one of the authors was involved.

◇◇◇ CASE EXaMPLE ◇◇◇◇◇◇◇◇◇◇◇◇◇◇◇◇◇◇◇◇◇◇◇◇◇◇◇◇◇◇◇◇◇◇◇◇◇

Two researchers from Durham University were commissioned to consult disabled people in a borough in northeast England about a number of planned service developments and, more particularly, to find out how disabled people wished to be consulted in the future. The study was jointly funded by health and social services. The funders initially invited a local voluntary organisation to carry out the study, but as members of the organisation felt they lacked the necessary research expertise and experience to undertake such work, they sought help from the university. The researchers, on the other hand, were concerned that they had no direct experience of disability and would have preferred the work to have been carried out by disabled researchers. After some weeks of negotiations, it was agreed that the researchers would work in partnership with a small group of disabled volunteers from the local agency. They formed a 'research team' that worked together for the duration of the project, with advice from a multi-agency steering group made up of funders, service providers and practitioners.

Clarifying stakeholder expectations

In preparing the ground for a piece of research, there are three key areas worth discussing with the main stakeholders in advance and these are discussed below.

Clarifying purposes

If the research has been commissioned, or there is a process of negotiating with a host agency or group of service users, it is important to identify the various stakeholders in the research and discuss what they want to get out of it. Discussion with potential research participants and other stakeholders can also help to clarify the purpose of the research, highlight differences in expectations and stimulate the rethinking of a project.

If undertaking an evaluation, it is important to be clear whether the key stakeholders agree on its main focus. Robson (2000) identifies four types of evaluation as follows:

1 *Evaluation of needs* – study of the extent to which the needs of an existing programme's target group are being met, or a needs analysis in preparation for planning a new programme
2 *Processes* – analysis of how the programme is working, who takes part, what happens on a day-to-day basis
3 *Outcomes* – analysis of the effect or impact of the programme on those taking part, or beyond
4 *Efficiency* – consideration of how the beneficial effects compare with the costs of running the programme.

An evaluation can also be formative/developmental – feeding in findings and ideas for improvement on an ongoing basis – or summative – making a judgement about the success of a project at the end. Action research projects may do both, but sometimes these roles fit together uneasily. Robson (2000) distinguishes the different emphases in formative and summative evaluations:

■ *Formative evaluations* tend to stress gathering information on processes, with the credibility of the evaluator depending on an understanding of the programme and rapport with the users/staff.

■ *Summative evaluations* may focus more on outcomes, with credibility depending on technical competence and impartiality.

Trying to do both, as inevitably happens in a two- or three-year ongoing evaluation, can be problematic for a researcher, who seeks acceptance as a semi-insider/critical friend, but also needs distance as an expert observer.

Clarifying principles

Having read a lot of literature on user empowerment, emancipatory research and research ethics, practitioner researchers should have an idea about the values they want to underpin the research and how these translate into practice principles. However, these should be discussed and debated with stakeholders to develop a mutually agreed set of principles. Compromises may need to be made as we cannot assume that a researcher's high-minded ideals for maximum participation, power-sharing and radical action for change will be shared by any or all the various stakeholders.

In the case example, the researchers and volunteers in the research team worked together to explore the most appropriate way they could achieve the aims of the project. Each member of the team brought to the discussions their knowledge, experiences, values and beliefs. The volunteers had a strong influence in establishing some general principles, which the researchers had to ensure were met by the research methods they proposed. In this way, the principles formed an important framework within which the methodology had to operate (Barnes and Kendall, 2001). The principles adopted were:

■ To work to a social model of disability, while respecting the important contribution that health services make to the lives of disabled people
■ To work towards the inclusion of all disabled people aged 18–65 who live in the borough, irrespective of whether they use health or social care services
■ To ensure reciprocity by recognising that learning is a two-way process
■ To aim for sustainability and continuation after the project
■ To respect differences, giving participants a choice of ways in which to engage with the project
■ To accept that the project provides a first stage towards empowerment
■ To encourage better understanding of local service users' experiences and expectations of services through the use of qualitative research methods
■ To value the knowledge, skills and expertise of all participants.

Clarifying roles and responsibilities

If the research design and process is to be a collaborative one, it is important to be as clear as possible at the outset what role the various stakeholders in the research will play. In the case example, five stakeholder groups were identified who wished to contribute to the study and therefore had to agree their roles and responsibilities, as described below:

1   *Commissioners* drew up a specification for the study and agreed to participate in an advisory group, which would meet for a fixed number of meetings to steer the project. They also made a commitment to taking action after the study had reported.

2   The *voluntary organisation* that had contracted the researchers agreed a substantial role in the project. The chief executive became a member of the advisory group. As the organisation and its staff were well known to disabled people in the town, they agreed to provide support for the volunteer researchers, administrative support and personal assistants for the focus groups and use of their database. For reasons of confidentiality, the research team could not have direct access to the database of names and addresses but the agency agreed to mail out a letter and questionnaire from researchers.

3   The *volunteer researchers* agreed to attend meetings to plan and manage the research. They only wished to have a small role in data collection because of limited energy and restricted mobility but they assisted in the focus groups and the survey administration. They also negotiated to attend the university to learn about data analysis and be involved in interpreting the findings. They did not wish to take responsibility for writing up the research but they agreed to read and comment on drafts. No powers of veto were discussed. However, recommendations were to be decided by the volunteers on discussion with the researchers and then presented locally by the volunteers. The volunteers also agreed to do what they could to ensure that the findings of the report were acted on.

4   The *researchers* agreed to take responsibility for seeing that the research was completed but their role was to be complementary to the volunteers. Expertise on disability issues and the locality would be provided by the volunteers, while research expertise would be provided by the researchers. In carrying out the research, the researchers would undertake the work that the volunteers did not wish or feel able to carry out.

5   *Service providers* gave the research team access to their services to meet service users. Managers of key services agreed to introduce their service plans to focus groups that were held to discuss the proposals but to withdraw after their presentation if that was the wish of the group. Should conflicts arise in the research team, the chief executive of the voluntary agency agreed to provide support for the volunteers while the professional researchers would access supervision at the university.

Negotiating ethical issues

There is an increasing concern with ethical issues in research. The majority of recent textbooks on social research methods include a chapter on this theme (for example Bulmer, 2001; Hammersley and Atkinson, 2007; Bryman, 2008) and there is a growing number of books with a specific focus on research ethics (for example Homan, 1991; Mauthner et al., 2002; Oliver, 2003; Israel and Hay, 2006; Long and Johnson, 2006) or that have an ethical slant (D'Cruz and Jones, 2004; Farrell, 2005). We cannot go into all the possible issues here, but will highlight several that are particularly important and may have added complexities in the context of participatory research with service users, to which many of the generic social research textbooks pay less attention (for useful examples relevant to social work, see McLaughlin, 2007; Munford et al., 2008).

Rights of the sponsors/commissioners

If your research is being funded by an external body, certain conditions might be placed on the research, and if the research has actually been commissioned, then the controls imposed in the contract may be tighter still. Contract researchers may be left with little choice – acceptance of the contract as presented or rejection of the research commission. However, there may be room for negotiation, so it is worth thinking through in advance the implications of some of the implicit and explicit agreements with sponsors to ensure that they do not attempt to control the research process and findings in a way that may stifle justified criticism of policy, organisations or practice. In the case example, the research questions, timescale, costs and format of the final report were found to be non-negotiable, but the use of a participatory method was accepted, with all the uncertainties it brought about how the study might be conducted and the methodologies used.

The commissioner of a piece of research may ask to see a draft copy of your report and exercise the right to suggest or make amendments. While Oliver (2003) suggests that this is not desirable, as they may wish to change findings that are inconvenient to them, the risk is reduced in the kind of research/evaluation that we are looking at in this chapter. The commissioner of the research may be part of a stakeholder advisory group (as in the case example) and will share the role of feeding in views and amendments with other stakeholders. The issue to determine in advance is whether they have the right of veto, or are just regarded as part of a broader decision-making group. It is also important to plan in advance how any steering group will operate – seeking consensus, voting if necessary, giving the right of veto to certain parties.

Gaining permission/access

If you wish to undertake a piece of research that involves accessing records, staff and/or service users in a social work, health or related setting, you are likely to have to seek permission from more than one body or gatekeeper. For research in a British health service setting, such as a hospital or clinic, or local authority social care services, a proposal outlining the full details of the research and methods to be used will have to be submitted to a research ethics committee (an institutional review board in the US and some other countries). Procedures for doing this are constantly being updated, so it is wise to consult relevant websites and organisations well in advance to find out what is required (in a British context, see DH, 2005; National Research Ethics Service/NHS National Patient Safety Agency, www.nres.npsa.nhs.uk).

Most universities also operate research ethics committees and, in some cases, university social work departments have their own committees that approve student dissertation proposals. The purpose of such committees is to ensure that researchers do not engage in practices that exploit or harm service users, or collect information that does not contribute to answering the research questions. They also see that the appropriate safeguards are in place for consent, confidentiality, anonymity and so on.

Gaining approval from a health service research ethics committee can be a lengthy process and may involve minor or substantial changes in your research proposal, or even its rejection. For pieces of social work research that are based on involving service users in research design and planning, the requirement to specify in advance details of the approach and methods can be restricting. Some research ethics committees may have little appreciation of the principles and methods of participatory action research, so it is important to justify the legitimacy of such an approach.

Once past this hurdle, it may be important to gain permission from 'gatekeepers', such as hospital consultants, project managers, directors of social care services or head teachers, in order to access the users of their services. It is then crucial to seek permission from the people you want to work with. Traditionally, they have been the last people to be asked about participating in the research, if, indeed, they are asked at all.

Asking for consent

The principle of seeking the informed consent of research participants is now a standard requirement in all social research. Seeking informed consent is particularly important in a social work context, in that it is a mark of respect to research participants and offers them the right not to participate. It also gives some protection to researchers from later complaints or litigation. However, gaining informed consent is not a straightforward matter. Homan (1991) offers a useful analysis of what might be meant by 'informed' and 'consent':

- *Informed*
  - That all pertinent aspects of what is to occur and what might occur are disclosed to the subject
  - The subject should be able to understand this information.
- *Consent*
  - The subject is competent to make a rational and mature judgement
  - The agreement to participate should be voluntary and free from coercion and undue influence.

This definition prompts the question of whether informed consent can ever really be given – often we do not know what might happen as a result of the research, especially in a social work context, when it is participatory, with others taking part and steering its direction. And how do we judge the 'competence' of someone to understand the nature of research? All we can do is think carefully about what information a potential participant needs to know and can understand.

There are particular issues in social work research, which may often be undertaken with people who are sick, young or vulnerable in other ways. It may be easy to manipulate or persuade people to agree to something they do not fully understand, especially if we already have a professional relationship with them. We have to decide when it is appropriate to seek 'proxy' consent from a guardian, parent or carer. On some occasions, we may need to seek consent from service users and family members/carers as the research may have an impact on both parties. With user-led and/or participatory social work research, it is important to consider whose responsibility it is to seek consent and whether and how to differentiate between researcher service users and users who are respondents or interviewees. Particular issues can arise in research that involves people who are part of a particular community (indigenous) collecting data, as they may have conflicting loyalties and different understandings of ethical priorities, as a study in the US by Alexander and Richman (2008) demonstrates.

There is also the question of whether it is ever ethical to undertake research into aspects of people's lives without informing them that you are doing so. This is an area of debate within the social research community – with some people arguing that covert research may be necessary to gain data that would not be otherwise available in order to further human knowledge, and others arguing that such research should never be done. There is an issue of what counts as 'covert research', how much 'deception' is involved and whether it is acceptable in public places. For example, it might be regarded as acceptable for a researcher to undertake observations of teacher–children interactions in a classroom without informing the participants that she is looking for differences in the way boys and girls are treated – because teachers may change their behaviour accordingly. However, it might be regarded as highly questionable for a researcher to disguise their identity and take on the role of lookout (or 'watch queen') in a men's public lavatory in order to gain information on 'impersonal sexual relations', as Humphreys (1975) did in his highly controversial study. In participatory and practitioner research in social work, the issue of hiding the researcher's identity is rarely feasible and would generally be regarded as unethical.

Maintaining privacy

The commitment on the part of researchers to respect the right to privacy of the research participants is particularly important in practitioner research in a social work context. According to Bok (1984: 10):

> privacy is the condition of being protected from unwanted access by others – either physical access, personal information, or attention.

If the research involves interviewing or observing people, it is important to be clear with participants, at the time their consent is sought, to what extent confidentiality and anonymity will be preserved. Confidentiality involves maintaining secrecy in relation to private information gained in the course of the research relationship that, if revealed, might be damaging to the person concerned. Obviously, the main reason for interviewing people is to find out information that can be used in the research and reported in any findings. So to make a blanket promise of confidentiality would be rather counter-productive. Usually what can be offered is anonymity, that is, removing identifying features so that the source of the information cannot be identified.

Particular thought may need to be given to issues around privacy in relation to participatory research in social work where service users may be interviewing other service users and may come to know sensitive information. When writing up the research, it may be hard to ensure anonymity, as members of the project, service or tightly knit community may easily recognise the turn of phrase used by people they know, or a description may only fit one person, for example chair of the management committee. As Woodman et al. (1995: 61) point out in relation to researching the lesbian community:

> even with the careful elimination of names in the write-up, it may be possible to iden-
> tify participants through demographic data published in the results.

Conclusion

When embarking on a piece of research/evaluation, particularly if the evaluation is intended to be participative, there are a number of preparatory questions that should be considered before detailed plans for the methodology can be drawn up. It is helpful to try to predict some of the potential difficulties in advance. This requires you to be flexible in your planning and allow plenty of time. Some of the issues for consideration include:

- Clarifying the purpose of the research, as this will guide the broad approach to be taken and the role you might play in the work
- Identifying who the stakeholders will be, the roles they might play and their lines of responsibility and accountability
- Negotiating the principles by which the research will be pursued with the stakeholders, such as reciprocity, open communication, respect for differ-ence, including reference to codes of practice/conduct (for example BASW, 2002; BSA, 2004)
- Negotiating acceptable constraints with funders or commissioners to ensure that the research can be conducted and reported as the participants would wish
- Identifying who might be the gatekeepers to the individuals and data required
- Considering what can/should be promised with respect to anonymity and privacy and how you will reach people not normally reached, for example deaf people.

Some of these considerations may have to be revisited when the research meth-odology has been agreed. Thinking about research is a constant process and research design is not a linear activity, but rather an iterative process in which issues are discussed and renegotiated until the best possible approach can be found. Inevitably, in participatory research, with a number of stakeholders to satisfy, the set-up phase can be challenging, but good preparation can help all participants to understand the research and therefore contribute to it and own its results.

For further discussion of aspects of ethics and values, see Adams et al., 2009a, Chapter 4.

Bryman, A. (2008) *Social Research Methods, 3rd edn*, Oxford, Oxford University Press. Comprehensive overview of research methods designed for students, including chapters on research designs, ethics and conducting a small-scale project.

Evans, C. and Fisher, M. (1999) 'Collaborative evaluation with service users', in I. Shaw and J. Lishman (eds) *Evaluation and Social Work Practice*, London, Sage. Thoughtful practical discussion of the issues surrounding user-led and user-controlled research.

Fuller, R. and Petch, A. (eds) (1995) *Practitioner Research: The Reflective Social Worker*, Buckingham, Open University Press. Good overview of the nature of practitioner research, with chapters covering examples of research by practitioners.

Israel, M. and Hay, I. (2006) *Research Ethics for Social Scientists*, London, Sage. Comprehensive account of ethical issues in social research, including coverage of ethical theories, codes of ethics and regulatory systems in different countries.

Oliver, P. (2003) *The Student's Guide to Research Ethics*, Maidenhead, Open University Press/McGraw-Hill Education. Accessible text with exercises covering practical aspects of research ethics from a rather traditional perspective.

Doing literature searches and reviews

22

Literature searches and reviews are an important starting point for all kinds of research and practice-based projects. This chapter shows you how to build on existing knowledge by defining your topic and searching the literature. It also discusses the value of reviews for systematically assessing the contribution of existing publications to our understanding.

Chapter overview

Literature searches and reviews: their importance

Literature reviews are analyses of information gained from a literature search. The review is an examination of the existing writing about a topic of interest; the search is the process of finding the literature so that you can examine it and write the review. Sometimes, doing a literature review is in itself a piece of research, which creates knowledge, because it puts together information in a new way. For example, it might highlight trends. Another form of research by literature review, called a 'systematic review', aggregates results so that they are more powerful because the results from several studies added together cover a larger or more diverse population.

The principle behind literature reviews is that the development of knowledge builds on what other people have found out before, which will be recorded in the literature, so all study or research projects start out from a review. Otherwise, they just repeat existing knowledge. It is also a waste of time doing research to find out something that is already known.

Since all investigation, research and study builds on previous work in this way, learning to do literature searches and reviews extends students' skills in ways that they will use throughout their professional careers. In practice, a literature review gives credibility to an important report about a client, for example, or as the basis for starting or getting funding for a work project. Literature reviews are essential to getting a research grant, starting a research project or doing effective teaching. Having carried out a literature review allows you to say things like:

- Research demonstrates that the best course of action to modify John's challenging behaviour is …
- Research shows that the services that should be available for a population this size are …
- While our service currently provides a wide range of facilities for people with dementia, this proposed project has been shown to be effective in similar areas in enabling people with dementia to be managed in the community successfully and in reducing costs …

Literature reviews in social work education

Most higher education, including professional courses such as social work programmes, includes small research projects, extended essays or dissertations that require students to complete a literature search and review. This builds on the skills developed in the early stages of a course in written work, using these skills to complete a longer and more comprehensive project. Often these are relevant to the 'real world' rather than just being an assessment exercise. In the early part of courses, students are given a topic and a reading list, and put together information from the reading list to demonstrate their understanding of the topic. The best essays result from reading more widely than the list provided, for example some alternatives or additional works, and from presenting the material in an interesting or novel way. In assessments during the early stages of a course, this might just demonstrate that they have read the relevant material about a subject. Looking for relevant literature at this stage of the course is a good preparation for more extensive literature searching later and you can use the first part of this chapter as a guide to doing this more systematically; it would be good practice for the time when you come to do a full literature review.

A literature search and review in the final year of an undergraduate course or as part of a masters course takes skills in finding literature and presenting it to a higher level. As well as looking at what students know about, or tutors have suggested, methodical literature searching enables the information used in an essay or research project to be comprehensive and convincing. Presenting and commenting on the outcomes of the search in the review allows students to clarify and extend the material and may enable them to express judgements that are firmer and more creative.

The three main reasons for doing a literature search or review are:

- To find out useful written information about an unfamiliar topic. This also helps you to see different points of view and later on will enable you to teach, write a publication or report and recommend useful and worthwhile publications to help other people's learning.
- As the basis for a research project, because any research needs to build on what we already know.
- As a research project in itself to bring together comprehensive information about a topic.

Literature reviews are particularly important at two stages:

- Formulating and writing a research or project proposal. At this early stage, you have to explore the literature to make sure that the topic is practicable, worthwhile and has not been done before, or if it has been done before, that it is worth replicating in your situation.
- As the basis for the project. At this later stage, the literature review will help to decide the research question, plan the project, avoid pitfalls, stimulate ideas for questions and issues to explore and identify the concepts and aspects of the world that the project will examine.

Some of the work will be done at the pre-proposal stage, to enable you to demonstrate that the project is worth doing. Often you can do this by hand searching and informal searches of known sources of information in texts or your academic library. Then, you build on this for a more considered and comprehensive review to inform the study, using more systematic searches.

Search methods

Literature searches begin from what you already know. This might include knowledge that you have acquired writing an essay or doing a previous project.

Identifying and defining the topic

The first stage is deciding what your review will cover. At this stage, you think this out in general; more detailed and technical definitions come later. Lectures, tutorials and reading lists provided by tutors, friends and colleagues might suggest a range of issues that are relevant to a topic. You may also be able to think of issues that concern you. You also need to be critical about the ideas that come up in the early stages and look for alternatives.

As an example, let us explore a project on 'child neglect':

1   What does this phrase mean? Focusing on the professional meaning – obviously, it does not refer to children neglecting to do important things in their lives – what kinds of behaviour might be neglectful? Who can be neglectful – is it just parents, or might it be older brothers and sisters, other members of the family, or members of the public who happen to come into contact with a child? How is it different from or related to child abuse?
2   What is your particular interest? Is there a particular slant that has come up in your reading or in a placement? This might guide some of your choices.
3   What kinds of information are you looking for? Are you looking for empirical research, professional commentary, personal experience – of neglecters or people who have been neglected? Are you looking for better knowledge about neglect, or information about assessment or possible interventions, or official policies?

4 Being critical means looking at alternative perspectives. Are we too worried about child neglect? Perhaps it is an example of current societies being risk averse. Does it arise because of poverty or untreated mental illness among parents? To take a feminist perspective, might child neglect as a concept be used officially as a way of blaming mothers for children's difficulties? To take an anti-racist perspective, is it a concept that might lead to criticising childcare practices that come from the culture of someone from a minority ethnic group?

Keeping notes

Before you start, an important bit of forward thinking is to plan how to keep notes of the literature you find. When you come to write the review, dissertation or report of your project, you will have to cite or refer to the publications. Most higher education institutions have a standard format for this; they all differ slightly and students are usually given a written guide or referred to an internet guide on how to do it. Usually, they are based on standards set for academic publication, or on recognised standards such as those produced by the British Standards organisation or the International Organization for Standardization (ISO). Journals, professional groups and university departments adapt these for their own use. If you look carefully in the bibliography of this book, you will find that every type of reference has been produced in an identical format; the same is true of any professionally edited publication. Anything less than this standard of citation will look slipshod and raise questions about the care you have exercised over other aspects of the work. Doing this well is about maintaining your professional standards.

People who regularly write for academic or professional purposes get in the habit of keeping notes that cover all the information they are likely to need when they come to use the reference. It is infuriating to know that you read something somewhere, or to have a photocopy of something you want to quote, but to have to go back to your library to find it again because some vital piece of information is missing.

There are some convenient ways of dealing with this. If your university or organisation has a standard, keep a copy of it by you and stick to it. If not, pick the most prestigious journal in your field and look on its website or in a copy of the journal for its authors' guidance and stick to that. In social work, this might well be a journal like the *British Journal of Social Work*. In the broader social sciences, the current *Manual of the American Psychological Association* (APA, 2001) is widely used. This fifth edition is 440 pages long, which shows how detailed and careful you have to be.

When to use citations

When should you use citations? You are probably aware of articles or books that include so many citations they are hard to read; on the other hand, you have probably been frustrated by some books where you would like to follow something up and there are no citations to what you are interested in. The three main reasons for citing another author's work are as follows:

■ To prove a potentially disputable fact; for example 'research shows' – whose? 'Jones says' – where? However, just because someone says something in a book does not make it a fact, so there is no need to cite someone expressing an opinion, unless you are trying to prove that at least one author has argued for a particular point of view.

■ To guide readers to the wider literature or to point to an example of literature that illustrates the point you are making: 'some writers argue (citations), but others (citations) dispute this'.

■ To give credit where it is due to the original work of the author for their research or having the idea or organising the knowledge in the particular way you have found helpful.

To avoid using too many citations, you have to use your judgement about what readers might be likely to want to know. Two points about this. First, if you are writing a piece of work for assessment, you might err on the side of including more citations, because your aim is to demonstrate to your tutor that you know about a wide range of issues; to some extent this is also true of literature reviews. You may not get credit for this unless you really integrate the material into your argument; the rule should be not to use citations unless, in your argument, you have to use this particular piece of writing to prove a point or give credit. Second, do not use textbooks as an example to follow. The task of writers of textbooks is to make people aware of knowledge that is available and to cover the topic in a way that meets the needs of a wide range of readers. Therefore, they are likely to use citations heavily in a way that is not necessary in an ordinary piece of writing.

Informal and hand searching

Students are usually given reading lists, and see professional and academic journals and books on professional topics. To build on these, you can visit an academic, professional or public library. Ask the librarian how to find the things you want. They are trained to do this and usually welcome an interesting inquiry, but they will leave you to do your own searching, because you have to take responsibility for it.

To start hand searching, find the most recent and comprehensive book or journal on your topic, list all the references that are of interest to you, and then go looking for these. Do the same with these, and carry on until you cannot find references to anything that you have not already seen. This is called 'hand searching' because you actually find the printed copy of the journal or book and hold it in your hand to check.

The problem with doing a literature search by following back from a known publication is that you may get stuck in a single track. I recently read a piece of writing by a nurse looking at the transition of seriously ill children into adulthood, across the division between children's and adults' services. She had assiduously found all the sparse healthcare literature about this topic. However, she did not realise that careers guidance professionals interpret their work as transition from school to work, and there is a huge literature, with concepts and research about that transition that would have helped her.

Therefore, you should try a little serendipity. This means finding things by accident, but it is one of those situations where you have to encourage accidents to happen. If you look at the library list of topics, pick some general subjects related to yours and check through the shelves on those topics to see if you can find anything of interest. For example, if you are interested in family therapy, you may be used to looking at the family sociology and psychotherapy shelves. You could try looking at education or economics to find material in related topics. Just wandering through the library and looking at unexpected shelves or journals you do not usually view may bring a new insight to you.

Computer searching

Computer databases automate the searching process. Two kinds exist:

- search engines, which give you access to information on the internet
- databases produced by academic institutions and libraries covering a specialist literature, such as *Social Work Abstracts* or ASSIA (Applied Social Sciences Index and Abstracts).

Search engines such as Google are familiar, although for doing research, you may find Google Scholar, the specialist engine for academic work, more useful than the general engine. It is important to evaluate the quality of the information, since anyone can put things on the internet. Edited journals have quality control because someone has evaluated the usefulness and relevance of the contribution to a particular topic. This is true of academic and professional journals if they are peer reviewed. This means that two or three people who know something about the topic have looked at the publications and agreed that it is worthwhile.

The specialist databases do, however, present problems. First, you have to identify the topic accurately in one or two words, because the computer indexes rely on 'keywords'. I once did some research on 'missing people', for example. I asked someone who had written a book about it and he said there was very little literature, so I was not surprised when I came across only a few articles and books, most of which I already knew. However, one of these mentioned the term 'runaways'. When I searched for this word, I found hundreds of articles, including some on runaway nuclear reactions, which gave me a conceptual sidelight that we could see 'running away' as 'going out of control' – going out of someone else's control, perhaps.

A second problem with computer searching is that it is mainly useful for articles. This is, again, because indexing relies on keywords or 'abstracts', the summaries written by the authors of articles. Longer pieces of writing are less fully summarised, and chapters of books are sometimes not included in indexes. For similar reasons, the most comprehensive indexes are about fairly concrete scientific topics.

There is very little detail on books in most specialised databases. However, most libraries have OPACs (online public access catalogues), which cover their whole collection, and can be accessed from the internet, allowing you to look for books. You can search most university library catalogues for books; a good choice is a university that you know has a course in the subject you are interested in. Also, on the internet, you can search the catalogues of major public libraries like the British Library (www.bl.uk/) or the (American) Library of Congress (catalog.loc.gov/).

The search process

Limiting your search

So far, I have been describing preparation for a literature search. The next stage is to take that preparation further by defining the topic precisely, setting criteria for the search and carrying it out. From the preparation stage, you have a preliminary general idea of the main factors you will be looking for. You have probably already accumulated books or photocopies of articles and papers or notes about them.

Complex searching of computer databases involves setting out carefully a series of keywords. Most journal articles list about five or six keywords describing the topics covered by the article; if not, the database will contain keywords drawn from the title or abstract of the article. To see some examples of potential keyword searches, you could look at some of the knowledge reviews published by the Social Care Institute for Excellence (SCIE), which are all available on the internet. For example, Marchant et al. (2007: Appendix 1) list the various searches carried out. In ASSIA, the first two terms they searched for were 'child*' and 'infan*'. The asterisk in both cases allows multiple uses of this word to come out: the first term would produce results that included children, and the second would bring results for infant, infancy and infantilisation.

The number of words you search for is a balance between getting too much material, some of which is irrelevant, or setting the criteria too tightly and not getting material that will be worthwhile. The SCIE reviews employ staff to carry out the work, and so tend to be comprehensive; doing a small project involves being more limited in your ambitions. On the other hand, SCIE reviews deal with very well-researched topics; you may find that two or three research terms in an area that is not well covered will produce results that you can handle. As in the SCIE examples, your eventual formal report or dissertation will include a statement of what you searched for and how many results you got.

Many databases will give you title, references or abstracts of the articles that may interest you. You can decide from these whether you want to retrieve the actual article to look at, probably erring on the side of caution. In this way, you winnow down the number of titles that your search has thrown up to the number you think might be relevant.

For the report, you will need to keep a record of what you keep, what you reject and why. Again, a SCIE example will show the number of items of literature that came out at each stage in a sort of flow chart. More important, it makes clear the criteria on which they have been selected. An important criterion may be date: you may only search for recent articles, say the last 10 years. You may also limit the search by geographical areas or specialist subject, looking only in social work databases, for example, rather than social science ones. You may only be interested in empirical studies, and so you might not include theoretical articles. Alternatively, you may want to include accounts of practice projects. These decisions, again, need to be clearly expressed in the final report. Many people do this by producing a table at each stage, with the criteria for acceptance of an article into the study at that stage, and the number of articles finally included.

The review process

Review topics

When you have completed the search, you need to decide how to analyse the material within it. This is partly a trial and error process. As you did the search, you probably came across a few articles that seemed particularly comprehensive or important, while others offered interesting sidelights but were not so important. Reading the important ones and combining them with your earlier thoughts about the overall topic, you can begin to create a list of topics to cover in the review.

Deciding on topics is a matter of judgement, because there will be many interconnections; you may need to point up some of these as you write. There are two approaches to sorting out the material according to topics. One way is to create a table, in which you list the relevant features of every article you are considering. The first column would have the citation of the article, which includes its date. Where there are empirical results, your columns would cover matters such as the size and nature of the sample, any problems with the methods used, with findings categorised in a way that is relevant to your study. For a more theoretical topic, you might note the issues covered, so that you can see the number of times a topic comes up. Where there is a debate between writers, you could categorise the articles according to the position they take in the debate.

An alternative approach is to start with your topics and list the articles that deal with each topic, perhaps with a summary of their point of view, or a cogent quotation. In the old days, people might have done this on index cards or sheets of paper; nowadays you might do this in a series of files on a computer. You might even begin to construct a narrative about each topic, which would contribute to the review.

Thinking critically about a publication

In deciding the role that each publication you find would play in your review, you will make a critical review of its value in general – as a contribution to knowledge and understanding – and also to your topic. Thinking about its relevance to your topic is important, because a publication may be worthwhile, but not say anything about your particular topic.

A useful start is to divide publications into those that contain empirical data and those that are theoretical in character. This would enable you to check the acceptability of the empirical material, using research methods expertise. Are there flaws in the methods that lead you to doubt the validity of the outcomes? Or does the research cover a small population or limited groups of people, for example from one agency, so that you have doubts about whether it applies to other groups of people. You can then look at whether the empirical outcomes are strong enough to justify the conclusions that the authors draw from them. When you have been through this process, you can move on to consider the authors' arguments based on the empirical results.

Another useful early process is to consider the authors and what interests they have. Does the writing or research team have all the areas of expertise to cover the topic, or does their background or the place they work for suggest a particular interest. For example, much of the research on helping with bereavement has been done by psychiatrists, counsellors and social workers, who mainly come across people who have problems with grief. They might therefore organise their thinking and carry out research on those problems, without balancing the problem focus with a view that this is a natural social process, and look at the social support that people have. Another area of interest is the practice, management or research role of the writer. For example, a researcher paid by the government to evaluate the efficiency of care management processes might look at whether all care managers are keeping costs down to the same level, whereas a service manager might be interested in whether care managers all carry out the assessment procedures according to the official guidance. A practitioner might look at whether they receive management support and supervision in their work and are able to help service users challenge official decisions. All these perspectives are legitimate areas of inquiry, but they only cover one aspect of the care management role. Thinking about this would help you to decide on its importance for your particular topic.

The main part of reviewing the publication will be looking at its content. You could compare it with your own experience: does it seem to make sense? If not, what particular features of its findings or argument do you quarrel with? In the same vein, you could compare it with other publications that you have read. Does it build a similar picture to them, adding a point or two perhaps, or are its findings or argument unusual? This might cause you to look at the strength of argument and findings, and also whether it reveals a useful different perspective.

You could also look at whether the publication is comprehensive. For example, if it contains empirical research, did the study cover all the aspects of it that provide you with a full explanation? If it is a theoretical argument, have the authors considered all the relevant material and possible alternative theoretical positions? Authors sometimes unwisely focus on just a few of the publications of which they are aware, rather than ensuring that they have covered the field. This is particularly common when they comment on policy issues or on theory. For example, Pease's account of radical and critical social work theory (Adams et al., 2009a, Ch. 17) discloses a number of strands of radical theory, but many writers base their comments on just one or two well-known texts. Have they dealt fairly with the material they discuss?

You should also look at the arguments to see whether they are constructed logically. This is a technical matter; there are rules of logic that people should follow (see Bowell and Kemp, 2002, for a good summary). However, you can see whether there are gaps in the argument or assumptions that the writers have made with which you do not agree.

Another important point is to ask whether there are alternative explanations that the authors have not mentioned, but which could explain the findings or argument just as well. For example, if the researchers tested older people and people in the twenties and suggest that older people are more forgetful, you could ask whether older people might be less motivated to do well on such tests.

Also, it is important that the various points in the literature or empirical evidence are treated in a balanced way. Is one strong point set against another, or do the authors only put up weak arguments or evidence? Is the complexity of the issues recognised?

A credible review will need to balance a complex range of points; the following example covers a number of these issues. A recent *British Journal of Social Work* article on social work history using archival study of a local organisation implies that the emphasis on religious motivation in that organisation questions the idea that secularisation was an important factor in the formation of social work in the nineteenth century espoused in many social work texts, although only one is mentioned. We might ask: does the fact that one local organisation has a religious motivation invalidate the general thesis? Or is it the people involved in it, which would be different and we would have to look carefully at the article for the evidence. No, a specific example does not invalidate a general idea; this is a logical fallacy. Second, if we look at a range of social work histories, we can see that the picture is complex. Over a fairly long period, the churches shifted away from active help to people in need towards more social and religious roles. Therefore, many Christians and Christian churches set up specifically welfare organisations, with Christian objectives but separate from the organised churches. These organisations became more secular and separated from the churches over time. The development of social work method in the Poor Law and avowedly secular organisations, such as the Charity Organisation Societies in the UK and America, emphasised rational 'scientific charity' rather than decision-making on religious grounds. Eventually, the state took over responsibility for general social welfare over a period of many years. All these points support a view that social work is a secularisation of welfare services that were formerly the preserve of the churches in the UK. Third, more complex still, there is a European history of shifts between state, individual, Church and collective charities over many hundreds of years, of which the origins of social work is just a specific example (Payne, 2005, Ch. 1). Only a complex understanding of the issues around secularisation would offer the full picture to a reader. You might want to achieve this if your review is about the secularisation of welfare, but this was not relevant to the author of this particular study, who just needed to draw attention to the way in which her study contributed evidence towards an assessment of the secularisation thesis.

Writing the review

Once you have analysed the materials, you write a narrative that sets out the arguments, differences in results and issues that you can identify from the notes you have made. An important aspect of doing this is to balance the material according to the weaknesses in it. For example, I recently did a study (Payne, 2008) on staff support in palliative care, for which I did a computer search of the relevant publications in the last five years. Many of these were about staff stress, what different organisations did to help their staff and what organisational factors seemed to prevent stress from arising. Some wider management studies showed that organisational interventions were not very helpful to people experiencing stress; a more interpersonal approach was required. I noticed that many of the empirical studies were of female nurses, self-reporting feelings of stress, sometimes using some well-known self-report scales, in organisations that did not seem to do much to help them. There was evidence that many staff who were not nurses did not experience stress in the same way. This connects with the literature on emotional labour, which says that people closely involved with physical care, such as nurses, take on more of the emotionally demanding work than others whose responsibilities are less immediate, such as doctors (James, 1993). This example illustrates how you may need to connect what you do with wider literature not in the search. There was also literature on legal responses to staff stress, which suggested that there were difficulties in disentangling work stress from other stresses in life and research that suggested that non-work issues often caused the most stress for most people. I also found commentary from (mainly male) doctors and writers about how the stress of dealing all the time with people who were dying was exaggerated. This mixture of views from different types of evidence needed to be balanced into an overall account of how seriously we need to take staff stress and what could be done about it. Overall, I was cautious about accepting apparent levels of self-reported stress, but argued for personal support to be an important part of caring organisations.

Some of the ways that you may find helpful in dealing with a complex collection of material like this is to think it through in different categories:

- What we clearly know
- What we don't know
- What ideas or theoretical concepts exist about the topic
- What comments have been made from which theoretical positions about what we know and don't know – this is important because it allows you to see where people may be accepting of the present situation or critical of it
- What is my judgement about the issue; in particular, does the debate represent all the possible elements of the argument or are critical perspectives missing from the contents?

In the case of particular articles, you can ask yourself:

- What does the article say about what we already know?
- What does it claim to add to what we already know?
- With what strength of evidence or argument?
- What is my judgement about the claim?

In each case, it is helpful to be clear about the main findings, and to separate your own judgement from these.

Many research reviews concentrate on empirical studies, but it is equally possible to cover policy or theoretical work. However, for academic credibility, it is important to be comprehensive in your coverage. Theoretical and policy reviews need to cover all the alternative positions fairly, even if you disagree with them. For example, I am working on end of life care policy at the moment, and as part of this, I am writing a series of documents on what the political parties say about this. It is necessary to look at least at the three main political parties, but it is also important to look at parties that are significant in particular areas, for example the Democratic Unionist Party and Scottish National Party in government in Northern Ireland and Scotland respectively, and Plaid Cymru in Wales. I also intend to look at minor parties: what does the Green Party or the British National Party say about end of life care?

Systematic reviews

Of course, you will want to be methodical about your own study, but the term 'systematic review' has a specialist meaning. It refers to reviews of empirical research that are so similar that the results can be added together to give stronger information. If, for example, there are studies of the effects of child neglect covering populations in Hong Kong, India, the US and France, none of these may be large enough for you to say clearly how neglect affects children. But if they were all similarly conducted, you may be able to combine the results to make one study. The results cover different countries and cultures, so any results that come out strongly from the combination of results may be expected to apply very widely. Differences, on the other hand, may tell you something about factors that might affect only one country or culture; you might then look for an explanation for the differences.

Systematic studies require careful statistical analysis, and to carry them out, you need specialist advice. They may be the subject of a PhD, but not usually a BA or MA dissertation. However, informally, you might want to look specifically at empirical studies that emerge from a literature search to comment on the total populations that have been studied. Thinking about this enables you to be cautious about any biases in the populations studied. For example, psychological experiments often use students as experimental subjects, so their results may not apply to the general population. Practice studies sometimes focus on people who come for help, or are carried out by practitioners with a focus on helping people, so, again, they may not tell us something valid about a wider population.

Conclusion

In this chapter, I have outlined the process of carrying out literature searches and reviews. A brief account such as this cannot cover every eventuality, for which I refer you to the books recommended in the Further reading, and the advice available from professional librarians. The most important point to emphasise, covering the whole process, is the requirement to be absolutely meticulous in keeping bibliographical records and maintaining a record of what you did. It is also important to separate empirical findings from opinions expressed in the literature and distinguish them both from your own opinions. Any judgement you make in choosing between one piece of literature rather than another needs to be justifiable in your mind, and one of the best ways of making it justifiable is to set up a search and review process that is consistently applied throughout.

For further discussion of particular areas of policy and practice with children, families and adults, see Adams et al., 2009a, Chapters 22 and 23.

www.scie.org.uk/index.asp The SCIE website has useful and clearly written information on many aspects of literature reviews and other research topics, much of it freely available.

www.google.scholar.co.uk The specialist engine for academic work.

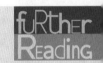

Aveyard, H. (2007) *Doing a Literature Review in Health and Social Care*, Buckingham, Open University Press. Less comprehensive that Hart's books, recommended below, this is practical and relates directly to health and social care issues.

Coren, E. and Fisher, M. (2006) *The Conduct of Systematic Research Reviews for SCIE Knowledge Reviews*, London, SCIE. Although a technical manual for conducting SCIE knowledge reviews and therefore about advanced literature reviewing, it is a clear, concise and detailed account of the process; the appendices give useful lists of relevant journals and databases for various social work reviews.

Hart, C. (1998) *Doing a Literature Review: Releasing the Social Science Research Imagination*, London, Sage; Hart, C. (2001) *Doing a Literature Search: A Comprehensive Guide for the Social Sciences*, London, Sage. Two excellent books on carrying out a literature review and literature search, covering everything you would want to know, with a broad focus on the humanities and social sciences.

23 Experiencing research as a practitioner

Chapter overview

In this chapter I explore how engagement in research practices, that is, actually doing the research, holds the potential to transform not just policy and practice but also the individuals who take part.

> Most of what we know, most of the knowing we do, is concerned with trying to make sense of what it is to be human and to be situated as we are. (Steedman, 1995: 58)

In this chapter, I would like to explore the meaning of 'transformation' within the context of research practice: what opportunities for growth might research offer to both researchers and participants and why this might be a valuable, but perhaps neglected, aspect. The central idea will be that doing research has the capacity to transform, to change permanently, the thinking, beliefs and attitudes of those who take it up. The changes brought about thus have the potential to bring about deeper and more personal understandings of social phenomena, in ways that the reported findings and outputs from research rarely seem to reflect or include.

There are a few eminent exceptions (most notably Bell and Newby, 1977; Roberts, 1995) to the dictum that research is largely presented in a sanitised and homogenised way, which fails to reveal its complexity, its untidiness, or the subjective experience of doing research. As a social work doctoral student in the 1990s, I found such texts to be reassuring about my experience of researching and also honest in their appraisal of the methodological and ethical dilemmas that research processes have a tendency to produce. But more importantly, they strongly emphasised the importance of critically reflecting on the process of conducting research, to question one's motives and methods and to view these reflections as an integral part of the data to be collected and analysed. My research was located within a qualitative paradigm and informed and enriched by a variety of feminist perspectives that supported the social work values I took into the research process. Coincidentally, these were the only sources that reflected a view of research that not only allowed for the subjectivity of the researcher (and the researched), but positively demanded that this element be incorporated as part of the narrative of the research. In this way, the deliberations and decision-making were revealed and consequently could be critically reviewed and scrutinised by readers, as part of judging the quality and validity of the research. At the time, it seemed that this was a trend that would continue to develop and enhance research quality across the board, but there has been little evidence of its presence, particularly in social work research, where the demands for 'best' evidence has meant 'clean, untouched (almost) by human hand or mind' evidence for practice and policy. The drive to publish journal articles has also influenced the shape and form of research writing, so that there is little room for reflection, critical or otherwise, on research methods and processes. Research reports serve many purposes and are written for a variety of audiences, so perhaps it is no surprise to find that reflective thinking is seldom found here, but importantly, this subject is rarely a prime focus in texts on research practice or research supervision.

While much has been written about the utility of social work research and the need for research to provide the evidence base for practice, the experience of doing and being involved in research has received little attention. Research is viewed as a means to an end, a way of providing the information needed to shape policy or direct practice, through the application of findings to the relevant field, group or problem. The drive for evidence-based practice (EBP) has also shifted the focus onto the outcomes or results of research (rather than the process or practice) in its insistence on providing strong, robust instructions about 'what works' in social work, as in other disciplines, for example health and education. EBP has strongly favoured a particular hierarchy of research methods, with randomised controlled trials and experimental methods being seen as the 'gold standard', and while strong critiques have been mounted against the whole philosophy (Trinder, 1996; Webb, 2001; Butler and Pugh, 2004) and its appropriateness for social work, the process of researching, research practice and its effects or impact have been neglected. In Chapter 1 of this book, the editors discuss the issue that EBP is just one form of research or knowledge-building and that research as the basis for social work practice incorporates critical reflection and critical commentary, partly because these techniques have the capacity to stimulate better practice, and partly because they put under critical scrutiny questions about what constitutes knowledge, as well as the evidence base from previous research (Chapter 1). This call extends much further than the demand for practitioners (and others) to be 'research minded' and not just critically reflective, but strongly suggests that we engage in what they have developed as 'thoughtfulness in practice' (Chapter 1):

> Thoughtfulness is, or should be, the six-sevenths of the iceberg of practice lying below the surface of visible actions. Thoughtfulness is a quality inherent in all good practice. It invariably accompanies action, reflection, decision-making and evaluation. (Chapter 1)

In the view of this book's editors, this quality of thoughtfulness can contribute to social work being transformational. They point out that the practitioner's research knowledge and expertise need to generate the capacity to pose critical questions that where necessary, for example, challenge an oppressive social reality (Chapter 1). It is this conceptualisation of practice as a space for transformation that I would now like to apply to research – not to the outcomes, but to the process or the heart of research practice; the doing of research, the engagement in a particular practice, which is located or situated within a complex profession and discipline with perceived values and ethics around such issues as social justice and equality, among others. I would postulate that engaging in research practice can be experienced as 'transforming' when the practice is approached with an open and inquiring mind by people who are capable and motivated to be critically reflective of the world they are engaged with, and reflexive and responsible about their actions and decisions throughout the process. I am talking here of experiencing learning and change at a personal level through engaging in research activities that extend beyond the results, findings and conclusions that might be drawn from the work about the research topic or subjects.

Meeting the methodological challenges in social work research

Research activity uses many of the same skills that are used in social work practice, such as collecting information as accurately as possible, analysing that information and drawing conclusions from those findings (Marlow, 2001: 25). Researchers also need to be skilled report writers who are able to present information and knowledge to a wide range of different audiences, if their work is to have an influence on practice or policy. Importantly, social work researchers also have a responsibility to think critically about the political and ethical elements of their work and should be guided by the same principles of 'rights, reciprocity, empowerment and anti-oppression' (Everitt et al., 1992: 85), which shape social work practice. This demands a critical awareness of the implications and consequences of the choices we make in research about methodologies and methods. The way that research questions are posed and the methods that are chosen to answer them reflect our view of the world, based on assumptions, pet theories and ideas, as well as the philosophical principles we might try to integrate. The wider debate about the philosophical roots of various methodological stances has been explored well in a variety of texts (see Fook, 1996; D'Cruz and Jones, 2004; Butler and Pugh, 2004 for examples) and is beyond the scope of this chapter, but the choices we make in our research practice reflect our own and others' views of how knowledge is generated, the nature of knowledge and the power dimensions of knowledge and research:

> If the fundamental purpose of social welfare is the pursuit of justice and equality, then practitioners have a professional responsibility to be alert to the ways in which power operates through ways of knowing. To be in a position to understand and name the needs and problems that others experience is to be powerful. To be in a position where others accord you the right to know and give credibility to your understandings, is also powerful. (Everitt et al., 1992: 17)

Social work researchers are no less bound to the ethics and values of the profession than practitioners and must demonstrate their understanding of these issues when they make explicit their methodological choices and follow through to select methods for the collection and analysis of information. Recent developments in the study of knowledge and its creation have highlighted the political nature of knowledge, its creation and its uses, and have, in particular, emphasised the importance of experience in relation to knowledge. Social work research has contributed to the growth in perspectives that privilege experience as a form of knowledge and value the voices of service users and experts by experience, as well as practitioners. Through this work we have come to understand that the world is shaped by multiple perspectives, often competing or conflicting, and that the social work task places us under an imperative to make sure that the voices and needs of those who are disadvantaged or marginalised within an increasingly fragmented and unequal society are heard and have influence on the policies and practices that shape everyday living:

> It is necessary for the researcher to make explicit his or her intellectual and ethical assumptions in justifying the methods as a way of demonstrating methodological rigour. We also emphasise the importance of reflexive and reflective practice in social work research to ensure that both paradigm and method are linked to account for the political and ethical dimensions in achieving social change. (D'Cruz and Jones, 2004: 57)

The challenge of social work researching means facing these methodological hurdles head on and creating a good fit between the research question and methodological stance the researcher occupies, leading to a clear exposition and justification of the methods chosen. To do this requires conscious effort on the part of researchers to identify their own world views and assumptions about how the world operates and the pervasive (but sometimes unrecognised) influence this can have on the research methods chosen and perhaps even the way that the research question is formed or constructed. As we shall see later in this chapter, critical reflection and reflexivity are important for research to be seen as rigorous and for releasing its transformatory potential.

Experiencing and practising research

It is only through doing research, through experiencing the process, that the potential personal growth opportunities become apparent and can be perceived by those involved and engaged in the quest for new knowledge. Of course, not all research activity (or all researchers) leads to change and transformation all of the time; nevertheless, these opportunities for growth do seem to present themselves and in this section I want to tease out what it is about researching that brings together certain key ingredients that might offer these possibilities. What happens on the research journey that enables those involved to take advantage of the situation? What is it about the practices they are carrying out that provide the circumstances and environment to enable researchers to grow? I will reflect on my own experiences in practising research and will also draw on the experiences of colleagues and students who I have supervised over a number of years, whose feedback has prompted my thinking and exploration of this subject. This is not empirical evidence, in the sense that data have been purposefully collected and analysed – indeed, some might be critical and consider these reflections anecdotal – but I hope they will be accepted in the spirit of exploration, where this chapter can be recognised as a preliminary stage that, of course, should be followed up using more empirical methods. I chose to use this 'anecdotal' evidence because this is what has sparked my own curiosity, very important in research practice, and encouraged me to investigate further and discover how little is written about the subjective experiences of doing research, let alone the positive effects that such activities might exhibit, in terms of the personal and professional growth of those involved. I offer this to readers in the hope of bringing the notion of transformative possibilities in social work research activity to wider attention.

So what do I mean exactly when I speak of the transformatory potential within research activities and processes? The first essential attribute for anyone engaging in research is curiosity, the desire or need to know something and to begin by admitting and accepting that one does not know. To be curious is to acknowledge a gap in knowledge and to be motivated to fill that gap, so that when we decide to research something, our approach should be open and inquiring and accepting of the deficit in our knowledge. This stance is essential to research that has the potential to be a transformatory experience for the researcher and possibly for others when they share this curiosity. In my own work I have conducted research that has been founded on just such curiosity, and equally premised by acknowledging that I did not have the answers and must do something to acquire them. Research that is self-initiated in this way almost always represents a personal quest for new information or knowledge and also a journey of 'finding out', of discovery and self-learning. There are other ways in which research might be initiated that are much more pragmatic and grounded in our responsibilities and practices as social workers and academics, where the need for research arises from practical issues (or role demands), where the question may already have been shaped and defined, as perhaps are the methods and the final purpose of any research endeavour. If we approach these more mundane activities with the same openness and drive to 'find out', we can often replicate the conditions within which change and possibly transformation of ourselves might still occur. Approaching areas of our knowledge with which we are familiar and apply frequently with an open mind can, in fact, produce the strongest personal challenges to our view of the world and can destabilise our certainties and existing ways of working and being:

> The process of researching is one of questioning, of generating and being open to evidence. It is about teasing out values and theoretical assumptions with a preparedness to engage in debate with those who may interpret the evidence differently. It contrasts with polemic, rhetoric and common sense. It disrupts routine and procedure. (Everitt, 1998: 107)

For example, as part of my doctoral research, I chose to study the childcare system and the experience of being in care. At the start of my research, I had been employed as a social worker in various roles for a number of years, mostly connected with children in care. One of the major personal challenges of this research was the need to articulate and actively critique what I thought I knew about being in care, which included a whole range of theoretical perspectives (for example attachment theories), policies and practices that I had internalised and taken for granted as a practitioner and manager in children's services for some years. Approaching these knowledge claims from a different perspective, that of a researcher committed to voicing the experiences of women who had been in care, provided a strong shift in my focus and enabled me to realise that knowledge is created and applied within specific historical, social and political contexts, which shape how knowledge is used and interpreted for practice. This was potentially a 'transforming moment', in the sense that the data collected from the women I interviewed conflicted with the theories and ideas – or at least, the way they had been applied in these circumstances – I had used and valued as powerful assessment tools for many years as a practitioner. I became intensely aware of the power they held in social work to mould and shape people's lives and actions, in contrast to the lack of power that the participants in my research possessed in terms of influencing 'knowledge'. The decision to privilege their knowledge on the basis of the experiences and expert status of the participants and to use this new perspective to critique the use of concepts and theories in this way was an ethical one. It was based on an understanding of how certain 'knowledges' (theories, ideas) had been used to make sense of the phenomenon of being a child, being female and being in care and to control and shape the lives of those who interacted with social work and particularly the care system at that time. This learning from my research activities brought about a shift in the way I understood the use of theories in social work and, importantly, how I had applied them in my practice as a social worker and in my teaching as a social work educator, which, in turn, changed how I perceived many areas of my life, professionally and personally.

The research provided the opportunity to become open to new and possibly conflicting ideas, but the most beneficial aspect was in removing me from the comfort zone of social work practice and in taking on a new role as a novice researcher. Recognising this new role placed me in a different location in relation to the information I received and also the body of knowledge that had been internalised as a practitioner. As a novice in this role, I felt obliged to accept that I did not 'know' and this sensitised me to the issues surrounding knowledge and its generation and made me vigilant in terms of ensuring that the claims I made about what I had found were clearly and robustly substantiated. This heightened sensitivity provided the motivation for a level and depth of questioning and analysis, including of myself as the researcher, that I had not encountered in such a way before, and accepting the challenges led to the transformatory potential being experienced. It goes without saying that this experience, the meaning and sense I made of it at the time, cannot be repeated because it was of its time and context. The research practice changed my views and ways of working (for the better, I would hope) in a transformatory way, that is, following this experience, it was impossible to revert back to the understandings of the world that I had had before I embarked on the research journey. While acknowledging therefore that we can never experience the same event or situation in the same way again because the person experiencing is changed, possibly transformed, by it, I have adopted ways of working that restore the sense of not knowing, of seeing things as if 'for the first time', and challenging the taken-for-granted aspects. I have learned that this frame of mind can be applied across the spectrum of my professional activities (and sometimes to my personal life) in beneficial ways, because it makes visible the judgements I make and demands that I analyse and reflect on them and thus become much more self-conscious and aware of my learning and the changes that emerge:

> From the reflexivity tradition, critical reflection might be seen as a way of researching personal practice or experience in order to develop our understanding of ourselves as knowers – this helps us to make the connections between ourselves as individuals and our broader social, cultural and structural environment. (Fook, 2004: 19)

Other colleagues have reported similar challenges from their research practices and I am aware that the students I have supervised over the years have also reported moments in the research process when the certainty of the social world they occupy has been strongly challenged by the information they have received or collected.

CASE EXAMPLE

Many years ago, I supervised a student, a team manager for a fostering team, undertaking a dissertation at MA level, who found that the dialogue his research allowed with foster carers challenged his assumptions about the nature of the work they did and the forms of knowledge that informed what they did. The decision to reflect on his own practice in managing services and people from what he felt was a false premise led him, initially, into what could be described as a 'crisis of confidence' in his role. It destabilised his former grip on his professional world and threatened his sense of professional identity. Choosing to follow through the implications of his new-found knowledge is what made this experience of the research process a transformational one for him, because he chose to critically reflect and integrate this new knowledge rather than reject it or confine its relevance to the topic. In reflecting, he was able to recognise that his motivation for conducting the study had been to know more about the experiences of caring for children from the perspective of foster carers and that in acknowledging this, he was accepting that his existing knowledge would be both added to and challenged. In his view, the crucial stance to occupy was one of being sensitised to new knowledge, being open to new ideas and understanding, and focusing this attention on an area of activity that he had been deeply enmeshed in for some years.

This reflects what Reissman (1994: 135) refers to as 'the outsider within', where making explicit one's own positioning in relation to one's research activities allows for a different perspective or focus in the research:

> Research is essentially all about seeing the world in fresh ways, about searching again, or re-searching the same territory and seeing it in a different light. (Darlington and Scott, 2002: 20)

Curiosity alone is clearly insufficient in terms of producing high-quality research, let alone for creating the conditions for research practice to have personal transformatory potential for those who embark on the research process. In this example, as in my own experiences, the researcher's initial curiosity, coupled with an open mind and an ability to be critically reflective and reflexive, meant that the research practices revealed their transformational potential. The fostering manager was able to turn this new knowledge back onto his own situation and challenge the existing discourses about managing such services within his dissertation and, indeed, within his role as a social work manager.

Transformation, then, seems to take place within the research milieu when curiosity can be combined with other key social work attributes, for example reflective practice, that are more readily found in the literature on social work practice, rather than in research texts. I have chosen therefore to go right back to some basic definitions so that I can understand how these terms are contextualised within research practice in social work. What does 'transformation' mean in this context and what role do critical reflection and reflexivity play in harnessing these opportunities for growth within research practice?

The concept of transformation

A dictionary definition of transformation from the online *Compact Oxford English Dictionary* defines transformation as 'a marked change in nature, form, or appearance', but it is necessary to adapt this to the current context, where what is being considered is the person, the 'self' who interacts with others and with the social world they occupy. This definition, therefore, does not do justice to a view of transformation as the essential quality of a human experience that leads to change which is permanent and irreversible. Consequently, in this context, I would see a transformatory experience as one that leads to change from which there is no going back: following such an experience, it is impossible to return to the self that was there before the experience and revert to the knowledge one had then. This experience literally changes the way one views the world and also the way one engages with the world, and changes the individual at a personal level, not just professionally. This wider interpretation has roots in psychoanalytic and philosophical/religious thinking, for example in Buddhism, and is aligned to a model of human development that sees the individual as in a state of continuous growth and learning, and life as a process of finding meaning and making sense of experience.

Critical reflection and transformation

The notions of transformation and transformatory learning have been around in the fields of nursing (Rolfe et al., 2001; Johns and Freshwater, 2005) and education (Mezirow, 1991; Crowther and Sutherland, 2005) for quite some time and are built on an understanding of critical reflection in practice settings (Schön, 1983; also see Gould and Taylor, 1996 for a social work perspective). The concept relates to the idea that personal growth and transformation can be nurtured through certain learning experiences, and that critical reflection – an activity that can also foster change or trans-formation at a personal level in the individual – is key to that learning. Of course, the main focus on critical reflection has been on promoting professional competence and skills, but the boundaries between the professional and the personal are fluid and not so clearly demarcated in roles that are concerned with working with people and where one of the principal tools used in supporting others and creating change is the 'self'. This requires more than just the critical appraisal of practice in a superficial sense and demands of practitioners that they are aware of their impact on others, their presenta-tion. They must also possess an acute awareness of the way their role is shaped by a variety of influences, including government and agency/organisational policy, and issues of care and control and social work values and ethics. It is at this boundary between the personal and the professional that the possibility of transformation exists and is made accessible through the processes of critical reflection and reflexivity. Jan Fook has given a clear exposition of these terms and the various ways they have been applied in a variety of disciplines and states that:

> Reflexivity involves the ability to recognise that all aspects of ourselves and our contexts influence the way that we research (or create knowledge). (Fook, 2004: 18)

These concepts are not usually associated with research and are not particularly evident in accounts of research practice, but it would be interesting to investigate this further and consider the 'doing' of research, that is, the subjective experience of being a researcher within a professional and disciplinary context that requires practitioners to be reflective and self-aware. Viewing the research process as interactive, weaving in and out of prac-tice and the subjective experiences of the researcher (and research participants), allows for possibilities for change outside the bubble of research activity and challenges the notion of research being a sealed off, separated world. Of course, research undertaken while studying for an MA or PhD might carry with it expectations of learning and the promotion of self-knowledge and growth and would also provide the supervision and support to enable the personal and professional challenges to be faced and tackled. Nevertheless, the advantages of viewing the world as if 'for the first time', combined with the ability and motivation for critical reflection are the essential and indispensable components necessary for transformatory research practice throughout academic or practice pathways. Paying attention to the sensitising effects of engaging in research in critically reflective ways has benefits for the outcomes of research and its impact on policy and practice, as well as for the individual researcher. It demands a deeper engagement between the researcher and the conceptual and ethical frameworks for social work research and can thereby strengthen the quality and rigour of our research.

Critical reflection revealed in a research account can add to, rather than detract from, the strength and authenticity of the research and this tends to shine through when the research is disseminated. Conference papers and journal articles – the traditional primary channels for the dissemination of research – tend to be more evocative and influential if they have been written not just by an 'expert' but include evidence of critical engagement with the context for the research and reflection of the researcher's ongoing dialogue with the subject or topic under investigation. In qualitative research accounts, the subjective thoughts and actions of the researcher are much more common and expected as part of the process of revealing 'the workings' (Holliday, 2002: 47) and enhancing the rigour of their research. It makes considerable demands on researchers to identify and justify the methodological and conceptual frameworks through which they view the research question and contextualise the methods chosen for the collection and analysis of data. Revealing these deliberations is the first stage in critically reflecting on the decisions one makes throughout the research process, and therefore releasing the transformatory potential of these activities, and should be adopted for all research activities for social work, not just those that fit the qualitative paradigm:

> Researchers bring their histories, biographies and subjectivities into every stage of the research process, and this influences the questions they ask, how they ask them and the ways in which they try to find answers. The subjectivity of the researcher should not be seen as a regrettable intrusion, but as a factor in the interactions of doing research. (Humphries and Martin, 2000: 79)

Critical reflection is not just the ability to be aware of our actions or decisions and look back on them after the event to identify the lessons that might be learned for the future. It is an active, fluid and ongoing process of understanding and being sensitive to the world around us and the tasks we might be completing. It is also about viewing ourselves and our work as if for the first time and giving this the level of attention that the new and exciting might demand of us. This 'making the familiar strange' (Holliday, 2002: 93) is what allows critical reflection to be used as a transformatory tool in both practice and research in social work. This is, however, not a neutral stance but one in which the researcher or practitioner is aware of their partial gaze and can identify the familiar and taken for granted and also be aware of other views and lenses through which the situation or task might be viewed or perceived. We need these skills not just to be reflective practitioners (and researchers) in everyday practice, but in order to critique the knowledge base informing practice and make sound decisions in a world of constant change, shifting perspectives and imperatives and relational working:

> If we are to encourage on the part of practitioners 'wise judgement under conditions of uncertainty' ... process knowledge and an ability to analyse practice may be equally or more important that the dissemination of formal knowledge. (Taylor and White, 2006: 948)

Taylor and White are clearly talking about social work education here but I would contend that social work research (and practice) also demand 'wise judgement', which can be best achieved through active critical reflection on the part of the researcher.

Conclusion

It will be clear from what I have said that I am an advocate for research activity that is meaningful and demands the same level of commitment to social justice and reflective practice that any other social work practice might. I have tried to identify clear benefits from approaching research practice in this way and would emphasise that the impact on the individual who researches in this way can be potentially transformative, not just for practice and knowledge production, but for themselves as individuals. Although it is clearly acknowledged that social work interventions can transform the lives and experiences of individuals, groups, families and communities, we rarely actively pursue the potential for change that research practices might offer, indeed, we shy away from discussing and debating the untidy and the subjective from our accounts in our striving to be objective, rational and 'scientific'. It is within these experiences and processes that the transformatory potential of research is revealed and it is only through the critical reflection and analysis of these experiences and their meanings that transformatory possibilities can be realised, not just for researchers but also for the participants and perhaps even those who read research reports and publications. By taking a more collaborative stance in research activities, not only do we extend these opportunities to a wider group but the active working together provides heightened critical reflection from a more diverse range of people.

In addition to this, I believe that social work has a clear duty to investigate issues of oppression and power, and within this, research activities and knowledge creation are not immune to power issues and dynamics. The critical consideration of these important ethical questions should be integral to good research practice. Social work has long been recognised as a political activity (Parton, 2000; Jordan and Jordan, 2000; Butler and Pugh, 2004), and it cannot avoid its responsibilities in respect of social justice in any area of activity, whether that be research or practice. To be effective, both must address issues of power and this applies equally to ourselves as individuals as to the profession or organisation to which we might belong. Critical reflection needs to be an integral part of how we conduct research for social work and we should reflect on the uses to which our findings might be applied.

As a work in progress, this chapter has encouraged me to think more widely than the impact on the research and to speculate that research practices that enable transformation might also have unsung benefits for those on the receiving end of our research. Using participatory and emancipatory methodologies allows the participants to have a much greater influence on the research process throughout and also on the research agendas, which so often are controlled not by social workers or service users but by others with a political motivation in mind. Participatory approaches also stimulate debate and communication, which, in turn, might intensify and deepen our critical reflection and thereby promote a transformatory environment for all involved, not just researchers.

So we must foster a culture of high-level critical reflection of our actions and our subjective responses throughout the research journey, from initial curiosity through to more imaginative and evocative ways of spreading the messages from research. We need to take advantage of the opportunities for transformatory practices within research and in engaging more closely with stakeholders in order to fulfil the social justice mandate we have for promoting a fairer, more egalitarian society. Transforming society and enabling individuals to fulfil their potential need transformatory social work to create the changes from which there will be no going back.

For further discussion of aspects of working with service users, see Adams et al., 2009a, Chapter 15.

D'Cruz, H. and Jones, M. (2004) *Social Work Research: Ethical and Political Contexts*, London, Sage. Explains the methodological issues and their relevance and draws links between practice and research.

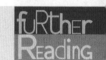

Fook, J. (1998) *The Reflective Researcher: Social Workers' Theories of Practice Research*, Sydney, Allen & Unwin. Excellent introduction to the use of reflection in research and practice for social work.

Johns, C. and Freshwater, D. (2005) *Transforming Nursing Through Reflective Practice*, 2nd edn, London, Blackwell. Nursing text but a good introduction to the notion of transformation in professional and caring practice.

24 Evaluating practice

Chapter overview

This chapter explores the practice of evaluation and how this relates to social work practice. The complex relationship between evidence and practice is explored. The author makes suggestions for good practice in relation to evaluation and the dissemination of findings. He concludes by proposing a model that relates evidence to practice and policy.

This chapter examines the problematic relationship between two forms of practice – social work practice and the practice of evaluation. The aim of the chapter is to explore the nature of this relationship and to suggest approaches to evaluation that maximise the relevance of evaluation as a practice for social work. The focus of the chapter is on evaluation, as opposed to research. By evaluation, we are referring to evaluation that aims to assess the effectiveness of interventions in terms of their aims and objectives – such evaluation can be undertaken by project workers, service users or external evaluators. Drawing on the author's practice, as a fieldworker, policy maker and evaluator, this chapter begins by confirming that evaluation is a form of practice, examines some issues, tensions and controversies involved in the evaluation process, and tentatively suggests a form of evaluative practice that addresses some of these difficulties.

Evaluation as a form of practice

A commitment to evaluation as a form of practice is central to the development of a critical perspective on social care initiatives. There is a danger that evaluation can be seen as a purely technical enterprise – the application of value-free 'instruments' that in some straightforward manner measure 'outcomes'. However, it is argued here that the evaluator necessarily has a value commitment to change within the project or topic with which they are working. Evaluators, be they internal or external, will bring with them values about, for example, listening to people and utilising findings as part of the change process. Evaluation is therefore at heart an ethical and value-driven process. It will challenge the practitioner who wishes to engage critically with their own practice.

The practice of evaluation 'has grown massively in recent years' (Pawson and Tilley, 1997: 1). Funders have become more demanding in requiring independent evidence of the outcomes of projects they fund:

> " The demand for social workers and their managers to identify the effectiveness of their work is now very great. (Cheetham et al., 1992: 3) "

Extensive evaluation programmes have been put in place in relation to a number of government policy strategies, including, for example, Sure Start and the various Youth Justice Board initiatives. These policy initiatives often involve specific individual project evaluations and overall national evaluations.

Additionally, there has been a stronger emphasis on the dissemination of findings. This sometimes takes an institutional form, involving the establishment of organisations such as Research in Practice (www.rip.org.uk). A related development has been the growth of publications promoting evaluative evidence as central to practice and professional development. A successful and extensive example of this is the Barnardo's 'What Works' series (see, for example, Stein, 1997). There can be little doubt that evaluation as a practice has grown and developed in recent years. Social workers and related practitioners are likely to have their practice evaluated at some time during their career, academics are likely to be approached about undertaking evaluations, and practitioners will be expected to evaluate their own practice as a continuing process, and to involve service users in this process.

Issues, tensions and controversies

In 1975, Stan Cohen wrote a chapter entitled 'It's all right for you to talk', in which he analysed some of the tensions between social work practice and practices whose primary aim is the production and dissemination of knowledge. In his title, Cohen (1975) neatly summarises the reservations that social workers may have about the research and evaluation community. Frontline practitioners and policy makers may question whether evaluators can grasp the complexity and shifting nature of the real world. More concretely, in the contemporary environment of a culture of targets and inspections, social workers may be concerned about the outcomes of an evaluation. Could it lead to the closure of a project, changes to existing practice, or criticism from management?

External evaluators will share some of these concerns and have some of their own. Will they be allowed unfettered access to the data? Is the evaluation budget sufficient for the task that needs to be undertaken? Are the methods robust enough for the task? Will the report gather dust once produced, rather than being a real contribution to the development of policy and practice?

Before moving on to examine creative approaches to evaluation, first we examine the underlying causes of some of the tensions and problems involved in evaluation. We need to be aware of the complex and inherently problematic relationship between practice and evidence. Three specific underlying issues will be addressed:

- the challenge of methods
- the application of evidence to practice
- the relationship between evidence and service users.

The challenge of methods

It is important to recognise that, as Trinder (1996: 233) suggests, 'the future direction of social work research is contested'. There is a great diversity of possible evaluative methods available and, within the research community, there are differences and controversies, sometimes referred to as the 'paradigm wars'. Some would argue that the randomised controlled trial (RCT) should set the 'gold standard' (Macdonald, 1996), while others would argue that the theoretical basis of RCTs is flawed (Pawson and Tilley, 1997). Some would advocate 'action research', quantitative, single case or ethnographic methods, for example. Others would propose solving these dilemmas by suggesting that an eclectic approach to methodology has much to recommend it (see Fuller, 1996).

The question of methods, then, is a controversial one: different methods will uncover different forms of evidence and analysis will interpret them differently. It is argued here that this debate should be exactly that – an open debate. It is not helpful to exercise some form of closure – to propose in an unproblematic way that some method should be privileged over another. Knowledge is not static and is enhanced through debate and critique. Later in the chapter, it will be argued that methods have to address the issues of relevance and 'fit' with the project that is being evaluated. This can be managed through the formation of advisory groups that include a range of stakeholders (see Frost and Ryden, 2001).

The application of evidence to practice

Let us, for the sake of argument, accept that evaluators are able to gather robust and reliable evidence. Even if this were possible, there remains a problematic relationship between the evidence gathered and social work practice. Pawson and Tilley (1997) argue convincingly that evidence tends to be situational and we should be wary of transferability. For example, much has been made of the Head Start projects in the US. While the evidence can be seen as 'rigorous', the transfer to a different context such as the UK or to a different time is problematic. One might be able to produce rigorous evidence on a given topic in year X but, inevitably, given the pace of legislative, policy and social change, the context for this work will change, quickly and sometimes fundamentally, year by year.

Thus, even if we could agree the basis for collecting evidence, we need to examine in detail its application to practice – without assuming that evidence can be transferred to instructing social work practice in some unproblematic way. To give a concrete example, children looked after by relatives generally do better than children looked after by foster carers they have never met before (Nixon, 2008). This seems to be a perfectly acceptable and unproblematic finding. However, how can we translate this into practice? All we can say is that, in general, a child is likely to do better if placed with a relative than another foster carer. It does not mean that placement of a particular child with their grandmother will necessarily be successful, or even generally better than placement with another foster carer. Thus, while the evaluative knowledge is contextual and informative for policy, it cannot be determinative of practice in given concrete situations.

A second problem in the application of evidence to practice is presented by the considerable volume of evaluation and research findings in circulation. The welcome expansion of the internet has given us easy access to a wide range of information. But this can also be overwhelming – we are always aware that we cannot be familiar with all the relevant literature. A Google search on family support, for example, generates over 77 million hits.

A third area for concern is that the pleas for practitioners to apply research and evaluation findings in practice should not undermine the role of 'tacit' knowledge. Educational theorists have identified knowledge as 'codified' (explicit) and 'tacit' (implicit) (see Polanyi, 1983). Codified knowledge is that which is written down, can be taught and assessed. In contrast, tacit knowledge is that which we pick up from doing the job, and is more difficult to communicate.

Let us take an example of a social work team leader who chaired the team meeting last week. She has 'tacitly' picked up that the team seem to be unmotivated and generally uninterested by the meeting. She makes a mental note to be more upbeat next week – perhaps to start and end the meeting on a positive note. While there may be some professional guidance on chairing meetings and some limited research, this is an example that relies on tacit knowledge, which is crucial to professional competence. Even if the topic has been extensively researched, the knowledge is clearly situational and specific. There remains a crucial role for 'tacit' knowledge (Anning et al., 2006).

The controversial nature of the debate is illustrated by the following two quotes. The first is from the Government Chief Social Researcher's Office (GCSRO, 2003: 3):

> The Government's commitment to evidence-based policy is matched by its drive to develop excellence in Government research and evaluation.

Contrast this with Sir Michael Rutter's (2007: 207) concluding comment in *The National Evaluation of Sure Start*:

> I am forced to admit that I doubt that [the government] has the slightest interest in research evidence when dealing with its own policies.

The contrast could hardly be clearer.

The relationship between evidence and service users

Adherents of evidence-led practice argue that social work practice should be led by rigorous evidence. For example, Newman et al. (1996) argue that:

> Practitioners who adopt a particular approach must be able to describe what evidence has led them to do, what the intended outcomes will be and what the probability is of such outcomes occurring.

While it might be that evidence-based practice (EBP) is applicable in technical areas such as engineering and medicine, it is more difficult in social work because of its human and relational nature. Social work is fundamentally about recognising human subjectivity and responding with some form of partnership and cooperation with the service user. Thus, most forms of practice need to be actually negotiated and agreed. Relationships are the key to social work practice – relationships that cannot be reduced by a formulaic 'evidence-based approach'. Even if in theory the evaluator and the practitioner 'know' that approach X is 'what works', the service user may not wish to cooperate and might indeed prefer Y as a form of intervention. This is the very complexity of social work – negotiation, conflict and compromise. It the human and relational nature of social work that makes the relationship between practice and evidence a complex and problematic one (Parton and O'Byrne, 2000).

It can be argued that a dogmatic adherence to EBP immediately dismantles the possibility of any partnership approach to working with service users: if I, as a professional, possess the evidence, then I have no choice but to implement it, even if you, as a service user, disagree. Thus the claim made by Newman et al. (1996) is spurious, when they argue that professionals have a duty to base their work with 'the poor' on evidence and that a failure to do this is a breach of trust. If we do indeed base all our practice on 'evidence', then by default, any room for negotiation, partnership and compromise with the service user is lost.

Indeed, the proponents of evidence-led practice tend to privilege RCTs (Macdonald, 1996), which by definition tend to exclude any user involvement in the research and evaluation process. In RCTs, the research subjects are allocated as recipients or non-recipients of the service to be evaluated and therefore excluded from full knowledge of and participation in the evaluative process. This can be contrasted to more inclusive forms of research and evaluation, which tend to be more qualitative in nature (Cree and Davis, 2007). In such research, the views and perspectives of the service user are privileged over researcher-imposed 'outcomes'.

Thus far we have identified three main problems in the relationship between evidence and social work practice. In summary, these are that:

- there is no universally agreed evaluative methodology
- there is no straightforward manner of applying evidence to practice
- there is an uneasy relationship between the application of evidence and working in partnership with service users.

Having recognised these problems, and having provided a critique of those who would see the evidence and practice relationship as more one dimensional, the chapter now goes on to examine a basis for establishing a positive, but critical, relationship between evaluation practice and social work practice.

A creative evaluation practice?

What might a creative approach to evaluation practice look like? Before concluding with a proposed model for the use of evaluation in social work and social care, we examine some of the micro-aspects of evaluation practice. The connecting thread is that power and knowledge should be shared between evaluators, managers, practitioners and service users, with the aim that evaluation becomes an empowering tool for change.

Spencer et al. (2003) identify the following four guiding principles for quality evaluation, that it should be:

- *contributory* – in advancing wider knowledge or understanding ...
- *defensible in design* – by providing a research strategy that can address the evaluation questions posed
- *rigorous in conduct* – through the systematic and transparent collection, analysis and interpretation of qualitative data
- *credible in claims* – through offering well-founded and plausible arguments about the significance of the data generated.

Establishing the task

Evaluation practice can only be as good as the task that has been agreed and established, thus agreeing exactly what the task is forms an important stage of the evaluation process. What is the context of the evaluation? How is it funded? Whose idea was it? What methods will be needed? Who will be involved in any steering group? And so on. Some of these are detailed and even mundane questions but they are crucial to the success of an evaluation.

It is possible for an entire evaluation to founder following a failure to address a question of detail. Take, for example, the issue of confidentiality. Let us say that the evaluators wish to undertake a postal survey of service users. Should service users' addresses be given to the evaluators? Should service users' permission be gained in advance? These are small but fundamental points – one mistake here and the credibility of the entire evaluation project could be undermined. Successful evaluation involves the detailed negotiation of ways of working, drawing on the expertise of the evaluator, the practitioners and, wherever possible, the service users.

Clear and regular liaison

As part of the process of clearly establishing the task, it is necessary to set up clear and regular points of liaison for the evaluation process. If power is to be shared, this involves sharing information and decision-making on a regular basis. There are a number of reasons for ensuring effective liaison:

- To help in the commitment of the organisation, its practitioners and service users to the evaluative process.

- To enable discussion of any changes to the evaluation methods or within the organisation. Inevitably, the detail of the evaluation process will change over time. Rarely is an evaluation plan delivered as initially envisaged.
- To allow the evaluator to check the micro-aspects of the evaluation process with the various stakeholders. As we have argued above, in evaluation practice, seemingly technical questions – such as when a set of interviews should take place – involve a series of complex issues in relation to timing, place, confidentiality and so on.

Effective liaison is central to sharing power in the evaluation process. Evaluation should not be seen simply as an 'expert-led' process; rather, evaluation can be undertaken by staff or service users – all will require support and training. Evaluation issues can be discussed in advisory groups, which are one form of empowering service users and other stakeholders.

Adopting methods appropriate to the organisation

As we have seen, there is a range of evaluative methods that may be adopted. It is important in any empowering approach to evaluation that the methods utilised are appropriate to the organisation. This issue has two specific dimensions:

1 The methods adopted in any study must be consistent with the value base of the organisation. For example, where an organisation holds partnership with service users as a central value, it would be inconsistent, to say the least, if the evaluation methods did not fully involve service users in the design, execution, writing up and dissemination of the evaluation.

2 The methods need to be appropriate to the organisation – in the technical, methodological sense. To take an obvious example, adopting largely quantitative methods in a small-scale organisation, with an emphasis, say, on counselling, would clearly be inappropriate.

Implicitly, this is an unapologetically eclectic, multi-method stance. The methods should be suitable to the nature of the organisation and the specific expectations of the evaluation. The methodological debate should be open and not closed, dynamic and not fixed. Indeed, many of the best evaluative studies will involve a variety of methods, such as surveys and questionnaires, face-to-face interviews, observation of practice, documentary study and so on (Spencer et al., 2003). Qualitative data, such as users' perspectives on the service, can often be supplemented by quantitative data such as statistics outlining the frequency a service is used.

Involving stakeholders

A creative approach to evaluation has to avoid assuming that the evaluator is the holder of some magical key that will unlock the 'truth'. The traditional 'expert' model would hold that the evaluator has a privileged position in relation to 'knowledge'. An alternative model would rather emphasise a process of evaluation that is empowering – it shares knowledge and expertise, and mobilises, for example, practitioners' and service users' perspectives on how the project works. Pawson and Tilley (1997: 160–1) identify distinctive roles in evaluation for the different participants:

- *Subjects or service users* 'are likely to be far more sensitized to the mechanisms in operation within a program'. These can be uncovered using in-depth, face-to-face interviews or through focus groups.
- *Practitioners* 'translate program theories into practice and so are to be considered the great "utility players" in the information game'. They can act as partners in the process or as self-evaluators.
- *Evaluators* 'carry theories into the encounter with the program'.

Each party to an evaluation then has a valuable and clear role. Moreover, effective evaluation can be carried out as part of an ongoing quality enhancement mechanism by staff, which is part of developing a continuous critical reflection on practice. Evaluation then becomes an element of practice in the same way that counselling or campaigning is seen as a form of practice.

Examples of methods of evaluation in practice

Evaluations of practice typically take place in settings somewhat constrained by the requirements of managers and other practitioners, who seek fairly urgent answers to questions about the usefulness and effectiveness of particular initiatives. These pressures tend to shape and limit the methods of evaluation that are commonly adopted. We can list these methods in an abstract way, or categorise them according to their applications. The following are examples of applications of different methods of evaluation:

- *Interview-based survey of group members' views:* this may be used where we require a small-scale snapshot of people's perceptions at a point in time
- *Questionnaire-based survey of service users' views:* this could be the chosen method where a fairly detailed profile is required, for example of the views of older people in a locality concerning local services
- *Outcome-based critical appraisal:* focus groups or in-depth individual interviews, or both, may be used to gather the views of people about the outcomes of a particular intervention or initiative
- *Observation-based evaluation of a service:* a service user-led or carer-led group may gather information from members placed in key vantage points, from which they can observe the way people are treated in a social work setting.

Dissemination

Of course, the evaluation process does not finish with the production of a 'report'. The dissemination process is essential and needs to build on the model outlined above, with all parties being involved. As Trinder (1996: 238) argues, dissemination is itself 'a political process'. Dissemination is about sharing knowledge and using information as part of a change process. Effective evaluation findings should be fed into a process by which current policy and practice are critically reflected upon. This is a cyclical process of 'critical reflection', and is an important aspect of being a 'reflective practitioner' (see Payne, 1998: 119–37). Imaginative methods of feedback need to be adopted. An evaluation in which the author was involved was disseminated as part of a 'fun day' involving jugglers and other entertainment (Frost and Ryden, 2001). (www.evaluation.org.uk/resources/guidelines.aspx)

In summary, the UK Evaluation Society (www.evaluation.org.uk/resources/guidelines.aspx) provides the following helpful guidelines.

Evaluators need to:

- *be explicit* about the purpose, methods, intended outputs and outcomes of the evaluation; be mindful of unanticipated effects and be responsive to shifts in purpose
- *alert commissioners* to possible adjustments to the evaluation approach and practice; be open to dialogue throughout the process informing them of progress and developments
- *consider* whether it is helpful to build into the contract forms of external support or arbitration (should the need arise)
- *have preliminary discussion/s with commissioners* prior to agreeing a contract
- *adhere to the terms agreed in the contract* and consult with commissioners if there are significant changes required to the design or delivery of the evaluation
- *demonstrate the quality of the evaluation* to other parties through progress reports, for example on development and financial accountability, and adhere to quality assurance procedures as agreed in the contract
- *be aware of and make every attempt to minimise any potential harmful effects* of the evaluation prejudicing the status, position or careers of participants.

Evaluators also need to:

- *demonstrate* that the evaluation design and conduct are transparent and fit for purpose
- *demonstrate comprehensive and appropriate use of all the evidence* and that the evaluation conclusions can be traced to this evidence
- *work within the Data Protection Act* and have procedures which ensure the secure storage of data
- *acknowledge intellectual property* and the work of others
- *have contractual agreement over copyright* of evaluation methodology, findings, documents and publication
- *write and communicate evaluation findings* in accessible language
- *agree with commissioners from the outset about the nature of dissemination* in order to maximise the utility of the evaluation.

In practice, evaluators need to:

- *demonstrate a commitment to the integrity of the process* of evaluation and its purpose to increase learning in the public domain
- *be realistic about what is feasible* to achieve and their capacity to deliver within the timescale and budget agreed
- *know when to refuse or terminate* an evaluation contract because it is undoable, self-serving, or threatens to undermine the integrity of the process
- *be prepared to argue the case* for the public right to know in evaluation in specified contexts
- *treat all parties equally* in the process of the evaluation and the dissemination of findings.

Utilising and integrating evaluative evidence: the RIPE model

Thus far, we have established that the practice of evaluation has increased significantly in recent years. It has been argued that the relationship between evaluative evidence and social work practice is complex and problematic. Having recognised these issues, detailed practice issues arising from evaluation were discussed. We conclude by proposing a model that places the evidence generated by evaluation within a wider context.

This model can be given the acronym RIPE. It demonstrates that policy, practice and professional development are determined by the combined influences of research and evaluation findings (R), ideological positions (I), politics (P) and economics (E). These are now briefly examined in turn:

- *Research-based evidence and evaluation* were explored above. In the real world, direct links between evidence and practice are far from straightforward. In reality, evidence enters a melting pot with other influential factors such as ideologies, politics and economics.
- *Ideology* means the values and perspectives that social work practitioners use to guide and steer their practice.
- *Politics* refers to disputes over the distribution of power and decision-making. Politics – organisational, local and national – is evidently central to the policy-making process. But again, the relationship between evidence and politics is contested. Sometimes politicians will ignore even the most robust of evidence for political reasons, an often quoted example being former Home Secretary Michael Howard's view that 'prison works', despite evidence to the contrary (Pawson and Tilley, 1997). In other cases, there may be political reasons for publicising and emphasising a particular element of evidence.
- *Economics* is also crucial to this debate. For example, robust evidence may suggest a particular policy direction, for which resources are not made available. Equally, there may be economic reasons for hanging on to a practice that evidence has questioned.

The RIPE model is an attempt to recognise the complex interaction of factors that influence social work practice. The reality of social work practice is that there is a role for clear and well-disseminated research and evaluation findings, but that they have to exist in a world of competing ideologies, political conflict and economic possibility and restraints. This complex mix forms the context in which reflective social work practitioners and managers practise. The evaluator then becomes part of the change process, contributing from a committed perspective to the process of change.

Conclusion

This chapter has examined the role of evaluation and its complex link with social work practice. Having examined a number of problems, we have explored the elements of evaluation practice that enjoy a creative partnership with social work practice. We have concluded by proposing the RIPE model of policy and practice formation that takes the role of evaluation seriously, but which recognises that, in the real world of policy and practice formation, evaluation has to take its place alongside ideology, politics and economics.

For further discussion of aspects of evaluation in practice, see Adams et al., 2009a, Chapter 21.

www.evidencenetwork.org Comprehensive website providing a wide range of material reflecting on the relationship between evidence and policy. Publishes the useful journal, *Evidence and Policy*.

www.evaluation.org.uk Provides a network for evaluators providing materials and organising events and conferences.

www.europeanevaluation.org Provides a European perspective on the theory, practice and utilisation of evaluation findings.

www.ness.bbk.ac.uk The National Evaluation of Sure Start website provides a number of papers relating to the evaluation of the Sure Start initiative. The materials are relevant to all those with an interest in evaluation as they raise wider methodological issues.

Belsky, J., Barnes, J. and Melhuish, E. (2007) *The National Evaluation of Sure Start*, Bristol, Policy Press. High-profile evaluation in a British context of recent years. Includes Rutter's devastating critique of the design of Sure Start.

Pawson, R. and Tilley, N. (1997) *Realistic Evaluation*, London, Sage. Sophisticated guide to the theory and practice of evaluation.

Robson, C. (1993) *Real World Research: A Resource for Social Scientists and Practitioner-researchers*, Oxford, Blackwell. Probably now the standard text for practitioner research – practical guidance on issues such as designing surveys, analysing data and so on.

Shaw, I.F. (1999) *Qualitative Evaluation*, London, Sage. Wide-ranging and detailed discussion of qualitative methodology and methods.

Spencer, L., Ritchie, J., Lewis, J. and Dillon, L. (2003) *Quality in Qualitative Evaluation: A Framework for Assessing Research Evidence*, London, Cabinet Office. Guide to quality and the expectations of government in terms of qualitative research and evaluation.

Stein, M. (1997) *What Works in Leaving Care*, Barkingside, Barnardo's. Good example of the 'What Works' series; it includes some interesting reflections on the relationship between social work practice and research evidence.

25 Critical social work research

Chapter overview

This chapter argues for the maintenance of research in social work as a critical and potentially contentious activity, proactive rather than reactive, taking sides in an independent and professional way and challenging accepted ways of thinking rather than simply following up and evaluating accepted practice.

Introduction

Neither social work nor social research is a neutral activity. Like other social practices, they are both subject to external and internal forces. That they are unambiguously a 'good' cannot be taken for granted. Their contested nature is made clear by the statements, on the one hand, from the International Federation of Social Workers (IFSW, 2000) that social work 'addresses the barriers, inequalities and injustices that exist in society', and, on the other hand, by a UK government minister that social work 'is a very practical job ... not about being able to give a ... theoretical explanation of why [people] got into difficulties in the first place' (quoted in Horner, 2003: 2). Its history is illustrative of the struggles for dominance of different versions at different moments.

Similarly, social work research reflects contemporary views of what constitutes social problems, whose interests are met by these definitions and what are seen as the desirable outcomes of intervention. Arguments continue about the merits of various research paradigms or methods but, however it is viewed, social research is not an impersonal activity. It is imbued with the values of researchers, institutions and governments, and its processes and findings reflect those values. This can have profoundly conservative consequences, for example in reinforcing diagnoses of schizophrenia in young black men, or it can have radical potential, for example in opening to the public gaze the extent of sexual harassment at work, the widespread nature of domestic violence and abuse of children in the home. All research is political, engaged in a moral struggle about what is 'normal', what is 'truth', what is legitimate 'knowledge' and who can be validated as a 'knower'.

As with all social practices, social work research needs to be interrogated concerning its origins, its purposes and the ends for which it is intended. In considering social work futures, we need to recognise the struggles for meaning that are involved and their impact on service users and the nature of social work. This chapter is concerned to embrace the premise that social justice is an aim of social work, and that practitioners should be informed about all research that is value laden and able to pursue models that do not perpetuate the disadvantage experienced by poor and relatively powerless people. The profession is therefore obliged to strive for a research practice that takes account of its moral purpose to engage with oppressive structures and action to change them.

There is currently an unprecedented interest in 'research-based practice' and both central and local government, as well as social care agencies of all sorts, have an energetic concern to carry out research that will influence practice and demonstrate the relevance of research studies to their work. Such studies, because they represent particular interests, are as much a site of conflict as other social activities and are therefore to be approached with an attitude of critical, reflexive caution. Indeed, Butler (2003: 20) warns that 'accommodations' among the government, local authorities and those delivering services may operate to the detriment of service users.

An orthodoxy has developed within social work research that focuses on outcomes, and a 'what works' pragmatism characterises many contemporary studies (Humphries, 2008). This is based on the scientific (and political) assumption that 'a formal rationality of practice based on scientific methods can produce a more effective and economically accountable means of delivering social services' (Webb, 2001: 60). A research approach that is able to demonstrate its utility, practicality and reliability in providing clear solutions to 'real' problems is a particularly attractive prospect for governments and a way of achieving prestige and credibility for the profession. This positivist orientation – that the world is predictable, knowable and measurable, behaviour can be explained in causal, deterministic ways and knowledge arises out of experiments and observations using quantitative methods – has driven social work research towards an agenda that focuses on practical means to change behaviour in order to achieve social control. Indeed, the manipulation of human behaviour is an explicit aim of such research and outcomes are measured in terms of changes in behaviour. The evidence-based practice movement emerging from this philosophy is popular with governments and researchers because it offers definitive answers to social problems, it claims to discover 'what works'. There are, however, fundamental problems concerning 'objectivity', being 'value free' and 'neutral', to say nothing about the processes of inference that lead from evidence to explanation, which the evidence-based movement still has to confront.

This narrow perspective tends to ignore the context in which particular behaviours take place, ignoring questions about how the behaviour came to be constructed as a problem, what standards it is measured against and their legitimacy, what contextual factors contribute to it and what are its meanings to the people targeted for change? These questions have been marginalised in a climate where the emphasis is on the technical, 'checking evidence' approach and a preoccupation with cause and effect or cost-effectiveness. In this 'politics of enforcement' (Parton, 2000: 461) of a model of research obsessed with measurement, outcomes and targets, the question becomes, is there a place for research that takes account of moral considerations, takes sides, makes anti-oppressive ideals fundamental to the conception and design of studies in social work, and shifts these concerns from margin to centre?

Social research as a moral and political activity

Such questions identify social research as an explicitly moral and political activity. As Beresford and Evans (1999) point out, one of the consequences of the drive for an evidence base has been that social research in the late twentieth century shifted from a role in initiating policy developments to one of evaluating, monitoring and legitimating them. It now occupies a reactive position, emphasising the 'effectiveness, efficiency and economy of policy ... reflected in its increasing preoccupation with managerially and professionally defined outcomes and outcome measurement' (Beresford and Evans, 1999: 672). Any role examining policies themselves has been removed (see also Humphries, 2004b). This move betrays a moral and political conservatism in the profession and risks social work being robbed of its transformatory potential. The problem is with emphasis. The questions that affect research can never concern only 'what works?' Ethical research is concerned also with the conditions that lead to or hinder the self-realisation of individuals and social groups, and is based on an examination of the ways that power regulates material and ideological realities. It is engaged with human suffering and injustice, and one of its basic aims is to bring to public notice realities that were previously hidden and new perspectives on worlds that have been taken for granted.

What is needed is research that is contentious, that does not separate itself from a critique of social policies or social struggles but assumes a praxis – a unity of thought and action – that has at its heart changes in the lives of oppressed peoples and in the way they are treated within the social care system (see Hayes and Humphries, 1999). Butler (2003: 27) argues for the embracing of social work research as a 'value based, politically aware and engaged form of endeavour'. This may bring it into conflict with conventional expectations of the roles of social work and social research, but then the battle for social justice has to be what Butler (2003: 28) calls 'unbiddable'.

With such an approach comes a 'positioning' of the researcher to take sides and to reframe questions about knowledge and truth. 'Taking sides' does not mean an undiscriminating approach that supports individuals, groups or communities whether right or wrong, even if they are oppressed. We all have partial knowledge that, although crucial to our survival, sometimes excludes other people's truths, for example we may recognise disablism and be antagonistic to anti-racism, or be anti-racist and homophobic at the same time. These truths need to be taken as 'valid' but never left unproblematised. Taking sides involves a commitment not to factions, but to a particular set of values:

> Research that is concerned to expose and challenge inequalities is entirely compatible with these values. Research that attempts solely to measure the impact of interventions regardless of their relationship to the social context is not value free. Rather it has taken the side of whatever values have inspired the interventions it uncritically evaluates. (Humphries, 2004b: 114)

This process depends on researchers taking a position of conscious partiality (Mies, 1993) that recognises our limited understanding of the experiences of oppression of others, but requires us to take sides in the realities of vulnerability and marginalisation. This positioning involves an imaginative leap beyond common-sense assumptions to ask different questions and seek different answers, unsettle established practices and surprise ourselves with the discovery that there are alternatives after all.

Critical social research

Any approach that addresses the aims described above needs to have features that characterise it as critical. This is to say:

> At the heart of critical social research is the idea that knowledge is structured by existing sets of social relations. The aim of a critical methodology is to provide knowledge which engages the prevailing social structures. (Harvey, 1990: 2)

The features of critical social research are broadly that:

- It regards social structures as oppressive, maintained through political and economic power, and supported by a range of legitimating strategies
- It seeks to make these legitimations visible for examination and identify the oppressive and exploitative practices they underpin
- By focusing on specific social phenomena, it aims to get beyond taken-for-granted understandings, to their relationship to wider social and historical structures
- A legitimate target for analysis is the concepts that define an area of inquiry
- It goes beyond simply identifying oppressive structures towards seeking ways to combat, resist and change them
- The critical researcher is flexible enough to engage with these power dynamics in specific situations.

Critical research may be based on a range (or a combination) of epistemologies, such as some Marxisms, feminisms, anti-racism theories, and poststructuralist, disability, age-related and sexuality approaches. Methods might be both qualitative and quantitative. The key criterion is that they demonstrate the above features. Some writers have offered useful frameworks. Leonard (1997) drew together Marxist and feminist critiques as well as postmodern deconstruction. Soper (1993) attempted a similar project in her efforts to construct a principled position from which to evaluate social theory.

From margin to centre

Lorde (1984) created a framework for analysing class, 'race', gender, sexuality, age and disability. Her writing is an impulse towards wholeness, theorising out of her experiences as a black woman, lesbian, feminist, mother, daughter of immigrants, educator, cancer survivor and activist. This does not mean that authentic knowledge is the property only of those who have had similar experiences. Others may achieve partial identification with oppressed peoples, as discussed above. Lorde (1984: 112) asserts that 'the master's tools will never dismantle the master's house', meaning that those who are concerned to bring genuine changes to the lives of poor and exploited groups need to find new methods and new ways of thinking about social problems. If they are occupied by dominant interests, their energies will operate in a framework defined for them by others. Within social work – statutory, voluntary or private – it is impossible to avoid 'the master's interests', but even there it is possible perhaps to bring different tools to bear to define and examine them.

Some of these issues are also addressed by hooks (1984) through her analysis of the condition of black women and men in relation to their exploitation, and in the case of black women, their relationship to white feminism. Using the metaphor of 'margin and centre', she analysed these features to displace issues regarded as important by dominant groups and bring into focus the concerns of those relegated to the margins. I use her approach here to consider how social work research, driven by a moral and political agenda, might challenge the normative concerns of dominant research approaches by asking different questions and centring the interests and experiences of those most affected by social work, rather than the interests of practitioners, researchers, government or organisations. In this way, I hope that practitioner researchers might practise 'making the invisible visible', revealing an oppositional world view that will raise different questions and provide different answers.

Much feminist theory, argued hooks (1984), emerges from privileged women who live at the centre and whose perspectives rarely include knowledge and awareness of the lives of women and men who live on the margin. As a consequence, such theory lacks wholeness, the broad analysis that could encompass a variety of human experiences. At its most visionary, an encompassing theory will emerge from individuals who have knowledge of both margin and centre. Marginalised people may have knowledge of the centre through close observation of the actions of powerful groups, or through their multiple positioning at both margin and centre. Others may gain such knowledge out of listening to and empathising with those at the margin. It is this insight that is key to a perspective that challenges top-down interpretations and seeks to bring to light other understandings.

Subjugated knowledges

One of the differences between traditional research and alternative perspectives revolves around who can be a knower and the status of different kinds of knowledges. Traditionally, the 'knower' is the researcher who brings scientific objectivity to their work, gathers information from 'informants', analyses and interprets such data and writes about them in a way that addresses the questions they had set out to answer. Interpretive approaches have not particularly challenged this notion of the 'knower', but did begin to recognise the knowledge of marginalised groups and the subjective elements of human experience, that is, the meanings attributed to events and behaviour by particular social actors. Other approaches to research, notably feminist and participatory, explicitly set out to bring to light what hooks called 'subjugated knowledges'. In other words, there is more than one kind of knower and there is a range of kinds of knowledges. Moreover, subjugated knowledges are legitimate forms of knowing. Dominant groups may dismiss their authenticity, but the aim of critical research is to assert their legitimacy and insist that they be heard and recognised.

The importance of this is illustrated by Anne Fadiman's remarkable book, *The Spirit Catches You and You Fall Down* (1997), about a Hmong child, her American doctors, and the doctors' dismissal of the cultural knowledge of the child's community in preference to the Western medical tradition. The book is a single case ethnographic study of the medical problems of Lia Lee, three months old when she and her parents arrived in the US as refugees from Laos, meticulously reported and deeply revealing. The problems hinged on the fact that the Hmong see illness and healing as spiritual matters linked to virtually everything in the universe, while the medical community marks a division between body and soul and concerns itself exclusively with the former. Lia Lee was diagnosed as an epileptic, caused by the 'misfiring of her cerebral neurons'. Her parents called her illness 'quag dab peg' – 'the spirit catches you and you fall down'.

Ideas within the two cultures about diagnosis, care and treatment could hardly have been more different, and the medical community tended to dismiss Hmong knowledge as superstitious and harmful. For its part, the Hmong community was fearful and suspicious of medical approaches that refused to recognise a holistic world view. After years of confusion, anger and misunderstandings, tragically Lia Lee died while still in her childhood. The stakes in how subjugated knowledges are valued are high, sometimes with life and death consequences. Fadiman's treatment of the case study captured both the dominant medical view and that of the minority culture, and she was not unsympathetic to either, although she had direct experience of neither. Of relevance to social work is her capturing of the frustration expressed by caring doctors about what they saw as uncooperative parents unconcerned about the dangers to their child, and the cushion of love and concern emanating from the Hmong community and the child's family.

Social workers often experience such frustration with service users, resulting in pathological perceptions of them. The time and effort needed to understand these cultural differences are a fundamental condition for negotiating the appropriate help. Fadiman's ethnographic research took place over a number of years and she immersed herself in both the cultures studied. Social work practitioners may see this as an unrealistic task, and in any case, the approach is alien to a culture of research that emphasises efficiency, effectiveness and definitive answers. Yet it seems entirely appropriate research for a practitioner to conduct as part of her practice over time, and as a way of resisting dominant, and often oppressive, approaches.

Fadiman's study involved a single case, but the researcher was able to theorise from this to analyse cultural difference, dominance and the workings of institutional racism. She explored the connections between this and the colonial history of the US and Laos. Starting from a single moment, she wove a tapestry that encompassed global political patterns. Her work demonstrated a critical approach that was grounded in but did not end with the experiences of an individual family, their community and the particular practitioners engaged with them. The study was used to construct a number of layers of analysis and provided lessons for how practice, organisational structures and indeed wider social institutions and even international activity need to change if they are to have an evidence base that is in the interests of service users.

Talking back

A way of ensuring that research practice shifts the margin to the centre is providing the opportunity for marginalised groups to 'come to voice', and particularly to 'talk back':

> those who understand the power of voice as a gesture of rebellion and resistance urge the exploited, the oppressed to speak. (hooks 1989: 14)

When people speak of their oppression it is a painful thing, requiring courage and daring. It is a dangerous thing, because what the voice has to say may not be heard, may be rejected, seen as threatening or irrational, or may be appropriated and exploited. It is an unsettling thing, because it disrupts polite social relationships and risks a loss of approval from friends, colleagues and acquaintances. Yet often the struggle out of silence is an essential one towards healing and wholeness.

Durham (2003) carried out a practitioner research study of young men living with child sexual abuse. He brought their voices into focus, allowing them to talk back to those who had abused them and a society that had neglected them. He interviewed seven young men using a methodology influenced by ethnographic (particularly life story approach), feminist, anti-oppressive and social work practitioner research. His analytic framework sought to reconcile poststructuralist and structuralist theories, one of which tends to dismiss the structural determinants of oppression in favour of localised explanations, while the other reduces all oppressions to economic causes. He argued that such a framework allows a socially contextualised analysis of the young men's experiences, emphasising the importance of narrative and discourse, centralises issues of power, gender and sexuality, and allows for an examination of the ongoing impact of widespread social oppression. Durham's article includes a potentially useful analytic framework, expressed in a diagram, encompassing power relationships at different interrelated levels of social interaction. This allows for a description of the vividness and horror of individual experiences of child sexual abuse, and for linking these to discourses of power and sexuality and prescribed gender roles. In these ways, the emphasis is shifted from entirely individualistic explanations of social problems to take account of factors that have been relegated to the margin.

Durham's (2003) report of the study has strengths and weaknesses. By centring the voices of the young men interviewed, he conveys the damage, confusion, contradictory feelings and ongoing injury experienced by them into adulthood. The reader is left in no doubt as to the long-term consequences of such abuse, and the urgency of understanding and developing strategies for overcoming the resulting trauma. Although Durham does not go on to explore how social work might respond to people such as those in the study, the article offers insights into thoughts and feelings not often made public, and is therefore of use to practitioners. It is a tribute to the methods chosen and the skills of the practitioner researcher that he was able to access and make available survivors' constructions of the events described – presumably he was using case material from his own practice and consent was given to the material being used in this way.

Nevertheless, the article might have gone further in making the links with wider discourses and going beyond widespread beliefs that child sexual abuse arises from individual pathology. This promised to be one of the most valuable elements of the piece. The opportunity was presented to explore how feminism and poststructuralism might offer theoretical insights into the sexual abuse of boys by men – and thus pursue their potential for contributing to wider social theory – yet these critiques are only marginally and superficially used in the analysis. Furthermore, Durham's (2003: 311) argument that 'no single aspect of social oppression is seen as an absolute determinant of social power' held out a possibility of progress from the reductionist, compartmentalised and hierarchical view of oppression still pervasive in social work. The analysis did not, however, achieve fluency among class, age, 'race' and ability. Indeed, these are virtually ignored in the discussion, the main focus of which was sexuality, with gender not directly addressed. Although a connection is made between the anxieties of the young men about the implications of the abuse for their masculinity and 'compulsory heterosexuality', the argument does not offer any critique of compulsory heterosexuality. Such a critique would identify compulsory heterosexuality as a normative practice in society, embodied in the assumption that the ideal identity is a heterosexual one, with clearly defined behaviours allocated to women and men. This failure to decentre heterosexuality results in the young men's anxieties, that they might be or might be seen to be 'queer', not being politicised, leaving the normative notion of heterosexuality unchallenged and therefore being queer as pathological. In other words, social structures that hold heterosexuality as the implicit point of reference remain intact, are not displaced from centre to margin, and the opportunity for a creative challenge to structures of power is lost.

These criticisms may appear to some readers to be unnecessarily pedantic and nitpicking. However, in making them, I am using the terms of reference of the author himself, in that Durham is claiming to demonstrate these elements in his article. It is not sufficient that the young men's voices are heard. They must be analysed in the light of insights about the nature of oppression. Also, where research claims to be antioppressive, not to carefully unpack normative assumptions is a serious omission.

Reframing knowledge

Part of the project of critical research is to identify the ways knowledge is produced. In social work, there has been a growth in faith in 'scientific' knowledge over what Usher and Edwards (1994: 158) call 'narrative' knowledge, creating an imperialist culture of research and practice that is concerned with criteria of efficiency rather than being governed by some vision of a just society.

Some of this is illustrated by research conducted by Robinson (2003) to test the hypothesis that an increase in 'technicality' (scientific knowledge) in probation practice results in a decrease in professionalism (narrative knowledge). In taking research in probation as an example, I recognise that comparisons between probation and social work have limitations, since probation is excluded from social work in England and Wales. However, they have both been subjected to the modernisation agenda in the shift to instrumentalism and managerialism. This has raised concerns within both professions of a deskilling process, a reduction in the scope for judgement and interpretation of regulations, and a move towards work that is mechanical and administrative (Jordan and Jordan, 2000).

To this extent, Robinson's (2003) research has relevance for social work, in that she addresses one of the central preoccupations in contemporary practice, the perceived assault on professional identity by managerialist and technicist models of practice and research. In the absence of research on the actual implementation and impact of 'technical' initiatives, Robinson wanted to know whether frontline staff are really being robbed of the 'last remnants of discretion' (Nellis, 1995: 28), how they understand the relationships between the concepts of technicality, indeterminacy and professionalism, and whether practitioners are able to avoid or subvert attempts to dictate the shape of practice.

Robinson's study examined the implementation of a risk/needs assessment instrument – the Level of Service Inventory-Revised, LSI-R – to establish its contribution to the erosion of discretion, and establish the relationship between the instrument's implementation and perceptions of 'professionalism'. Scores allocated to a number of risk factors are said to predict the possibilities of reconviction. This in turn informs decisions about the type or 'level of service' appropriate to individual offenders.

Robinson used two area probation services, where the instrument had been in use for some time, to develop a case study approach. She adopted a 'stakeholder' model, so that the experiences and perceptions of the full range of personnel within the two organisations could be taken into account. She conducted 29 in-depth interviews, with personnel ranging from administrative staff to senior managers, and analysed the data by quantitative methods. She carried out an analysis of organisational documents to augment the data. She examined correlations across the data and concluded that both the technical properties of the instrument and the policies established in the two area services regarding the use of LSI-R indicated a high level of technicality or prescription of the assessment process and the post-assessment resource allocation decisions. However, Robinson's work questioned the easy assumption of a significant erosion of indeterminacy, discovering a more complex process at work.

First, the way the LSI-R was sold to practitioners by managers emphasised not only the technical skill needed to use the instrument, but also the professional skills necessary – 'it doesn't and never was intended to take completely away from professional judgement' (a manager quoted in Robinson, 2003: 598). Furthermore, a number of practitioners themselves saw the instrument as a reflection of or a supplement to their own assessment, not an alternative to it. And importantly, Robinson's examination of practice revealed that the LSI-R scores were far from pivotal in allocation decisions. Professional judgement and negotiation still had an important part to play. The most significant barrier to a purely actuarial approach ('government-by-numbers', p. 599) was in fact the offender population. Many of those offenders deemed suitable for intensive probation programmes by virtue of high LSI-R scores were not good candidates because of issues such as mental health, drug use or a history of failure to complete programmes. In addition, magistrates were resistant to the instrument, perceiving it as a threat to their discretion in sentencing. Robinson concluded that claims for the 'technical' profile of contemporary probation and social work practice may have been exaggerated, the experience of technical innovations may be shaped to a significant extent by context or perceptions of purpose, and the experience of deprofessionalisation may depend on the maintenance of an acceptable degree of indeterminacy.

One of the lessons from this research points to the limitations of methods led by apparently scientific knowledge that do not take account of narrative knowledge. Had Robinson's study counted the number of times the instrument had been used, and measured its routine technical application and the outcomes of scores and their influence on decisions about the level of service, she might have produced knowledge that concluded that indeed the probation task is dominated by technicality. She might also have concluded that the LSI-R 'works'. However, she found that the perceptions of those administering it did not suggest that they viewed it as a threat to their professional skills, but saw it as an aid that supplemented a professional clinical assessment. This suggests that they were able to resist and subvert the technical process by insisting on the role of professional judgement, ensuring that factors other than solely auditing techniques influenced the process.

The study is also evocative of decades of debates about the 'scientific method' versus interpretive approaches to social research. One of the key epistemological issues this debate addresses is whether it is appropriate to apply similar principles to the study of people to those applied in the physical sciences about the nature of reality and the rules that govern it. The implicit hypothesis that the application of a particular instrument will measure suitability for and identify appropriate treatment could not take account of the context of offenders' lives. In dealing with human beings, it is not possible to control variables as in a laboratory experiment, because of the unpredictability and contingency of lived experience and factors such as (in this case) illness and drug use, which are not conducive to measurement. Robinson rightly identified the offender population as the most significant barrier to a purely actuarial approach. This rather undermines the aim of the experiment, since 'offenders' or 'service users' are the raison d'être of the professions involved and cannot easily be dispensed with as inconvenient intrusions.

Robinson's tentative conclusion, that a professional future lies in a 'balance' between technicality and indeterminacy, may be that of a cautious researcher who realistically cannot envisage a future free of increasingly technical applications to social problems. At the same time, her agreement with a senior manager that the ultimate guardians of indeterminacy are not likely to be practitioners or their managers, but rather the clients with whom professionals work, is confirmation of the need for a research approach that does not take anything for granted and opens up spaces for contesting and relocating definitions of power and the purposes of intervention.

Nevertheless, unanswered questions concern the legitimacy of the knowledge constructed out of Robinson's research. Will the belief among practitioners that their professional discretion is not fundamentally threatened by galloping technicality make any difference at the end of the day? Or is it convenient for managers to patronise them by asserting no threat to their professionalism, while pursuing the technical route and rendering practitioners' views inauthentic and irrelevant? Do subjective meanings make a difference, beyond being an interesting 'finding'? What are the advantages and drawbacks of 'professional judgement' in any case? Are clients benefited or disadvantaged by them?

Robinson (2003) believes that the complexity described in her research may confound attempts to render probation practice a wholly technical enterprise. If so, this is to be welcomed, in order to recapture notions of uncertainty and ambiguity in professional practice, as urged by Parton (1998). Nevertheless, a critical research perspective would go beyond identifying oppressive structures and the activities that sustain them, to take action to combat and challenge them, in contrast to Robinson's uncommitted positioning. Analysed within the framework I have suggested for critical research, there are other points to be made. First, Robinson's positioning is unreflexive, in that she does not say anything about her own standpoint and attempts to maintain the illusion of the 'neutral' researcher. We are not told what her beliefs are about the topic under examination and how these might have influenced the aims and methods of the study. She does not share her views about notions of professionalism and its relation to modernisation plans. She does not concern herself with the impact the changes might have on probationers themselves.

Some clues are discernable in what she omitted to address in the study. Robinson did not set out to study the experiences or the 'bringing to voice' of people convicted of crimes, but the professional power of probation officers. This is not a criticism of the study as such, since clear and manageable parameters have to be set for any research, and Robinson's focus is a relevant and legitimate one. It is simply to make the point that the basic concern was not with the 'empowerment' of probationers. In this respect, her article did not address ethical questions about, for example, whether informed consent was sought and gained from probationers to take part in the LSI-R experiment or whether it was assumed this was not necessary; although the issue of whether genuine consent could be gained where people are subject to legal authority is a moot point.

Moreover, even within its own terms of reference, the study might have addressed the wider structures impacting on the work of professionals, as for example in the surveillance and disciplining of the self as an essential part of governmentality, a crucial aspect of the regulatory practices of a range of modern institutions (see Usher and Edwards, 1994). Robinson's suggestion of a 'balance' between technicality and indeterminacy evades the issue of the hegemony of managerialism and technicism as disciplinary practices. From this perspective, what appears to be resistance from professionals can be viewed as no more than an accommodation to a regime where 'power is hidden from the awareness of those through whom it circulates' (Usher and Edwards, 1994: 97). The study does not transgress, disrupt, challenge and change the material and ideological realities.

Conclusion

The degree in social work emphasises three characteristics of professionalism: theory, practice and research. What I have argued for here is the tracing of a seamless connection among these elements, by adopting a moral and political position to critique theory and inform practice, whether it is defined as 'research' or not. This perspective centres the experiences of those who are oppressed by social institutions, facilitates a description of the processes by which this happens, and provides the language to argue for an ultimate research focus on the working of the institutions of power in order to construct a holistic understanding of the forces impacting on service users' lives.

Research and practice that isolate individual behaviour and experience from the wider social and political context and focus narrowly on outcomes and effectiveness are blinkered and limited. In that model, 'objectivity' (ironically valued highly in constructing research designs) is sacrificed in a climate where 'outcomes' hold the dominant value and questions are not asked about origins, aims, motives, ideology and context. A critical approach does not mean that service users should themselves always be the objects of research. The workings of power can just as well be examined by a focus on elites, or on the mediators of power, as in Robinson's study of probation officers.

This is not to ignore the fact that oppressed groups can themselves be oppressors, or to romanticise the working class, women, black people or whoever. It is to reveal the links between their exploitation and social structures, and influence research practice towards more informed and effective ways of confronting their problems. My choice of studies examined in this chapter does not privilege any particular methodology, and I would argue that there are few methods that do not lend themselves to a critical approach. It is the desire to make the invisible visible, the urge to centre issues of justice, equality and empowerment that constitute the radical potential of social work research. The resultant focus is not only on how 'deviant' individual behaviour can be changed, but also on policies and institutional practices and their impact on the poor and the marginalised. It is on how such policies and practices are or can be challenged by those affected by them. The futures of social work can include an attitude to research that sets its critical sights on policies, institutions and structures as targets for change, rather than a meek acceptance that these are irrelevant to an individualistic and often demeaning practice. The motivation for such a shift in research focus – and a legitimate role for social work – is social transformation.

For further discussion of contemporary critical perspectives of relevance to research, see Adams et al., 2009b, Chapters 17 and 20.

D'Cruz, H. and Jones, M. (2004) *Social Work Research: A Political and Ethical Practice?*, London, Sage. Introductory research text for students on the degree in social work. Regards research as another social work method and is informed by social work's 'emancipatory' goals. Also a useful practical guide to the design, methods and processes of carrying out a research project. Structured around exercises to reinforce learning.

Fook, J. (2002) *Social Work: Critical Theory and Practice*, London, Sage. Explores a theoretical framework that attempts to integrate classic critical and postmodernist perspectives to produce a framework for social work. Also advocates an approach to social work theory, practice and research as a seamless whole. Grounded in examples and exercises from everyday practice.

Humphries, B. (2008) *Social Work Research for Social Justice*, Basingstoke, Palgrave Macmillan. Sets out a framework for social justice in research and examines a number of research approaches in the light of the framework. Considers a variety of examples, contains exercises for learning and suggests further reading.

Developing social work research

26

This chapter examines the role of social work research in practice and the different ways of understanding the relation between research and practice. It looks at the nature of research as a means of knowledge production and considers the different forms of knowledge that research can generate. Finally, it discusses the research process, choice of methods and the role of the researcher as both expert and facilitator.

Chapter overview

What is the purpose of social work research?

While there are many different approaches to social work research, there is a widely held view that the primary purpose of any research is to promote the development and improvement of social work practice. This is evident in the document *A Social Work Research Strategy for Higher Education 2006–20* (JUC SWEC, 2006), where it states:

> Our commitment to raise the quality and quantity of social work research is based on the difference that good research evidence can make to the lives and well-being of people who come into contact with social workers and with social care services.

This statement clearly suggests that social work research is indeed a resource for social workers to make use of in their day-to-day practice. It also underlines a close relationship between social work research and social work defined as a profession that

> promotes social change, problem solving in human relationships and empowerment and liberation of people to enhance well-being' (IFSW, 2000).

Despite this growing awareness of the potential contribution of research to practice, the relationship between social work practice and social work research remains problematic in various ways.

Making use of research

Over the past decade or more, there has been increasing emphasis on the utilisation of research in social work and social care. This drive towards creating a more systematic relationship between research knowledge and practice is a key feature of the modernisation agenda of the UK's successive Labour governments and is seen as a means of ensuring consistent standards of professional practice and service delivery (Trevillion, 2008). Government policy to promote or enhance the quality of practice in this way is evident in a range of initiatives in the social care sector, most notably the setting up of the Social Care Institute for Excellence (SCIE), whose remit is 'to raising standards of practice across the social care sector, through the better use of knowledge and research (Fisher, 2002a: 7). This call for more awareness and use of research is also evident in the requirements for both qualifying and post-qualifying training in social work, in the Quality Assurance Agency for Higher Education (QAA, 2000) benchmark statement for expected standards of degrees in social work and the more widely applicable National Occupational Standards for Social Work (Topss England, 2002).

The burgeoning interest in social work research in many countries has developed under the generic title of evidence-based practice (EBP). Increasingly, professionals engaged in social work and social care have appeared to embrace this approach as the basis for developing 'best practice'. However, as Butler (2003) suggests, what might be regarded as this pragmatic adoption of EBP requires closer examination. Arguably, social work has always been a research-informed practice and social work practitioners have always been urged to make use of research as a valuable resource. Social work in its early years as a formally recognised activity had a close relationship with social research through the work of many of the great reformers of the late nineteenth and early twentieth century. An involvement in the collection and application of social data has long been regarded as an integral part of social work practice and its professional identity (Lorenz, 2004).

Nevertheless, the nature of the relationship between social work and research has been and continues to be a much disputed area. For many practitioners, research has often seemed irrelevant and unconnected with the day-to-day realities of practice. For others, research that seeks to categorise and quantify people's 'lived experience' is regarded with suspicion, as it masks the complexity and uniqueness of individual experience and can operate as a further exploitation of already vulnerable people. Over many years, a range of initiatives has been introduced to address the perceived problem of the relevance of research to practice. These activities, which include the organisations Research in Practice and Making Research Count (see web links), have undoubtedly promoted greater awareness of research and increased its use by social workers, and contributed to the development of the 'research-minded practitioner'.

The term 'research-mindedness' has become a widely adopted term, although it can be used in various ways. Everitt et al. (1992) have made a strong argument for understanding research-mindedness as more than closing the gap between research and practice. Being a research-minded practitioner should involve using research as a way of opening up practice to critical scrutiny and incorporating the principles of practice into research. This view of research-mindedness challenges the notion that the utilisation of research is a straightforward linear process of implementation. Rather, it suggests a complex interplay of factors, a finding evident in a recent study of the use of research in social care practice undertaken by Walters et al. (2004). A key recommendation from this study was the need for a more systemic approach to research utilisation that takes account of the individual practitioner as having a responsibility to keep up to date with research and apply it to practice, and the organisation as a place for generating a culture of learning that supports research-mindedness.

This recognition of a more dynamic relationship between research and practice challenges more traditional understandings of this relationship, where research and theory are given the status of 'real' or universally applicable knowledge based on facts that are gathered independently of how people interpret them, and practice is seen as the application or translation of this knowledge into a set of skills and competences. An alternative understanding proposed here is that good practice, research and theorising are interdependent and inform each other in the development of knowledge for and about social work. These different conceptions of the nature of the relationship between research and practice reflect different underlying assumptions about the nature and purpose of social work research and merit closer examination.

Trends in social work research

Much social work research adopts what might be described as a 'strongly pragmatic approach' (Trinder, 2000), which is supported by the long-held and widely shared view that social work research should be seen as methodologically robust and relevant to practitioners. The focus is on the use of an appropriately chosen method in any given context. Every effort is made to take account of differences of views and the need to work in ways that facilitate partnership rather than patronage on the part of the researcher. Alongside this characterisation of social work research, Trinder (1996) identified two distinct approaches:

1   There is empirical EBP, which, although not new, has regained much ground in the US and the UK. Within the UK, this approach has become increasingly prominent through its explicit linking with initiatives within the NHS, where the emphasis is on EBP and clinical effectiveness (MacDonald, 1999; Thyer and Kazi, 2004). As noted earlier, this approach, broadly conceived as grounding professional judgements in evidence drawn from research findings, has wide acceptance, and appropriately so. However, when narrowly limited to particular research methods and practice interventions, it remains highly contestable as the only, or an exclusive, form of knowledge creation for practice (Trinder, 2000). By favouring the use of randomised controlled trials as the 'gold standard', this approach places a high value on research that is deemed valid in terms of its objectivity and clinical relevance (Webb, 2001). A further source of unease with this approach stems from its close association with managerial agendas and an emphasis on cost-effectiveness

and performance measurement at the expense of other, equally legitimate interests, most notably those of service users (Trinder, 2000).

2   There is the participatory or critical approach, with an emphasis on the potentially empowering role of research (Everitt and Hardiker, 1996). This approach has been described as the 'progressive response' by Beresford and Evans (1999). They set this 'new paradigm' of collaborative research in opposition to 'the reactionary response'. In tracing the origins of this approach, Beresford and Evans (1999) point to a range of sources, including the significant contributions arising from disability and feminist research and other movements engaged in emancipatory goals. Research strategies during the 1970s were associated with community development initiatives and social action (Holman, 1987). Typically, this knowledge is used to challenge more dominant or privileged forms of knowledge held by politicians, policy makers or professionals as a means of achieving change, generally at a local level. It is no accident that in today's world of deepening inequality, poverty and social exclusion, there is growing interest in such approaches as a means of resisting management-oriented research agendas (Dullea and Mullender, 1999).

These different approaches within social work research reveal the contested nature and purpose of social work research and social work practice in an increasingly managed environment. Exchanges within the pages of the *British Journal of Social Work* are evidence of this debate. While Sheldon (2001) remains a strong advocate of EBP as a means of promoting social work effectiveness, Webb (2001) sees the impact of both managerialism and narrowly conceived evidence-based approaches as leading towards an increasingly regulatory form of social work activity. While these debates may be of greater interest to those engaged in doing research, they highlight the importance of developing a form of research-mindedness that allows critical engagement with research in terms of the outcomes of research and the processes whereby knowledge is produced. In developing its approach towards establishing a research evidence base, SCIE has drawn attention to a range of knowledge used by social workers and, in doing so, has developed a more inclusive approach to the identification of different sorts and sources of knowledge for practice (Fisher, 2002a). As Humphries (2003) suggests, there is a need for research to generate different sorts of knowledge for understanding the complexities of social work practice. This signals the need for further exploration of the nature of research evidence as knowledge.

Research as knowledge production

Research involves finding out about the world and is therefore unavoidably about making knowledge claims. Put slightly differently, research can be seen as a form of systematic inquiry in the pursuit of knowledge. Underlying such apparently simply statements are bigger questions and matters of dispute. These involve claims and counterclaims concerning how the knowledge has been or should be produced and by whom, what counts as knowledge, and on what grounds are such claims being made.

As observed earlier, much social work research has traditionally focused on issues relevant to practice rather than the development of more conceptual or theoretical work. The emphasis on studies of effectiveness has come from a longstanding professional commitment to improve and enhance practice, and a more recent need to demonstrate a careful utilisation of public resources (Fisher, 1999). Alongside this more explicitly evaluative research primarily located within traditional research methodologies, other studies, while equally concerned with developing and improving practice, have focused less on outcome and more on developing an understanding of the processes involved. Much of this work has built on the seminal research of Mayer and Timms (1970), and service users' views have now become an integral part of many evaluative studies of social work and social care services. Exploring the various accounts of those involved in social work from the practitioners' perspective has also contributed to a more informed understanding of the dynamics of social work relations and the delivery of services in the wider organisational and policy context. Other studies have sought to explore service users' accounts alongside those of social work practitioners, and setting these various perceptions alongside each other has created many rich descriptions of social work practice.

Thus, recognising the diversity of interests of those involved in the process provides a means of visualising and exploring the contradictions and tensions inherent within social work practice. Such accounts offer a way of understanding more about the complexities of practice and generate new forms of knowledge. As Jones and Jordan (1996: 267) wrote:

> The real integration of theory and practice will not come about from a ponderous, rigid body of knowledge, but from the humility to learn from practitioners' experiences.

As this view of the relationships between social work theory, practice and research indicates, there is no intention to privilege practice over theory or indeed the reverse. The emphasis here is on exploring the different ways in which social work research can contribute to knowledge for practice and theory development. This is in contrast with traditional ways of making a clear distinction between different types of research, most notably as either 'pure' or 'applied' (Hammersley, 2003). A range of research strategies are needed to embrace different forms of knowledge as complementary and interconnected. Knowledge is not conceived abstractly but is viewed as a dynamic process in which theory and practice are interrelated.

It is inevitable then that research as a process of knowledge generation is inescapably a value-laden activity within which the researcher plays a significant role in this process. Over two decades ago, Wallace and Rees (1988: 59) argued for the importance of making values explicit within the research process:

> On the contrary, the pretence that values do not influence the choice of research interests and methods is more likely to produce bias than the explicitness that we have documented.

The view of social work research held here is that social work research, like social work, is best understood as a practical-moral rather than a technical-rational activity: it is not a matter limited to mere techniques and methods. Moral and political issues lie at the heart of both activities (Butler and Pugh, 2004). When discussing the development of a code of ethics for social work and social care research, Butler (2002) referred to the notion of the 'morally active practitioner'. This term was originally used by Husband (1995) when discussing ethics and anti-racist social work practice and it is equally relevant here. By emphasising the virtues or good character of the practitioner, Husband emphasises the personal and political nature of the role and the need for 'self-conscious reflection'. In the research context, this continual process of reflexivity requires professional expertise similar in many respects to that associated with social work practice, where the skills of reflexivity are seen as integral to the task. Fook (2000: 117) usefully distinguishes this form of reflexivity as:

> the ability to locate oneself squarely within a situation, to know and take into account the influence of personal interpretation, position and action within a specific context. Expert practitioners are reflexive in that they are self-knowing and responsible actors, rather than detached observers.

In the research context, this reflexive stance is central to the conduct of the activity and to the ways in which data are generated and analysed. Traditionally, reflexivity has been seen as a problem to be minimised through careful scrutiny and rigorous use of the scientific method. An alternative view is to see reflexivity as a resource to be acknowledged and valued. Rather than privileging the pursuit of objectivity and detachment at the expense of acknowledging their values and biases, critical reflection on feelings and assumptions can lead to research practice that is systematic and rigorous. With this emphasis on the role of critical reflection on the part of the researcher, we now turn our attention to the actual process of undertaking social work research.

Research as process

Earlier, we used a simple definition of research as a process of systematic inquiry in the pursuit of knowledge. Having given some consideration to the outcome of research in terms of the knowledge produced, we now need to examine this 'process of systematic inquiry' and the role of the researcher in carrying out this activity. A key question concerns the distinctive nature of social work research and its use of particular methods or approaches. It has been argued here that social work research can be characterised by its common concern for relevance to practice, its attention to multiple constituencies, and its acknowledgement of different ways of knowing. Shaw et al. (2006) suggest that it is a common concern for relevance to practice that animates the distinctiveness of social work research rather than its commitment to any particular paradigm or choice of methods. Others claim that research methods must be consistent with a vision of social work as an empowering form of practice. However, the extent to which social work research might wish to align itself with social science research or to argue that it is largely inseparable from social work practice itself remains a matter of continuing debate (Trevillion, 2000).

Nevertheless, it is important to understand these tensions within social work research as they inevitably are played out in the day-to-day practice of the researcher. While they are shaped by both the purpose(s) and context(s) of the particular research situation, how these are negotiated and managed by the researcher, whether a practitioner, service user or academic researcher, forms an integral part of the researcher's role and tasks. The primary task for the researcher is to consider what methods and activities are most likely to meet the purpose(s) of the research and what ways the purpose(s) will impinge on those methods. At all stages of carrying out the research, choices have to be made in the specific context and there are inevitably 'trade-offs' that have to be negotiated. There is a balance to be struck between adequate attention to social work's multiple constituents and interests alongside continuous attention to issues of methodological rigour.

Irrespective of the particular choice of method(s), careful attention to the power relations within the research process is required and any built-in inequalities challenged rather than re-enforced. A multiplicity of interests and accountabilities can be foregrounded rather than ignored, and continuously scrutinised and (re)negotiated. Of central importance is how the researcher sustains a critical approach to what constitutes participation in the research process while continuously examining the relative merits of different methods and techniques. Methodological diversity – as distinct from random eclecticism – is important in addressing the complexity of interests within the social work (research) community and the need for different forms of knowledge. This diversity and variety is inevitably mirrored in the broad range of methods adopted within social work research, where the emphasis on 'fit for purpose' becomes a central concern.

It is important to note that all methods have the potential to exploit or empower research participants. Value is often placed on the use of qualitative methods in promoting more inclusive practices. However, an uncritical use of methods that facilitate 'storytelling' and narrative accounts can undermine any real sense of involvement if 'abstracted from their contexts of production, stripped of language, and transformed into brief summaries' (Reissman and Quinney, 2005: 398). Equally relevant here is the use of large-scale surveys undertaken in ways that genuinely reflect the interests of the less powerful and still meet the demands of policy makers for relevance (Truman, 1999). The continuing development of mixed methods approaches is worth noting here in addressing the complexity of interests within the policy and practice arenas, a point usefully made by Humphries (2003) in the context of EBP, where a range of methods can be used to pursue service users' interests.

Alongside the creative use of existing methods, there is a need to develop innovative approaches to data production and alterative ways of involving groups previously excluded from having 'a voice' (Gibbs, 2001b; Whitmore, 2001; Sanders and Munford, 2005). Relevant here is Fook's (2003) argument for approaches that promote inclusion and participation of indigenous groups that include Australian Aborigines, and attend to the colonising functions of many traditional research designs (Smith, 1999). It is beyond the scope of this chapter to discuss the use of particular methods of data-gathering and analysis. Some useful texts are indicated in the Further reading below that consider these issues in more detail. Here, we reiterate the need for critical reflection on the part of the researcher as a means of ensuring the appropriate use of any particular method, old or new, in addressing the complexity of social work practice and its multiple constituencies.

Partnership working

Adopting a more participatory approach within the research process challenges the status of the researcher and their role as expert with overall control of the research methodology. For those actively engaged in promoting the wider involvement of participants in the research process, the researcher plays a more facilitative role, with expertise to share in the joint process of knowledge construction. When research is conceived in this way, it may involve discussion not only about the relative merits of different research approaches and possible methods to be employed, but also the carrying out of data-gathering and analysis. Where the researcher is working with a diverse range of participants to promote such discussion, which may also include the formulation of research questions, the task extends to facilitating the reflective and reflexive skills of those involved. All participants, including the researcher, become engaged in reflection and learning (Fisher, 2002b; Smith, 2004). Conceived in this way, social work research remains focused on the goal of knowledge creation but in ways that are consistent with an approach congruent with social work's commitment to participation and empowerment (Beresford, 2000).

Managing the complexity of the research process in ways that facilitate a more inclusive approach underlines the centrality of self-reflexivity on the part of the researcher. Certain groups can be supported or privileged, not least those whose interests have received insufficient attention or been ignored. Adopting an empowering stance can be seen as pursuing a commitment to social justice through the inclusion of a particular group previously excluded or unheard. At the same time, identifying various categorised groupings and privileging one against the other does not always adequately address the ways in which different constituent groups pursue their interests and at what costs to other groups. Emancipatory knowledge claims also generate their own power relations and cannot escape the contradiction that the privileging of any form of knowledge over another creates a hierarchy whereby some forms of knowledge become devalued and are afforded low status. As Humphries (2004b) argues, what is important for the social work researcher is a commitment to values rather than 'to factions (regardless of whether right or wrong)'. She advocates taking sides against oppression by using research to critically reflect on the nature and impact of societal structures and processes on the lives of individuals, rather than making claims to be on the side of 'the oppressed'.

This emphasis on the role of critical reflection in the research process and how reflexivity on the part of the researcher can be a resource are central to promoting the democratisation of the research process. Combined with skills in negotiation, the researcher can facilitate adequate discussion and debate of research methodologies and ensure greater transparency in the use of all research methods. Much can be gained from a careful examination of all methods and their potential use in ways that take account of the purpose and context of social work research. The systematic documentation of the methods employed for data collection and analysis is also important in demonstrating how the various constituent interests have been addressed throughout the research process. This reporting of the negotiations and trade-offs forms part of ensuring the transparency of the process and provides a basis for assessing the quality of the research.

Critical engagement with research – as users of research and research practitioners – requires close scrutiny of the outcomes of any research and the processes employed. Some key questions here are: 'Who benefits from the research, either directly as a research user or indirectly as a beneficiary of potentially more effective practice?' Of what value is the research for these intended users or beneficiaries? Who is the judge of quality in social work research? Recent work by Shaw and Norton (2007) identifies a number of potential criteria for judging the quality of research. These mirror the concerns within social work research to address relevance for practice and methodological rigour in ways that are congruent with social work's commitment to empowering forms of practice.

Conclusion

This chapter began by emphasising the role of research as a resource for practice. At the same time, it has been shown that making use of research is not a straightforward application of research to practice but requires a more critical engagement with research as not the only source of knowledge. To be able to make best use of research, there is a need to understand more about the diverse nature and purposes of research and its complex relationship with social work practice, itself a contested activity. The focus of the chapter has been on using research or becoming research minded – a practitioner who is sufficiently aware of research to be able not only to identify and access it, but also to understand how it has been produced and for what purpose. It has not been the remit of this chapter to consider in any detail the actual methods of collecting or analysing data. Rather, the emphasis has been on understanding the research process as a moral and political activity, where there is a need for careful scrutiny of power relations at all stages in the research process. Attention has also been drawn to the role of the researcher as negotiator and facilitator and the importance of critical reflection and self-reflexivity as a key resource. Hopefully, the issues raised here have encouraged you to inquire further into the world of research. It is only through our critical engagement with research that it will become embedded in social work practice and realise its potential in making a difference to the lives of those who come into contact with social workers.

For further discussion of ongoing aspects of personal and professional development, see Adams et al., 2009a, Chapter 26.

www.uea.ac.uk/menu/acad_depts/swk/MRC_web/public_html/ Making Research Count is a national research dissemination network based regionally in the social work departments of nine English universities.

www.rip.org.uk Research in Practice supports evidence-informed practice with children and families.

www.ripfa.org.uk Research in Practice for Adults supports evidence-informed practice and policy.

www.scie.org.uk Social Care Institute for Excellence.

Becker, S. and Bryman, A. (eds) (2004) *Understanding Research for Policy and Practice: Themes, Methods and Approaches*, Bristol, Policy Press. Provides a broad overview of social research from a range of perspectives that locates social work research within the wider field of social sciences.

D'Cruz, H. and Jones, M. (2004) *Social Work Research: Ethical and Political Contexts*, Sage, London. Excellent introductory text that provides an overview of research in the context of professional social work.

Humphries, B. (2008) *Social Work Research for Social Justice*, Basingstoke, Palgrave Macmillan. Takes further the issues raised in this chapter concerning the nature and role of social work research as an empowering form of practice.

McLaughlin, H. (2007) *Understanding Social Work Research*, Sage, London. Useful text that covers a range of issues, including EBP and service user involvement, in more detail.

Concluding comment

This final book in our social work trilogy has continued the journey of practice development in social work. Continued professional development in the complex world of social work depends on social workers coming to grips with the uncertainties and complexities of practice. Interwoven with these themes is that of integration. The further theme we have continued from our two previous books (Adams et al., 2009a, 2009b) is that of connectedness, as practice involves working across disciplinary, professional and organisational boundaries. We have argued that the challenges of practice require practitioners to adopt an integrative style of working in different settings, as they undertake management and leadership roles and develop a research focus. This book has been structured around these three aspects: Part 1 has dealt with major areas of practice, Part 2 with leadership and management and Part 3 with research.

Integrating critical practice

It is vital that critical practitioners retain a creative style of working that is open to continuous refinement and improvement. By its nature, criticality is ongoing and never finished. When we bring this notion of criticality together with the goal of integrating practice, it is apparent that integrating is also a continuing activity. It would be a lost opportunity to regard any piece of practice as having achieved full integration, since critical practitioners would then be unable to revisit it and pose the important question: 'What could I have done differently and better?' It is not a sign of weakness that we continue to have second, even third thoughts about our practice. On the contrary, the more we can bring our learning, experience, thoughts and emotions to bear on what we have done, the greater our potential for continued improvement. This process of continual self-questioning is helped by continuing to discuss with other people and keeping up to date with reading in areas of particular interest as practitioners. It is made much more systematic and potentially revitalising by developing a research interest in an aspect of current practice being undertaken. We have given research in practice its anchoring position at the end of this third book in our trilogy to emphasise the fact that practitioner research makes a particularly vital contribution to continuing professional development.

In this book, integrative social work has been concerned with creating something new and different from aspects – theories, approaches, methods, skills – that exist on their own. Notions such as 'complexity' and 'boundary crossing' enable us to appreciate how we can bring different dimensions to bear holistically on our practice. We can appreciate that there are differences in kind between the different types of material we have encountered in the three parts of this book. Embedded in these differences are questions and debates about various aspects of these. As examples of this, from the last part of this book, which has dealt with research, we can identify three important questions, which it is easier to raise than to answer: What counts as knowledge? What counts as evidence? What counts as social work? There are no simple answers to such questions. We are likely to keep returning to them as we study and practise within particular aspects of social work.

Continuing professional development

The process of critical reflection on practice does not stop short at the end of work with a particular case, or at the end of a day's work. The processes of analysis and action, continually deconstructing and reconstructing to reflect constantly changing circumstances, are open-ended. We have deliberately avoided implying that critical practice is an end point, but have presented it within the traditions of social criticism and critiques of practice.

In a similar vein, professional and personal development continually interweave. Criticality is not a concept that can be contained in the office without it affecting our thoughts, feelings and actions more widely. The processes of personal and professional development interact. In much the same way, personal development is a continuing process and is affected by life events as well as by work. It is fashionable to attach terms such as 'lifelong learning' and 'ongoing practice' to the discussion of practice development. However, we would attach the aim of developing critical practice in social work to any programme of continuing professional development. It is significant that there is a lack of closure in our statements about the level of expertise that critical practice requires. Becoming a critical practitioner is easier to recognise than it is to accept somebody's claim to have achieved being a critical practitioner, as though it is a once-in-a-lifetime accomplishment.

The critical practitioner constantly strives towards the accomplishment of developing the habit of criticality. There is an acceptable level of expertise, but whether there are 'experts' in critical practice is another matter. It is probably more realistic to assert that criticality continues to be affected by the major critiques of power and those hierarchical structures of division and oppression – racism, sexism and class – which generate continually changing frameworks for critical analysis and action. Of course it is also affected by personal matters such as the level of energy a practitioner can apply today. The people we work with also have an impact on the degree of criticality we apply. Colleagues, subordinates and managers, service users, carers and members of a multiprofessional team may all have a place in determining the extent of our criticality at any time and in any situation. Being critical means responding thoughtfully to the relationships we are working within, while also holding on to the idea that those relationships should not prevent the criticality that is necessary for ... what? We must critically decide.

Managing uncertainty, complexity and tensions

We have illustrated how uncertainties, complexities and tensions are embedded in practice. There are aspects of our experience that are solidly grounded in the continuity of the past with the present. There are other aspects where we are pushing beyond what we already know from experience and prior learning. These create gaps and discontinuities for us, which can leave us feeling uncertain but also provide opportunities for transformation in the future.

The problems that service users and therefore practitioners face are complex, because of our own uncertainties and because people's vulnerabilities and problems are complex. There are always different potential choices for action and these always become more extensive if we are critical. Being critical creates dilemmas for us, but offers a wider range of opportunities. Being a critical practitioner is difficult in these circumstances because it involves accepting constraints and freedom, in the context of everyday realities. While critical practice is emancipatory because it should transform lives and social structures and empower workers and clients, it takes place in the context of the oppressive structures of racism, sexism and class, which have their impact at every turn on the efforts of the practitioner. The tensions of practice are compounded by legal, organisational and practice requirements that further constrain the worker. Social work is more difficult because creative practice is possible in these circumstances, than if prohibitions existed against any such initiatives. It is part of the uniqueness of social work that such difficulties exist and that, paradoxically, they also present opportunities to resist oppression.

The pace of change in social work is such that this book, too, becomes part of social work's history, even in the period between its writing and publication. However, the notion of critical practice is like a template, which can be brought to bear on any situation, enabling us as practitioners to remain optimistic and in control of our practice, in the face of the tensions.

Moral hope for practitioners

We have seen how social workers subscribe to a code of ethics, which reflects the fact that social work is a moral activity. We are not referring here to moralising, but to the need to maintain professional values in practice. The challenge for practitioners is to avoid being ground down by the constraints and becoming so undisciplined that they lose their moral bearings. The persistence of oppression in all its forms reinforces the need for an optimistic critical practice, which is not defensive or nihilistic in the face of prevailing social structures, but engages with them. Moral hope (Leonard, 1997) is a way of thinking that enables practitioners to do that by providing alternative ways of considering problems and possible solutions or ways forward. It provides a guarded optimism that is rooted in the belief that resistance and survival strategies can be utilised to formulate alternatives to what is currently available. Without moral hope, there is only burnout and despair. This book provides ammunition for this, in the form of ideas, knowledge and experiences. Carole Smith (2001) has written of the need not to abandon the traditional values of social work – the qualities of sensitivity, concern, reassurance, compassion and warmth – in striving to achieve the morally good. This offers a prospect beyond a view of practice advancing on the basis of evidence alone, where social work may be merely the tool of instrumental rationality.

Critical practice is transformational

In various ways, critical practice is a transformational activity. We suggested above that moving from understanding to criticality is an essential stage in moving eventually towards action. This is because deciding to intervene necessarily requires us to think that the present situation requires transformation, not just maintenance or change. Criticality must, therefore, be transformational. However, it does not in itself transform: the final stage is to act on the critical decision. When we can practise critically, we can use these skills to advance our practice, for the benefit of those we work with and for the benefit of better social work and better services.

The diversity of fields for practice means that transformations can take place in various domains and at different levels. Advancing social work practice means helping the achievements in those fields to interact, so it is more generic in its progress. Initially, when the worker transforms understanding by making it critical, it becomes relocated in its wider contexts. Subsequently, understandings are continually revisited. This is not a one-off event, segregated from practice. But it may gain in emancipatory and empowering potential as the practice develops. The worker makes links with other areas of practice, in the light of analysis and action, and puts clients in touch with others in comparable situations, in a liberating fashion.

Critical analysis enables the practitioner to perceive oppressive features beyond ideologies and reconceptualising, which is integral to continuing critical action. In this sense, critical practice is political, not in the party political sense but in the sense that it engages with debates about how scarce resources are allocated and where the power to make decisions about them is located. Critical practice, therefore, deploys social work values in challenging inequalities and social justice.

An example of the fusion between political and moral commitment that is embedded in professional values is the People's Inquiry into Detention in Australia (Briskman et al., 2008), which was sponsored by the Australian Council of Heads of Social Work (referred to in Adams et al., 2009b, Ch. 5). This demonstrates how social workers can act to uphold the values of social justice. It also shows how necessary it is to develop and use research skills in practice. Without the gathering of evidence and rigorous analysis, it would not be possible to construct a credible case for change. This illustrates how the role of critical practitioners depends on their expertise as well as on their commitment.

This theme of commitment is part and parcel of maintaining criticality. We need to be engaged positively in our practice. The critical practitioner is at the opposite pole from the alienated worker. In this sense, critical practice is akin to a belief that has penetrated the ideological masking of oppressive features of the social situation. Critical practice engenders a sense of hope in the values that the worker seeks to establish and confirm, and in their application. Just as we have engaged in dialectical and reflexive processes in writing and editing this book, so we invite you, the reader, as a critical practitioner, to try using the chapters in this way and endorse this fundamentally critical approach to practice.

As editors, we are committed to exposing and challenging oppression, rather than presenting this book as a stock of already fixed knowledge. Both we and you, as critical practitioners in our own ways, are active participants in the development of this critical awareness, actions and practice. In pursuing this, we maintain the hope that social work practice may be transformed through its own actions to improve its helpfulness. In our first book together, *Social Work: Themes, Issues and Critical Debates* (Adams et al., 2009a), we focused on understanding – what some people call 'knowledge for'. In the second book, *Critical Practice in Social Work* (Adams et al., 2009b), we focused on expertise – what some people call 'skills' or 'knowledge how to' – in applying our analysis to practice. In this third book, we have pushed the boundaries of our expertise as critical practitioners in different directions – towards more complex situations and problems, into leadership and management and practice-based research. These are all challenging tasks in their own different ways. They are unending tasks, in that the constantly changing variety of practice means that we have to act creatively and innovatively to develop our practice, so as to transform social work and its actions in positive ways.

www.iassw-aiets.org International Association of Schools of Social Work.

www.socialworkaction.org The activist network of social work academics, practitioners, students and others.

www.basw.co.uk The British Association of Social Workers is the professional body representing social workers.

www.gscc.org.uk The General Social Care Council sets standards for social work and registers practitioners.

www.sssc.uk.com The Scottish Social Services Council regulates standards and registers practitioners in Scotland.

www.ccwales.org.uk The Care Council for Wales regulates standards and registers practitioners in Wales.

www.niscc.info The Northern Ireland Social Care Council regulates standards and registers practitioners in Northern Ireland.

Bibliography

Abbott, A. (1988) *The System of Professions*, Chicago: University of Chicago Press.

Abbott, S. and Lewis, H. (2002) 'Partnership working and eligibility criteria: what can we learn from the implementation of guidance on continuing health care?', *Social Policy and Administration*, **36**(5): 532–43.

ACMD (Advisory Council on the Misuse of Drugs) (2003) *Hidden Harm: Responding to the Needs of Children of Problem Drug Users*, London: Home Office.

ACMD (Advisory Council on the Misuse of Drugs) (2007) *Hidden Harm: Three Years On*, London: Home Office.

Adair, A. (1986) *Effective Teambuilding*, London: Pan.

Adams, J. (1995) *Risk*, London: UCL Press.

Adams, R. (1991) *Protests by Pupils: Empowerment, Schooling and the State*, Basingstoke: Falmer.

Adams, R. (1998a) 'Social work processes', in R. Adams, L. Dominelli and M. Payne (eds) *Social Work Themes, Issues and Critical Debates*, 2nd edn, Basingstoke: Macmillan – now Palgrave Macmillan.

Adams, R. (1998b) *Quality Social Work*, Basingstoke: Macmillan – now Palgrave Macmillan.

Adams, R. (1998c) 'Empowerment and protest', in B. Lesnik (ed.) *Challenging Discrimination in Social Work*, Aldershot: Ashgate.

Adams, R. (2000) 'Quality assurance', in M. Davies (ed.) *The Blackwell Encyclopaedia of Social Work*, Oxford: Blackwell.

Adams, R., Dominelli, L. and Payne, M. (eds) (2009a) *Social Work: Themes, Issues and Critical Debates*, 3rd edn, Basingstoke: Palgrave Macmillan.

Adams, R., Dominelli, L. and Payne, M. (eds) (2009b) *Critical Practice in Social Work*, 2nd edn, Basingstoke: Palgrave Macmillan.

Adams, R., Dominelli, L. and Payne, M. (eds) (2009c) *Practising Social Work in a Complex World*, 2nd edn, Basingstoke: Palgrave Macmillan.

ADSS (Association of Directors of Social Services) (2005) *Safeguarding Adults: A National Framework of Standards for Good Practice and Outcomes in Adult Protection Work*, London: ADSS.

Alaszewski, H. and Alaszewski, A. (1998) 'Professional and practice: decision making and risk', in A. Alaszewski, L. Harrison and J. Manthorpe (eds) *Risk, Health and Welfare*, Buckingham: Open University Press.

Aldridge, J., Parker, H. and Measham, F. (1999) *Drug Trying and Drug Use across Adolescence: A Longitudinal Study of Young People's Drug Taking in Two Regions of Northern England*, DPAS Paper No.1, London: Home Office.

Alexander, L. and Link, B. (2003) 'The impact of contact on stigmatising attitudes towards people with mental illness', *Journal of Mental Health*, **12**(3): 271–90.

Alexander, L. and Richman, K. (2008) 'Ethical dilemmas in evaluations using indigenous research workers', *American Journal of Evaluation*, **29**(1): 73–85.

Anning, A., Cottrell, D., Green, J. et al. (2006) *Developing Multiprofessional Teamwork for Integrated Children's Services*, Buckingham: Open University Press.

APA (American Psychological Association) (2001) *Publication Manual of the American Psychological Association*, 5th edn, New York: APA.

Appleby, G.A. and Anastas, J.W. (1998) *Not Just a Passing Phase: Social Work with Gay, Lesbian, and Bisexual People*, New York: Columbia University Press.

Askeland, G.A. and Payne, M. (2008) *Globalization and International Social Work: Postmodern Change and Challenge*, Aldershot: Ashgate.

Avery, G. (2004) *Understanding Leadership: Paradigms and Cases*, London: Sage.

Bailar, J.C. and Bailer, A.J. (1999) 'Risk assessment – the mother of all uncertainties: disciplinary perspectives on uncertainty in risk assessment', *Annals of New York Academy of Sciences*, **895**: 273–85.

Balding, J. (2001) *Young People in 2000*, Exeter: Schools Health Education Unit.

Balloch, S., Pahl, J. and McLean, J. (1998) 'Working in social services: job satisfaction, stress and violence', *British Journal of Social Work*, **28**: 329–50.

Bandalli, S. (1998) 'Abolition of the presumption of doli incapax and the criminalisation of children', *Howard Journal of Criminal Justice*, **37**(2): 114–23.

Banks, S. (2003) 'From oaths to rulebooks: a critical examination of codes of ethics for the social professions', *European Journal of Social Work*, **6**(2): 133–44.

Banks, S. (2006) *Ethics and Values in Social Work*, 3rd edn, Basingstoke: Palgrave Macmillan.

Barnes, C. (1991) *Disabled People in Britain and Discrimination: A Case for Anti-discrimination Legislation*, London: Hurst.

Barnes, C. and Mercer, G. (eds) (1997) *Doing Disability Research*, Leeds: Disability Press.

Barnes, C., Mercer, G. and Shakespeare, T. (1999) *Exploring Disability*, Cambridge: Polity Press.

Barnes, D. and Kendall, M. (2001) 'Working with disabled people in consultation and research', *Research Policy and Planning*, **19**(1): 17–24.

Barr, A. (2003) 'Participative planning and evaluation skills', in S. Banks, H. Butcher, P. Henderson and J. Robertson (eds) *Managing Community Practice: Principles, Policies and Programmes*, Bristol: Policy Press.

Barr, A. and Hashagen, S. (2000) *ABCD Handbook: A Framework for Evaluating Community Development*, London: Community Development Foundation.

BASW (British Association of Social Work) (2002) *A Code of Ethics for Social Work*, Birmingham: BASW.

Bateman, N. (2000) *Advocacy Skills for Health and Social Care Professionals*, London: Jessica Kingsley.

Bauld, L., Chesterman, J. and Judge, K. (2000) 'Measuring satisfaction with social care amongst older service users: issues from the literature', *Health and Social Care in the Community*, **8**(5): 316–24.

Bayley, J. (1999) *Iris and the Friends*, London: Abacus.

Bayliss, K. (2000) 'Social work values, anti-discriminatory practice and working with older lesbian service users', *Social Work Education*, **19**(1): 45–53.

Beattie, A. (1994) 'Healthy alliances or dangerous liaisons? The challenge of working together in health promotion', in A. Leathard (ed.) *Going Inter-professional: Working Together for Health and Welfare*, London: Routledge.

Beck, U. (1992) *Risk Society: Towards a New Modernity*, London: Sage.

Beck, U. (1998) 'Politics of risk society', in J. Franklin (ed.) *The Politics of Risk Society*, Cambridge: Polity Press.

Beck, U. (1999) *World Risk Society*, Cambridge: Polity Press.

Becker, S. (1997) *Responding to Poverty: The Politics of Cash and Care*, Harlow: Longman.

Beckett, C. (2003) *Child Protection*, London: Sage.

Belenky, M., Clinchy, M., Goldberger, N. and Tarule, M. (1997) *Women's Ways of Knowing: The Development of Self, Voice and Mind*, New York: Basic Books.

Bell, C. and Newby, H. (1977) *Doing Sociological Research*, Allen & Unwin: London.

Ben-Ari, A.T. (2001) 'Homosexuality and heterosexism: views from academics in the helping professions', *British Journal of Social Work*, **31**: 119–31.

Bennett, K., Heath, T. and Jeffries, R. (2007) *Asylum Statistics*, Home Office, www.homeoffice.gov.uk/rds.

Beresford, P. (2000) 'Service users' knowledges and social work theory', *British Journal of Social Work*, **30**(4): 489–503.

Beresford, P. (2008) 'Fast food nation', *Guardian Society*, 28 May, p. 4.

Beresford, P. and Evans, C. (1999) 'Research note: research and empowerment', *British Journal of Social Work*, **29**(5): 671–7.

Berger, R.M. (1983) 'What is a homosexual? A definitional model', *Social Work*, **28**(2): 132–5.

Berridge, V. ([1981]1999) *Opium and the People: Opiate Use and Drug Control Policy in Nineteenth and Early Twentieth Century England*, London: Free Association Books.

Biehal, N. (2007) 'Reuniting children and their families: reconsidering the evidence on timing, contact and outcomes', *British Journal of Social Work*, **37**(5): 807–23.

Bilson, A. and Ross, S. (1999) *Social Work Management and Practice: Systems Principles*, 2nd edn, London: Jessica Kingsley.

Bindel, J. (2006) 'Absent enemies', *Guardian*, 21 November.

Blaug, R. (1995) 'Distortion of the face to face: communicative reason and social work practice', *British Journal of Social Work*, **25**: 423–39.

BMA (British Medical Association) (2007) *Domes-*

tic Abuse, London: Science and Education Department, BMA.

Bok, S. (1984) *Secrets: Concealment and Revelation*, Oxford: Oxford University Press.

Bottoms, A.E. (1995) 'The philosophy and politics of punishment and sentencing', in C. Clark and R. Morgan (eds) *The Politics of Sentencing Reform*, Clarendon Press: Oxford.

Bowell, T. and Kemp, G. (2002) *Critical Thinking: A Concise Guide*, London: Routledge.

Boyne, G., Gould-Williams, J., Law, J. and Walker, R. (2001) 'The impact of best value on local authority performance: evidence from the Welsh pilots', *Local Government Studies*, **27**(2): 44–68.

Bradley, G., Penhale, B., Manthorpe, J. et al. (2000) *Ethical Dilemmas and Administrative Justice: Perceptions of Social and Legal Professionals towards Charging for Residential and Nursing Home Care*, Hull: University of Hull.

Bradley, R. (1987) 'Workload management in an area team', in B. Glastonbury, R. Bradley and J. Orme (eds) *Managing People in the Personal Social Services*, Chichester: Wiley.

Brewer, C. and Lait, J. (1980) *Can Social Work Survive?*, London: Temple Smith.

Bridgen, P. and Lewis, J. (1999) *Elderly People and the Boundary between Health and Social Care 1946–1991*, London: The Nuffield Trust.

Brigham, L. (2000) 'Understanding segregation from the nineteenth to the twentieth century: re-drawing boundaries and the problems of "pollution"', in L. Brigham, D. Atkinson, M. Jackson et al. (eds) *Crossing Boundaries: Change and Continuity in the History of Learning Disability*, Kidderminster: British Institute of Learning Disabilities.

Briskman, L., Latham, S. and Goddard, C. (2008) *Human Rights Overboard: Seeking Asylum in Australia*, Carlton North, Victoria: Scribe.

Broad, B. and Fletcher, C. (eds) (1993) *Practitioner Social Work Research in Action*, London: Whiting & Birch.

Brockbank, A. and McGill, I. (1998) *Facilitating Reflective Learning in Higher Education*, Buckingham: SRHE/Open University Press.

Brooker, D. (2006) *Person-centred Dementia Care: Making Services Better. Bradford Dementia Group Good Practice Guides*, London: Jessica Kingsley.

Brown, A. and Bourne, I. (1996) *The Social Work Supervisor*, Buckingham: Open University Press.

Brown, C. (2004) 'Social work intervention: the deconstruction of individuals as a means of remaining in the UK', in D. Hayes and B. Humphries (eds) *Social Work, Immigration and Asylum*, London: Jessica Kingsley.

Brown, H.C. (1991) 'Competent child-focused practice: working with lesbians and gay carers', *Adoption and Fostering*, **15**(2): 11–17.

Brown, H.C. (1992) 'Lesbians, the state and social work practice', in M. Langan and L. Day (eds) *Women, Oppression and Social Work: Issues in Anti-discriminatory Practice*, London: Routledge.

Brown, H.C. (1998) *Social Work and Sexuality: Working with Lesbians and Gay Men*, Basingstoke: Macmillan – now Palgrave Macmillan.

Brown, L., Tucker, C. and Domokos, T. (2003) 'Evaluating the impact of integrated health and social care teams on older people living in the community', *Health and Social Care in the Community*, **11**(2): 85–94.

Brownlee, K., Sprakes, A., Saini, M. et al. (2005) 'Heterosexism among social work students', *Social Work Education*, **24**(5): 485–94.

Bryman, A. (2008) *Social Research Methods*, 3rd edn, Oxford: Oxford University Press.

BSA (British Sociological Association) (2004) *Statement of Ethical Practice*, www.britsoc. co.uk/equality.

Buchanan, D. and Huczynski, A. (2004) *Organizational Behaviour*, 5th edn, London: Prentice Hall.

Buckle, J. (1981) *Intake Teams*, London: Tavistock.

Bulmer, M. (2001) 'The ethics of social research', in N. Gilbert (ed.) *Researching Social Life*, 2nd edn, London: Sage.

Burnes, B. (2004) *Managing Change*, 4th edn, London: Prentice Hall.

Burnett, A. and Fassil, Y. (2002) *Meeting the Health Needs of Refugees and Asylum Seekers in the UK*, London: NHS Publications.

Burney, E. (1999) *Crime and Banishment: Nuisance and Exclusion in Social Housing*, Winchester: Waterside Press.

Burton, J. and van den Broek, D. (2008) 'Accountable and countable: information management systems and the bureaucratization of social work', *British Journal of Social Work*, Advance Access, doi:10.1093/bjsw/bcn027.

Butler, I. (2002) 'A code of ethics for social work and social care research', *British Journal of Social Work*, **32**: 239–48.

Butler, I. (2003) 'Doing good research and doing it well: ethical awareness and the production of social work research', *Social Work Education*, **22**(1): 19–30.

Butler, I. and Drakeford, M. (2003) *Social Policy, Social Welfare and Scandal: How British Public Policy is Made*, Basingstoke: Palgrave Macmillan.

Butler, I. and Pugh, R. (2004) 'The politics of social work research', in R. Lovelock, K. Lyons and J. Powell (eds) *Reflecting on Social Work: Discipline and Profession*, Aldershot: Ashgate.

Butler, J. (2004) *Undoing Gender*, New York: Routledge.

Butler-Sloss, E. (2003) *Are we Failing the Family? Human Rights, Children and the Meaning of Family in the 21st Century*, www.led.gov.uk/judicial/speeches/ dbs030403.htm.

Butt, R. (2005) 'The trials of living with the "feral youths" of Salford', *Guardian*, 21 May.

Byatt, A.S. (2000) *The Biographer's Tale*, London: Chatto & Windus.

Bywater, J. and Jones, R. (2007) *Sexuality and Social Work*, Exeter: Learning Matters.

Cable, S. (2002) 'The context: why the current interest?', in S. Glen and T. Leiba (eds) *Multiprofessional Learning for Nurses: Breaking the Boundaries*, Basingstoke: Palgrave Macmillan.

Caddick, B. and Watson, D. (1999) 'Rehabilitation and the distribution of risk', in P. Parsloe (ed.) *Risk Assessment in Social Care and Social Work*, London: Jessica Kingsley.

Cameron, A. and Lart, R. (2003) 'Factors promoting and obstacles hindering joint working: a systematic review of the research evidence', *Journal of Integrated Care*, **11**(2): 9–17.

Camilleri, P. and Ryan, M. (2006) 'Social work students' attitudes toward homosexuality and their knowledge and attitudes toward homosexual parenting as an alternative family unit: an Australian study', *Social Work Education*, **25**(3): 288–304.

Campbell, J. and Oliver, M. (1996) *Disability Politics: Understanding our Past, Changing our Future*, London: Routledge.

Carpenter, V. (1988) 'Amnesia and antagonism: anti-lesbianism in the youth service', in B. Cant and S. Hemmings (eds) *Radical Records: Thirty Years of Lesbian & Gay History, 1957–1987*, London: Routledge.

Carroll, M. and Holloway, E. (eds) (1999) *Counselling Supervision in Context*, London: Sage.

Carroll, S. (2008) *NHS Drug Availability: An Evaluation of the National Institute for Health and Clinical Excellence*, London: The Bow Group.

Carson, D. (1996) 'Risking legal repercussions', in H. Kemshall and J. Pritchard (eds) *Good Practice in Risk Assessment and Risk Management*, London: Jessica Kingsley.

Cashmore, J. and Paxman, M. (2006) 'Predicting after-care outcomes: the importance of 'felt security', *Child and Family Social Work*, **11**: 232–42.

Castel, R. (1991) 'From dangerousness to risk', in G. Burchell, C. Gordon and P. Miller (eds) *The Foucault Effect: Studies in Governmentality*, Hemel Hempstead: Harvester Wheatsheaf.

Challis, D., Stewart, K., Donnell, M. et al. (2006) 'Care management for older people: does integration make a difference?', *Journal of Interprofessional Care*, **20**(4): 335–48.

Chambon, A.S. and Irving, A. (1999) 'Introduction', in A.S. Chambon, A. Irving and L. Epstein (eds) *Reading Foucault for Social Work*, New York: Columbia University Press.

Charing, G., Deswardt, P., Henry, M. et al. (eds) (1975) *Case Con – Gay Issue 18*.

Cheek, J. (2000) *Postmodern and Poststructural Approaches to Nursing Research*, Thousand Oaks, CA: Sage.

Cheetham, J., Fuller, R., McIvor, G. and Petch, A. (1992) *Evaluating Social Work Effectiveness*, Buckingham: Open University Press.

Ciuccarelli, P., Ricci, D. and Vaisecchi, F. (2008) *Handling Changes through Diagrams: Scale and Grain in the Visual Representation of Complex Systems*, Milan: Politecnico di Milano, Design Knowledge Research Unit.

Clarke, A. (1999) *Evaluation Research: An Introduction to Principles, Methods and Practice*, London: Sage.

Clarke, C.L. (2000) *Social Work Ethics: Politics, Principles and Practice*, Basingstoke: Macmillan – now Palgrave Macmillan.

Clarke, J. and Glendinning, C. (2002) 'Partnership and the remaking of welfare provision', in C. Glendinning, M. Powell and K. Rummery (eds) *Partnerships, New Labour and the Governance of Welfare*, Bristol: Policy Press.

Clarke, J., Gewirtz, S. and McLaughlin, E. (eds) (2000) *New Managerialism, New Welfare?*, London: Sage.

Cohen, M. and Mullender, A. (eds) (2003) *Gender and Groupwork*, London: Routledge.

Cohen, S. (1975) 'It's all right for you to talk', in R. Bailey and M. Brake (eds) *Radical Social Work and Practice*, London: Edward Arnold.

Cohen, S. (2001) *Immigration Controls, the Family and the Welfare State*, London: Jessica Kingsley.

Cohen, S. (2003) *No-one is Illegal: Asylum and Immigration Control, Past and Present*, London: Trentham Books.

Cohen, S. and Hayes, D. (1998) *They Make you Sick: Essays in Immigration Control and Health*, Manchester: Greater Manchester Immigration Aid Unit/Manchester Metropolitan University.

Community Care (2002) 'Council loses fight over cancer sufferer', *Community Care*, **1445**: 6.

Cooper, J. and Kapur, N. (2004) 'Assessing suicide risk', in D. Duffy and T. Ryan (eds) *New Approaches to Preventing Suicide*, London: Jessica Kingsley.

Coote, A. (1994) 'Performance and quality in public services', in A. Connor and S. Black (eds) *Performance Review and Quality in Social Care*, London: Jessica Kingsley.

Cope, S. and Goodship, J. (2002) 'The Audit Commission and public services: delivering for whom?', *Public Money and Management*, **22**(4): 33–40.

Corden, J. and Preston-Shoot, M. (1987) *Contracts in Social Work*, Aldershot: Gower.

Corrigan, P., Edwards, A., Green, A. et al. (2001) 'Prejudice, social distance and familiarity with mental illness', *Schizophrenia Bulletin*, **27**(2): 219–25.

Corrigan, P.W. and Penn, D.L. (1999) 'Lessons from social psychology on discrediting psychiatric stigma', *American Psychologist*, **54**(9): 765–76.

Coulshed, V., Mullender, A., Jones, D.N. and Thompson, N. (2006) *Management in Social Work*, Basingstoke: Palgrave Macmillan.

Council of Europe (2005) Report by Mr Alvaro Gil-Robles, Commissioner for Human Rights on his visit to the UK, 4–12 November 2004, CommDH (2005), Strasbourg: Council of Europe.

Couture, S.M. and Penn, D.L. (2003) 'Interpersonal contact and the stigma of mental illness: a review of the literature', *Journal of Mental Health*, **12**(3): 291–306.

Craig, G. (2002) 'Poverty, social work and social justice', *British Journal of Social Work*, **32**: 669–82.

Cree, V. (2000) *Sociology for Social Workers and Probation Officers*, London: Routledge.

Cree, V. and Davis, A. (2007) *Social Work: Voices from the Inside*, London: Routledge.

Crotty, M. (1998) *The Foundations of Social Research: Meaning and Perspective in the Research Process*, London: Sage.

Crowther, J. and Sutherland, P. (eds) (2005) *Lifelong Learning: Concepts and Contexts*, Routledge: London.

CSCI (Commission for Social Care Inspection) (2006) *The State of Social Care in England*, London: CSCI, www.csci.org.uk/PDF/state_of_social_care.pdf.

Cupitt, S. (1997) 'Who sets the agenda for empowerment?', *Breakthrough*, **1**(2): 15–28.

Daily Mail (1991) 'The little tearaways: police start a war on crime with the four year olds', 15 February.

Darlington, Y. and Scott, D. (2002) *Qualitative Research in Practice: Stories from the Field*, Maidenhead: Open University Press.

Davey, B., Levin, E., Iliffe, S. and Kharicha, K. (2005) 'Integrating health and social care: implications for joint working and community care outcomes for older people', *Journal of Interprofessional Care*, **19**(1): 22–34.

Davies, C. (1995) *Gender and the Professional*

Predicament in Nursing, Buckingham: Open University Press.

Davis, A. (1996) 'Risk work and mental health', in H. Kemshall and J. Pritchard (eds) *Good Practice in Risk Assessment and Risk Management*, London: Jessica Kingsley.

Dawson, C. (2000) *Independent Successes: Implementing Direct Payments*, York: York Publishing Services.

D'Cruz, H. and Jones, M. (2004) *Social Work Research: Ethical and Political Contexts*, London: Sage.

DCSF (Department for Children, Schools and Families) (2007) *The Children's Plan: Building Brighter Futures*, London: TSO.

DCSF (Department for Children, Schools and Families) (2008) *Youth Task Force Action Plan*, London: TSO.

Deacon, A. (2002) *Perspectives on Welfare*, London: Open University Press.

Decrescenzo, T.S. (1984) 'Homophobia: a study of the attitudes of mental health professionals toward homosexuality', in R. Schoenberg, R. Goldberg and D. Shore (eds) *Homosexuality and Social Work*, New York: Haworth Press.

Deegan, P.E. (1994) 'Recovery: the lived experience of rehabilitation', in L. Spaniol and M. Koehler (eds) *The Experience of Recovery*, Boston: Center for Psychiatric Rehabilitation.

Desforges, D.M., Lord, C.G., Ramsay, S.L. et al. (1991) 'Effects of structured co-operative contact on changing negative attitudes towards stigmatised groups', *Journal of Personality and Social Psychology*, **60**(4): 531–44.

DfES (Department for Education and Skills) (2003) *Every Child Matters*, Green Paper, London: TSO.

DfES (Department for Education and Skills) (2004) *Every Child Matters: Change for Children*, London: TSO.

DH (Department of Health) (1998) *Modernising Social Services: Promoting Independence, Improving Protection, Raising Standards*, White Paper, Cm 4169, London: TSO.

DH (Department of Health) (1999) *National Service Framework for Mental Health*, London: TSO.

DH (Department of Health) (2000a) *No Secrets: Guidance on Developing and Implementing Multi-agency Policies and Procedures to Protect Vulnerable Adults from Abuse*, London: TSO.

DH (Department of Health) (2000b) *Framework for the Assessment of Children in Need and Their Families*, London: TSO.

DH (Department of Health) (2000c) *The NHS Plan*, London: TSO.

DH (Department of Health) (2002a) *Requirements for Social Work Training*, London: TSO.

DH (Department of Health) (2002b) *Fair Access to Care Services,* London: TSO.

DH (Department of Health) (2004) *Protection of Vulnerable Adults Scheme in England and Wales for Care Homes and Domiciliary Care Agencies: A Practice Guide,* London: TSO.

DH (Department of Health) (2005) *Research Governance Framework for Health and Social Care,* 2nd edn, London: TSO.

DH (Department of Health) (2006) *Our Health, Our Care, Our Say: A New Direction for Community Services,* White Paper, Cmnd 6737, London: TSO.

DH (Department of Health) (2007) *10 Steps to your SES: A Guide to Developing a Single Equality Scheme,* London: TSO.

DHSS (Department of Health and Social Security) (1988) *Community Care: Agenda for Action,* Griffiths Report, London: HMSO.

Dingwall, R. (1989) 'Some problems about predicting child abuse and neglect', in O. Stevenson (ed.) *Child Abuse: Public Policy and Professional Practice,* Hemel Hempstead: Harvester Wheatsheaf.

Dingwall, R., Eekelaar, J. and Murray, T. (1983) *The Protection of Children: State Intervention and Family Life,* Oxford: Basil Blackwell.

Dobash, R.E., Dobash, R.P. and Cavanagh, K. (1985) 'The contact between battered women and social and medical agencies', in J. Pahl (ed.) *Private Violence and Public Policy: The Needs of Battered Women and the Response of the Public Services,* London: Routledge & Kegan Paul.

Dobash, R.E., Dobash, R.P., Cavanagh, K. and Lewis, R. (2000) *Changing Violent Men,* London: Sage.

Doel, M. (2005) *Using Groupwork,* London: Routledge.

Dombeck, M. (1997) 'Professional personhood: training, territoriality and tolerance', *Journal of Interprofessional Care,* **11**(1): 9–21.

Dominelli, L. (1996) 'Deprofessionalising social work: anti-oppressive practice, competencies and post-modernism', *British Journal of Social Work,* **26**: 153–7.

Dominelli, L. (2004) *Social Work: Theory and Practice for a Changing Profession,* Cambridge: Polity Press.

Dominelli, L. (2005) 'Social inclusion in research: reflections upon a project involving young mothers', *International Journal of Social Welfare,* **14**(1): 13–22.

Dominelli, L. and Holloway, M. (2008) 'Ethics and governance in social work research in the UK', *British Journal of Social Work,* **38**(5): 1009–24.

Dorn, N. and Lee, M. (1999) 'Drugs and policing in Europe: from low streets to high places', in N.

South (ed.) *Drugs: Cultures, Controls and Everyday Life,* London: Sage.

Dorn, N., Murji, K. and South, N. (1992) *Traffickers: Drug Markets and Law Enforcement,* London: Routledge.

Douglas, M. (1992) *Risk and Blame: Essays in Cultural Theory,* London: Routledge.

Dowie, J. (1999) 'Communication for better decisions: not about "risk"', *Health, Risk and Society,* **1**(1): 41–53.

DRC (Disability Rights Commission) (2002a) *Response to Draft Mental Health Bill, England and Wales,* London: DRC.

DRC (Disability Rights Commission) (2002b) *Public Attitudes Survey,* conducted by BMRB, London: DRC.

DRC (Disability Rights Commission) (2003) *Disability Equality: Making it Happen. A Review of the Disability Discrimination Act 1995,* London: DRC.

DRC (Disability Rights Commission) (2004) *Strategic Plan 2004–7,* London: DRC.

DRC (Disability Rights Commission) (2006a) *Equal Treatment: Closing the Gap,* London: DRC.

DRC (Disability Rights Commission) (2006b) *Closing the Gap DVD,* London: DRC.

DRC (Disability Rights Commission) (2007a) *The Disability Agenda,* London: DRC.

DRC (Disability Rights Commission) (2007b) *Maintaining Standards, Promoting Equality,* London: DRC.

DRC/HSE (Disability Rights Commission/Health and Safety Executive) (2003) *Review of UK Case Law on the Use of Health and Safety Requirements as a False Excuse for Not Employing Sick or Disabled Persons,* London: DRC/HSE.

Dulaney, D.D. and Kelly, J. (1982) 'Improving services to gay and lesbian clients', *Social Work,* **27**(2): 178–83.

Dullea, K. and Mullender, A. (1999) 'Evaluation and empowerment', in I. Shaw and J. Lishman (eds) *Evaluation and Social Work Practice,* London: Sage.

Durham, A. (2003) 'Young men living through and with child abuse: a practitioner research study', *British Journal of Social Work,* **33**(3): 309–23.

Dustin, D. (2008) *The McDonaldization of Social Work,* Aldershot: Ashgate.

DWP (Department for Work and Pensions) (2001) *Recruiting Benefit Claimants: Qualitative Research with Employers in ONE Pilot Areas,* Research Series Paper No. 150, London: DWP.

DWP (Department for Work and Pensions) (2003) *Housing Benefit Sanctions and Anti Social Behaviour: A Consultation Paper,* London: DWP.

DWP (Department for Work and Pensions) (2008) *Working for a Healthier Tomorrow: Dame Carol Black's Review of the Health of Britain's Working Age Population*, London: TSO.

Eadie, T. and Canton, R. (2002) 'Practising in a context of ambivalence: the challenge for youth justice workers', *Youth Justice*, 2(1): 14–26.

Earle, R., Crawford, A. and Newburn, T. (2003) 'Referral orders: some reflections on policy transfer and "what works"', *Youth Justice*, 2(3): 141–50.

Edmunds, M., Hough, M., Turnbull, P.J. and May, T. (1999) *Doing Justice to Treatment: Referring Offenders to Drug Services*, DPAS Paper No.2, London: Home Office.

Edmunds, M., May, T., Hearden, I. and Hough, M. (1998) *Arrest Referral: Emerging Lessons from Research*, Drugs Prevention Initiative Paper 23, London: Home Office Central Drugs Prevention Unit.

Egeland, C. and Gressgard, R. (2007) 'The "will to empower": managing the complexity of the others', *Nordic Journal of Feminist and Gender Research*, 15(4): 207–19.

Elshtain, J.B. (ed.) (2002) *Jane Addams: A Reader*, New York: Basic Books.

Employers Forum on Disability (1998) *Practical Guide to Employment Adjustments for People with Mental Health Problems*, London: Employers Forum on Disability.

Englander, D. (1994) *A Documentary History of Jewish Immigrants in Britain 1840–1920*, Leicester: Leicester University Press.

Epstein, S. ([1987]1998) 'Gay politics, ethnic identity: the limits of social constructionism', in P. Nardi and B. Schneider (eds) *Social Perspectives in Lesbian and Gay Studies: A Reader*, London: Routledge.

Etzioni, A. (ed.) (1969) *The Semi-professions and their Organization*, New York: Free Press.

Evans, C. and Fisher, M. (1999) 'Collaborative evaluation with service users', in I. Shaw and J. Lishman (eds) *Evaluation and Social Work Practice*, London: Sage.

Evans, D. (1999) *Practice Learning in the Caring Professions*, Aldershot: Ashgate.

Everitt, A. (1998) 'Research and development in social work', in R. Adams, L. Dominelli and M. Payne (eds) *Social Work: Themes, Issues and Critical Debates*, 2nd edn, Basingstoke: Macmillan – now Palgrave Macmillan.

Everitt, A. and Hardiker, P. (1996) *Evaluating for Good Practice*, Basingstoke: BASW/Macmillan – now Palgrave Macmillan.

Everitt, A., Hardiker, P., Littlewood, J. and Mullender, A. (1992) *Applied Research for Better Practice*, Basingstoke: Macmillan – now Palgrave Macmillan.

Evetts, J. (2006a) 'Introduction: trust and professionalism: challenges and occupational changes', *Current Sociology*, 54(4): 515–31.

Evetts, J. (2006b) 'Short note: the sociology of professional groups: new directions', *Current Sociology*, 54(1): 133–43.

Ewald, F. (1991) 'Insurance and risk', in G. Burchell, C. Gordon and P. Miller (eds) *The Foucault Effect: Studies in Governmentality*, Hemel Hempstead: Harvester Wheatsheaf.

Fadiman, A. (1997) *The Spirit Catches You and You Fall Down*, New York: Farrar, Strauss & Giroux.

Fannin, A., Fenge, L.-A., Hicks, C. and Lavin, N. (2008) *Social Work Practice with Older Lesbians and Gay Men*, Exeter: Learning Matters.

Farrell, A. (ed.) (2005) *Ethical Research with Children*, Maidenhead: Open University Press.

Fauth, R. and Mahdon, M. (2007) *Improving Social and Health Care Services*. London: SCIE.

Featherstone, B. and Green, L. (2008) 'Judith Butler', in M. Gray and S.A. Webb (eds) *Thinking about Social Work: Theories and Methods for Practice*, London: Sage.

Fell, P. and Hayes, D. (2007) *What Are They Doing Here? A Critical Guide to Asylum and Immigration*, Birmingham: Venture Press.

Ferris, D. (1977) *Homosexuality and the Social Services: The Report of an NCCL Survey of Local Authority Social Services Committees*, London: National Council for Civil Liberties.

Feuerstein, M.T. (1986) *Partners in Evaluation: Evaluating Development and Community Programmes with Participants*, London: Macmillan – now Palgrave Macmillan.

Fisher, M. (1999) 'Social work research, social work knowledge and the research assessment exercise', in B. Broad (ed.) *The Politics of Social Work Research and Evaluation*, Birmingham: Venture Press.

Fisher, M. (2002a) 'The Social Care Institute for Excellence: the role of a national institute in developing knowledge and practice in social care', *Social Work and Social Sciences Review*, 10(2): 6–34.

Fisher, M. (2002b) 'The role of service users in problem formulation and technical aspects of social research', *Social Work Education*, 21(3): 305–12.

Fook, J. (1996) *The Reflective Researcher: Social Workers' Theories of Practice Research*, Sydney: Allen & Unwin.

Fook, J. (2000) 'Deconstructing and reconstructing professional expertise', in B. Fawcett, B. Featherstone, J. Fook and A. Rossiter (eds)

Postmodern Feminist Perspectives, London: Routledge.

Fook, J. (2002) *Social Work: Critical Theory and Practice*, London: Sage.

Fook, J. (2003) 'Social work research in Australia', *Journal of Social Work Education*, **22**(1): 45–57.

Fook, J. (2004) 'Critical reflection and transformational possibilities', in L. Davies and P. Leonard (eds) *Social Work in a Corporate Era*, Aldershot: Ashgate.

Foreman, M. and Quinlan, M. (2008) 'Increasing social work students' awareness of heterosexism and homophobia: a partnership between a community gay health project and a school of social work', *Social Work Education*, **27**(2): 152–8.

Foster, P. and Wilding, P. (2000) 'Whither welfare professionalism?', *Social Policy and Administration*, **34**(2): 143–59.

Foucault, M. (1972) *Discipline and Punish*, Harmondsworth: Penguin.

Foucault, M. (1978) *The History of Sexuality*, vol. 1: *An Introduction*, New York: Random House.

Foucault, M. (1980) *Power/Knowledge: Selected Interviews and Other Writings, 1972–1977*, ed. C. Gordon, Brighton: Harvester Press.

Foucault, M. (1981) 'The order of discourse', in R. Young (ed.) *Untying the Text: A Post-structuralist Reader*, London: Routledge & Kegan Paul.

Foucault, M. (1988) 'Technologies of the self', in L. Martin, H. Gutman and P. Hutton (eds) *Technologies of the Self: A Seminar with Michel Foucault*, London: Tavistock.

Foucault, M. (2000) 'Foucault', in J.D. Faubion (ed.) *Essential Works of Michel Foucault 1954–1984*, vol. 2: *Aesthetics, Method, and Epistemology*, London: Penguin.

Franklin, B. and Parton, N. (1991) *Social Work, the Media and Public Relations*, London: Routledge.

Fraser, H. (2004) 'Doing narrative research: analysing person stories line-by-line', *Qualitative Social Work*, **3**(2):179–201.

Freeth, D. (2001) 'Sustaining interprofessional collaboration', *Journal of Interprofessional Care*, **15**(1): 37–46.

Freidson, E. (1970) *Professional Dominance: The Social Structure of Medical Care*, New York: Atherton Press.

Freidson, E. (2001) *Professionalism: The Third Logic*, Cambridge: Polity Press.

Freire, P. (1972) *The Pedagogy of the Oppressed*, Harmondsworth: Penguin.

Frost, N. (2002) 'A problematic relationship? Evidence and practice in the workplace', *Social Work and Social Sciences Review*, **10**(1): 38–50.

Frost, N. and Ryden, N. (2001) *An Evaluation of the South Lakeland Family Support Service*, Barkingside: Barnardo's.

Frost, N., Robinson, M. and Anning, A. (2005) 'Social workers in multidisciplinary teams: issues and dilemmas for professional practice', *Child and Family Social Work*, **10**: 187–96.

Fuller, R. (1996) 'Evaluating social work effectiveness: a pragmatic approach', in P. Alderson, S. Brill, I. Chalmers et al. (eds) *What Works? Effective Social Interventions in Child Welfare*, Barkingside: Barnardo's.

Fuller, R. and Petch, A. (eds) (1995) *Practitioner Research: The Reflective Social Worker*, Buckingham: Open University Press.

Furedi, F. (2002) *Culture of Fear*, London: Continuum.

Gallagher, G. (2003) 'Refugee treatment the world's harshest: Ozdowski', *The Age*, 10 October.

Galvani S. (2007) 'Refusing to listen: Are we failing the needs of people with alcohol and drug problems?', *Social Work Education*, **26**(7): 697–707.

Garland, D. (2001) *The Culture of Control: Crime and Social Order in Contemporary Society*, Oxford: Clarendon Press.

GCSRO (Government Chief Social Researcher Office) (2003) *Quality in Qualitative Evaluation: A Framework for Assessing Research Evidence*, London: Cabinet Office.

Gibbons, A. (1999) *A Fight to Belong*, London: Save the Children.

Gibbs, A. (2001a) 'Partnerships between the probation service and voluntary sector organizations', *British Journal of Criminology*, **31**(1): 15–18.

Gibbs, A. (2001b) 'The changing nature and context of social work research', *British Journal of Social Work*, **31**: 689–701.

Giddens, A. (1998) 'Risk society: the context of British politics', in J. Franklin (ed.) *The Politics of Risk Society*, Cambridge: Polity Press.

Gilgun, J. (1994) 'Hand into glove: the grounded theory approach and social work practice research', in E. Sherman and W.J. Reid (eds) *Qualitative Research in Social Work*, New York: Columbia University Press.

Gillespie, D. and Glisson, C. (eds) (1992) *Quantitative Methods in Social Work: The State of the Art*, Binghamton, NY: Haworth Press.

Gilman, M. (2000) 'Social exclusion and drug using parents', in F. Harbin and M. Murphy (eds) *Substance Misuse and Child Care: How to Understand, Assist and Intervene When Drugs Affect Parenting*, Lyme Regis: Russell House.

Ginsberg, N. (1989) 'Institutional racism and local authority housing', *Critical Social Policy*, **8**(3): 4–19.

Glasby, J. (2001) 'Money talks: the role of finance in social work education and practice', *Social Work Education*, **20**(4): 493–98.

Glasby, J. and Glasby, J. (2002) *Cash for Caring: A Practical Guide to Social Services Finance*, Lyme Regis: Russell House

Glaser, B. and Strauss, A. (1967) *The Discovery of Grounded Theory*, Chicago: Aldine.

Glastonbury, B., Bradley, R. and Orme, J. (eds) (1987) *Managing People in the Personal Social Services*, Chichester: Wiley.

GLC Women's Committee (1986) *Tackling Heterosexism: A Handbook of Lesbian Rights*, London: GLC.

Glennerster, H. (2003) *Understanding the Financing of Welfare*, Bristol: Policy Press.

Goldson, B. and Jamieson, J. (2002) 'Youth crime, the "parenting deficit" and state intervention: a contextual critique', *Youth Justice*, **2**(2): 82–99.

Golombok, S. (2000) *Parenting: What Really Counts?*, London: Routledge.

Gondolf, E. (2002) *Batterer Intervention Programs: Issues, Outcomes and Recommendations*, Thousand Oaks, CA: Sage.

Gondolf, E. (2004) 'Evaluating batterer counseling programs: a difficult task showing some effects', *Aggression and Violent Behavior*, **9**(6): 605–31.

Gordon, P. and Newnham, A. (1985) *Passport to Benefits: Racism in Social Security*, London: CPAG/Runnymede Trust.

Gorman, H. (2000a) 'Collaboration in community care and primary care', in M. Davies (ed.) *The Blackwell Encyclopaedia of Social Work*, Oxford: Blackwell.

Gorman, H. (2000b) 'Winning hearts and minds? Emotional labour and learning for care management work', *Journal of Social Work Practice*, **14**(2): 149–58.

Gorman, H. (2003) 'Which skills do care managers need? A research project on skills, competency and continuing professional development', *Social Work Education*, **22**(3): 245–61.

Gorman, H. and Lymbery, M. (2007) 'Continuous professional development', in M. Lymbery and K. Postle (eds) *Social Work: A Companion to Learning*, London: Sage.

Gorman, H. and Postle, K. (2003) *Transforming Community Care: A Distorted Vision?*, Birmingham: Venture Press.

Gould, N. and Taylor, I. (1996) *Reflective Learning for Social Work*, Aldershot: Ashgate.

Gramick, J. (1983) 'Homophobia: a new challenge', *Social Work*, **28**(2): 137–41.

Grant, L. (2000) 'Disabled people, poverty and debt: identity, strategy and policy', in J. Bradshaw and R. Sainsbury (eds) *Experiencing Poverty*, Aldershot: Ashgate.

Gray, P. (2002) *Disability Discrimination in Education: A Review of the Literature on Discrimination Across the 0–19 Age Range Undertaken on Behalf of the Disability Rights Commission*, London: DRC.

Green, J. (1992) 'The community development project revisited', in P. Carter, T. Jeffs and M. Smith (eds) *Changing Social Work and Welfare*, Buckingham: Open University Press.

Greenland, C. (1987) *Preventing CAN Deaths: An International Study of Deaths due to Child Abuse and Neglect*, London: Tavistock.

Grice, A. (2007) 'Crackdown to prevent the young falling into life on state benefits', *Independent*, 29 December.

Grier, A. and Thomas, T. (2003) 'Out of order', *Young People Now*, 16–22 July.

GSCC (General Social Care Council) (2004) *Code of Practice for Social Care Workers and Code of Practice for Employers of Social Care Workers*, London: GSCC.

GSCC (General Social Care Council) (2008) *Social Work at its Best: A Statement of Social Work Roles and Tasks for the 21st Century*, London: GSCC.

Guardian (2001) 'Welcome to Britain', compilation of articles originally published 20–3 May.

Hagell, A. and Newburn, T. (1994) *Persistent Young Offenders*, London: Policy Studies Institute.

Hague, G. and Malos, E. (2005) *Domestic Violence: Action for Change*, 3rd edn, Cheltenham: New Clarion Press.

Hague, G., Mullender, A. and Aris, R. (2003) *'Is Anyone Listening?' Accountability and Women Survivors of Domestic Violence*, London: Routledge.

Hague, G., Mullender, A., Aris, R. and Dear, W. (2001) *Abused Women's Perspectives: Responsiveness and Accountability of Domestic Violence and Inter-Agency Initiatives*, End of Award Report to the ESRC, Bristol: University of Bristol, School for Policy Studies.

Hague, G., Thiara, R.K., Mullender, A. and Magowan, P. (2008) *Making the Links: Disabled Women and Domestic Violence. Final Report*, Bristol: University of Bristol, School for Policy Studies.

Hales, L. (2002) 'Do drug testing and treatment orders really work?', *Criminal Justice Matters*, **47**: 18–19.

Hall, C. (1997) *Social Work as Narratives: Storytelling and Persuasion in Professional Texts*, Aldershot: Ashgate.

Hall, C., Slembrouck, S. and Sarangi, S. (2006) *Language Practices in Social Work: Categorisation and Accountability in Child Welfare*, London: Routledge.

Hall, M., Maclennan W. and Lye M. (1993) *Medical Care of the Elderly,* Chichester: John Wiley.

Hamer, S. (2002) 'It takes two to tango', *Criminal Justice Matters,* **47**: 14–15.

Hammersley, M. (2003) 'Social research today: some dilemmas and distinctions', *Qualitative Social Work,* **2**(1): 25–44.

Hammersley, M. and Atkinson, P. (2007) *Ethnography: Principles in Practice,* 3rd edn, London: Routledge.

Harbin, F. and Murphy, M. (2000) *Substance Misuse and Child Care: How to Understand, Assist and Intervene When Drugs Affect Parenting,* Lyme Regis: Russell House.

Hardiker, P. and Barker, M. (1988) 'A window on child care, poverty and social work', in S. Becker and S. MacPherson (eds) *Public Issues, Private Pain,* London: Social Services Insight Books.

Harding, S. (1991) *Whose Science? Whose Knowledge? Thinking from Women's Lives,* Milton Keynes: Open University Press.

Hardman, K. (1997) 'Social workers' attitudes to lesbian clients', *British Journal of Social Work,* **27**(4): 545–63.

Harman, K. and Paylor, I. (2002) 'A shift in strategy', *Criminal Justice Matters,* **47**: 8–9.

Harris, D.J., O'Boyle, M., Warbrick, C. et al. (2005) *Law of the European Convention on Human Rights,* 2nd edn, London: LexisNexis UK.

Harris, J. (2003a) '"Businessology" and social work', *Social Work and Society,* **1**(1), www.socwork.net/2003/1/debate/400.

Harris, J. (2003b) *The Social Work Business,* London: Routledge.

Harris, J. and Roberts, K. (2002) *Disabled People in Refugee and Asylum Seeking Communities,* Bristol: Policy Press/Joseph Rowntree Foundation.

Hart, E. and Bond, M. (1995) *Action Research for Health and Social Care: A Guide to Practice,* Buckingham: Open University Press.

Hart, S.D., Michie, C. and Cooke, D.J. (2007) 'Precision of actuarial risk assessment instruments: evaluating the "margins of error" of group v. individual predictions of violence', *British Journal of Psychiatry,* **190**: s60–5.

Harvey, L. (1990) *Critical Social Research,* London: Unwin Hyman.

Hawkins, P. and Shohet, R. (2000) *Supervision in the Helping Professions,* 2nd edn, Buckingham: Open University Press.

Hayes, D. (2002) 'From aliens to asylum seekers: a history of immigration controls and welfare in Britain', in S. Cohen, B. Humphries and E. Mynott (eds) *From Immigration Controls to Welfare Controls,* London: Routledge.

Hayes, D. and Humphries, B. (1999) 'Negotiating contentious research topics', in B. Broad (ed.) *The Politics of Social Work Research and Evaluation,* Birmingham: Venture Press.

Hayes, D. and Humphries, B. (2004) *Social Work, Immigration and Asylum: Debates, Dilemmas and Ethical Issues for Social Work and Social Care Practice,* London: Jessica Kingsley.

Hayter, T. (2000) *Open Borders: The Case against Immigration Controls,* London: Pluto Press.

Healy, K. (2000) *Social Work Practices: Contemporary Perspectives on Change,* London: Sage.

Healy, K. and Meagher, G. (2004) 'The reprofessionalization of social work: collaborative approaches for achieving professional recognition', *British Journal of Social Work,* **34**(2): 243–60.

Heath, S. (1982) *The Sexual Fix,* London: Macmillan – now Palgrave Macmillan.

Heather, N. and Robertson, I. (2003) *Problem Drinking,* 3rd edn, Oxford: Oxford University Press.

Henkel, M. (1995) 'Conceptions of knowledge in social work education', in M. Yelloly and M. Henkel (eds) *Learning and Teaching in Social Work: Towards Reflective Practice,* London: Jessica Kingsley.

Henwood, M. and Hudson, B. (2008) *Lost to the System? The Impact of Fair Access to Care,* London: CSCI.

Hepworth, M. (2000) *Stories of Ageing,* Buckingham: Open University Press.

Hester, M. (2005) 'Making it through the criminal justice system: attrition and domestic violence', *Social Policy and Society,* **5**(1): 79–90.

Hewstone, M. (2003) 'Intergroup contact: panacea for prejudice?', *The Psychologist,* **16**(7): 352–5.

Hicks, S. (1996) 'The "last resort"? Lesbian and gay experiences of the social work assessment process in fostering and adoption', *Practice,* **8**(2): 15–24.

Hicks, S. (1997) 'Taking the risk? Assessing lesbian and gay carers', in H. Kemshall and J. Pritchard (eds) *Good Practice in Risk Assessment and Risk Management 2: Protection, Rights and Responsibilities,* London: Jessica Kingsley.

Hicks, S. (2000) '"Good lesbian, bad lesbian …": regulating heterosexuality in fostering and adoption assessments', *Child & Family Social Work,* **5**(2): 157–68.

Hicks, S. (2003) 'The Christian right and homophobic discourse: a response to "evidence" that lesbian and gay parenting damages children', *Sociological Research Online,* **8**(4), www.socresonline.org.uk/8/4/hicks.html.

Hicks, S. (2006) 'Maternal men: perverts and deviants? Making sense of gay men as foster carers and adopters', *Journal of GLBT Family Studies*, **2**(1): 93–114.

Hicks, S. (2008a) 'Gender role models ... who needs 'em?!', *Qualitative Social Work*, **7**(1): 43–59.

Hicks, S. (2008b) 'Thinking through sexuality', *Journal of Social Work*, **8**(1): 65–82.

Hicks, S. (2008c) 'What does social work desire?', *Social Work Education*, **27**(2): 131–7.

Hicks, S. and McDermott, J. (eds) (1999) *Lesbian and Gay Fostering and Adoption: Extraordinary Yet Ordinary*, London: Jessica Kingsley.

Hicks, S. and Watson, K. (2003) 'Desire lines: "queering" health and social welfare', *Sociological Research Online*, **8**(1), www.socresonline.org.uk/8/1/hicks.html.

Hidalgo, H., Peterson, T.L. and Woodman, N.J. (eds) (1985) *Lesbian and Gay Issues: A Resource Manual for Social Workers*, Silver Springs, MD: NASW.

Hill, M. (2000) 'Social services and social security', in M. Hill (ed.) *Local Authority Social Services: An Introduction*, Oxford: Blackwell.

Hillin, A. (1985) 'When you stop hiding your sexuality ... ', *Social Work Today*, **4**: 18–19.

Hirschman, A.O. (1998) *Crossing Boundaries: Selected Writings*, New York: Zone Books.

HM Government (2007) *Putting People First: A Shared Vision and Commitment to the Transformation of Adult Social Care*, London: TSO.

HM Government (2008) *Drugs: Protecting Families and Communities – the 2008 Drug Strategy*, London: HM Government.

HM Prison Service (1998) *Tackling Drugs in Prison: The Prison Service Drugs Strategy*, London: HM Prison Service.

Holliday, A. (2002) *Doing and Writing Qualitative Research*, London: Sage.

Holman, B. (1987) 'Research from the underside', *British Journal of Social Work*, **17**(6): 669–83.

Holwerda, O. (2002) 'Love and sex: homosexuality', in C. Gruber and H. Stefanov (eds) *Gender in Social Work: Promoting Equality*, Lyme Regis: Russell House.

Homan, R. (1991) *The Ethics of Social Research*, London: Longman.

Home Office (1996) *Exchange of Information with the IND of the Home Office*, ref. IMG/96 1176/1193/23, circular to local authorities.

Home Office (1999) 'Home Secretary Urges Councils to Use New Powers to Protect the Vulnerable', press release, 15 October.

Home Office (2001) 'Hard-hitting New Programme to Tackle Persistent Young Offenders Goes Live', press release, 17 July.

Home Office (2002a) 'Blunkett: New Powers to Tackle Youth Crime', press release, 13 September.

Home Office (2002b) *Protecting the Public: Strengthening Protection against Sex Offenders and Reforming the Law on Sexual Offences*, Cm 5668, Norwich: Trading Standards Office.

Home Office (2002c) 'Secure Remands Extended Nationally', press release, 13 September.

Home Office (2003) *Youth Justice: The Next Steps Companion Document to Every Child Matters*, London: Home Office.

Home Office (2005a) *DNA Expansion Programme 2000–2005: Reporting Achievement*, London: Forensic and Pathology Unit, Home Office.

Home Office (2005b) *Drugs Act 2005*, www.drugs.gov.uk/drugs-laws/drug-act2005/.

Home Office (2007) *Planning Better Outcomes and Support for Unaccompanied Asylum Seeking Children*, Consultation Paper, London: Immigration and Nationality Directorate, Home Office.

Home Office (2008) *Drugs: Protecting Families and Communities – 2008–2018 Strategy*, www.drugs.homeoffice.gov.uk/publication-search/drug-strategy/drug-strategy-2008-2018?view=Binary.

Home Office/DH/DES/Welsh Office (1991) *Working Together under the Children Act 1989: A Guide to Arrangements for Inter-agency Cooperation for the Protection of Children from Abuse*, London: HMSO.

Home Office/Scottish Executive (2001) *Consultation Paper on the Review of Part I of the Sex Offenders Act 1997*, London: HMSO.

Home Office/Youth Justice Board (2002) *Final Warning Scheme: Guidance for the Police and Youth Offending Teams*, London: Home Office.

hooks, b. (1984) *Feminist Theory: From Margin to Center*, Boston: South End Press.

hooks, b. (1989) *Talking Back*, Boston: Sheba.

Horder, W. (2002) 'Care management', in M. Davies (ed.) *Companion to Social Work*, Oxford: Blackwell.

Horner, N. (2003) *What is Social Work?*, Exeter: Learning Matters.

Hough, G. (1999) 'Social work in the customer culture', in B. Pease and J. Fook (eds) *Transforming Social Work Practice*, London: Routledge.

Hough, G. and Briskman, L. (2003) 'Responding to the changing socio-political context of practice', in J. Allan, B. Pease and L. Briskman (eds) *Critical Social Work: An Introduction to Theories and Practices*, Sydney: Allen & Unwin.

Hough, M. (1996) *Drug Misuse and the Criminal Justice System: A Review of the Literature*, Drugs Prevention Initiative Paper No.15, London: Home Office Central Drugs Prevention Unit.

House of Commons (1993) *Juvenile Offenders*, Home Affairs Select Committee, Session 1992–3.

House of Commons (2005) *Anti Social Behaviour*, Home Affairs Select Committee, Fifth Report of Session 2004–5, vols 1–3, TSO: London.

House of Commons Health Committee (2008) *National Institute for Health and Clinical Excellence*: First Report of Session 2007–08', vol. 1, London: TSO.

Houston, S. and Griffiths, H. (2000) 'Reflection on risk on child protection: Is it time for a shift in paradigms?', *Child and Family Social Work*, **5**(1) 1–10.

Howe, D. (1987) *An Introduction to Social Work Theory*, Aldershot: Gower.

Howe, D. (1992) 'Child abuse and the bureaucratization of social work', *Sociological Review*, **40**(3): 491–508.

Howe, D. (1998) 'Adoption outcome research and practical judgement', *Adoption and Fostering*, **22**(2): 6–15.

Hudson, B. (2002) 'Interprofessionality in health and social care: the Achilles' heel of partnership', *Journal of Interprofessional Care*, **16**(1): 7–17.

Hudson, B. (2007) 'Pessimism and optimism in inter-professional working: the Sedgefield integrated team', *Journal of Interprofessional Care*, **21**(1): 3–15.

Hudson, B., Young, R., Hardy, B. and Glendinning, C. (2001) *National Evaluation of Notifications for Use of the Section 3 Partnership Flexibilities of the Health Act 1999*, Second Interim Report, Leeds/Manchester: Nuffield Institute of Health/Primary Care Research and Development Centre.

Hughes, K., Bellis, M.A. and Kilfoyle-Carrington, M. (2001) *Alcohol, Tobacco and Drugs in the North West of England: Identifying a Shared Agenda*, Liverpool: Liverpool John Moores University.

Hughes, L. and Pengelly, P. (1997) *Staff Supervision in a Turbulent Environment*, London: Jessica Kingsley.

Hugman, R. (1998) *Social Welfare and Social Value*, Basingstoke: Macmillan – now Palgrave Macmillan.

Humphreys, C. (2000) *Social Work, Domestic Violence and Child Protection: Challenging Practice*, Bristol: Policy Press.

Humphreys, C. and Stanley, N. (eds) (2006) *Domestic Violence and Child Protection: Directions for Good Practice*, London: Jessica Kingsley.

Humphreys, C. and Thiara, R. (2003) 'Domestic violence and mental health: "I call it symptoms of abuse"', *British Journal of Social Work*, **33**(2): 209–26.

Humphreys, C., Hester, M., Hague, G. et al. (2000) *From Good Intentions to Good Practice: Mapping Services Working with Families Where There is Domestic Violence*, Bristol: Policy Press.

Humphreys, L. (1975) *Tearoom Trade: Impersonal Sex in Public Places*, Chicago: Aldine.

Humphries, B. (1997) 'From critical thought to emancipatory action: contradictory research goals', *Sociological Research Online*, **2**(1), www.socresonline.org.uk/socresonline/2/1/3.html.

Humphries, B. (1999) 'Feminist evaluation', in I. Shaw and J. Lishman (eds) *Evaluation and Social Work Practice*, Buckingham: Open University Press.

Humphries, B. (2003) 'What else counts as evidence in evidence-based social work?', *Social Work Education*, **22**(1): 81–91.

Humphries, B. (2004a) 'The construction and reconstruction of social work', in D. Hayes and B. Humphries (eds) *Social Work, Immigration and Asylum*, London: Jessica Kingsley.

Humphries, B. (2004b) 'Taking sides: social work research as a moral and political activity', in R. Lovelock, K. Lyons and J. Powell (eds) *Reflecting on Social Work: Discipline and Profession*, Aldershot: Ashgate.

Humphries, B. (2008) *Social Work Research for Social Justice*, Basingstoke: Palgrave Macmillan.

Humphries, B. and Martin, M. (2000) 'Disrupting ethics in social research', in B. Humphries (ed.) *Research in Social Care and Social Welfare: Issues and Debates for Practice*, London: Jessica Kingsley.

Hunt, B. (2003) *The Timid Corporation: Why Business is Terrified of Taking Risk*, Chichester: John Wiley.

Hunt, G. (1995) *Whistleblowing in the Health Service: Accountability, Law and Professional Practice*, Florence, KY: Singular Publishing/Delmar/Cengage.

Hunt, G. (1998a) 'Whistle-blowing', *Encyclopaedia of Applied Ethics*, **4**: 525–35.

Hunt, G. (ed.) (1998b) *Whistle Blowing in the Social Services: Public Accountability and Professional Practice*, London: Arnold.

Hunter, N. and Polikoff, N. (1976) 'Custody rights of lesbian mothers: legal theory and litigation strategy', *Buffalo Law Review*, **25**: 691–733.

Hunter, S., Shannon, C., Knox, J. and Martin, J. (1998) *Lesbian, Gay, and Bisexual Youths and Adults: Knowledge for Human Services Practice*, Thousand Oak, CA: Sage.

Huntington, A. (1999) 'Child care social work and the role of state employees', *Child and Family Social Work*, **4**(3): 241–8.

Huntington, J. (1986) 'The proper contributions

of social workers in health practice', *Social Science and Medicine*, **22**(11): 1151–60.

Husband, C. (1995) 'The morally active practitioner and the ethics of anti-racist social work', in R. Hugman and D. Smith (eds) *Ethical Issues in Social Work*, London: Routledge.

IFSW (International Federation of Social Workers) (2000) *The Definition of Social Work*, Berne: IFSW, www.ifsw.org/.

Independent (2005) 'The dangers of criminalising children', editorial, 20 June.

Israel, M. and Hay, I. (2006) *Research Ethics for Social Scientists*, London: Sage.

Jackson, S. and Scott, S. (eds) (1996) *Feminism and Sexuality: A Reader*, Edinburgh: Edinburgh University Press.

James, N. (1993) 'Divisions of emotional labour: disclosure and cancer', in S. Fineman (ed.) *Emotions in Organizations*, Newbury Park, CA: Sage.

Jenkins, P. (1992) *Intimate Enemies: Moral Panics in Contemporary Great Britain*, New York: Aldine de Gruyter.

Jerrom, C. (2003) 'Anti-social behaviour: Blunkett's plans leave social workers in quandary over "enforcement" role', *Community Care*, 20–26 March: 18–19.

Jeyasingham, D. (2008) 'Knowledge/ignorance and the construction of sexuality in social work education', *Social Work Education*, **27**(2): 138–51.

Johns, C. (2000) *Becoming a Reflective Practitioner*, Oxford: Blackwell.

Johns, C. and Freshwater, D (2005) *Transforming Nursing through Reflective Practice*, 2nd edn, London: Blackwell.

Johnson, G., Scholes, K. and Whittington, R. (2005) *Exploring Corporate Strategy*, 7th edn, Harlow: Prentice Hall.

Johnson, P., Wistow, G., Schulz, R. and Hardy, B. (2003) 'Interagency and interprofessional collaboration in community care: the interdependence of structures and values', *Journal of Interprofessional Care*, **17**(1): 69–85.

Johnson, T. (1972) *Professions and Power*, Basingstoke: Macmillan – now Palgrave Macmillan.

Johnstone, G. (2002) *Restorative Justice: Ideas, Values, Debates*, Cullompton: Willan Publishing.

Jones, A. and May, J. (1992) *Working in Human Service Organisations*, Melbourne: Longman.

Jones, K., Cooper, B. and Ferguson, H. (eds) (2008) *Best Practice in Social Work: Critical Perspectives*, Basingstoke: Palgrave Macmillan.

Jones, K.B. (1993) *Compassionate Authority: Democracy and the Representation of Women*, London: Routledge.

Jones, L., Holmes, R. and Powell, J. (2005) *Early Childhood Studies: A Multiprofessional Perspective*, Maidenhead: Open University Press/ McGraw-Hill Education.

Jones, M. and Jordan, B. (1996) 'Knowledge and practice in social work', in M. Preston-Shoot (ed.) *Social Work Education in a Changing Policy Context*, London: Whiting & Birch.

Jordan, B. (1989) *Social Work in an Unjust Society*, London: Routledge.

Jordan, B. and Jordan, C. (2000) *Social Work and the Third Way: Tough Love as Social Policy*, London: Sage.

JUC SWEC (Joint University Council Social Work Education Committee) (2006) *A Social Work Research Strategy in Higher Education, 2006–20*, London: Social Care Workforce Research Unit, King's College.

Kadushin, A. (1976) *Supervision in Social Work*, New York: Columbia University Press.

Karstedt, S. and Farrall, S. (2007) *Law-abiding Majority? The Everyday Crime of the Middle Classes*, London: Centre for Crime and Justice Studies, King's College.

Keene, J. (1997) 'Drug misuse in prison: views from inside: a qualitative study of prison staff and inmates', *The Howard Journal*, **36**(1): 28–41.

Kelly, N. (2000) Decision Making in Child Protection Practice, unpublished PhD thesis, Huddersfield: University of Huddersfield.

Kemshall, H. (1997) *Reviewing Risk: A Review of Research on the Assessment and Management of Risk and Dangerousness: Implications for Policy and Practice in the Probation Service*, London: Home Office.

Kemshall, H. (2002a) *Risk, Social Policy and Welfare*, Buckingham: Open University Press.

Kemshall, H. (2002b) *Risk Assessment and Management of Serious Violent and Sexual Offenders: A Review of Current Issues*, Edinburgh: Scottish Executive Social Research.

Kemshall, H. and Maguire, M. (2001) 'Public protection, partnership and risk penalty', *Punishment and Society*, **3**(2): 237–64.

Kendall, G. and Wickham, G. (1999) *Using Foucault's Methods*, London: Sage.

Kirk, S.A. and Reid, W.J. (eds) (2002) *Science and Social Work: A Critical Appraisal*, New York: Columbia University Press.

Knapman, J. and Morrison, T. (1998) *Making the Most of Supervision in Health and Social Care*, Brighton: Pavilion.

Knight, J., Heaven, C. and Christie, I. (2002) *Inclusive Citizenship: The Leonard Cheshire Social Exclusion Report*, London: Leonard Cheshire.

Kohli, R. (2007) *Social Work with Unaccompanied Asylum Seeking Children*, Basingstoke: Palgrave Macmillan.

Langan, M. and Lee, P. (eds) (1989) *Radical Social Work Today*, London: Unwin Hyman.

Langley, J. (2001) 'Developing anti-oppressive empowering social work practice with older lesbian women and gay men', *British Journal of Social Work*, **31**: 917–32.

Larson, M.S. (1977) *The Rise of Professionalism: A Sociological Analysis*, Berkeley, CA: University of California Press.

Lart, R. (1997) *Crossing Boundaries: Accessing Community Mental Health Services for Prisoners on Release*, Bristol: Policy Press.

Lawson, H. (ed.) (1998) *Practice Teaching: Changing Social Work*, London: Jessica Kingsley.

Leadbeater, C. (2004) *Personalisation through Participation: A New Script for Public Services*, London: Demos.

Leathard, A. (2003) *Interprofessional Collaboration: From Policy to Practice in Health and Social Care*, Hove: Brunner-Routledge.

Lee Nelson, M. and Holloway, E. (1999) 'Supervision and gender issues', in M. Carroll and E. Holloway (eds) *Counselling Supervision in Context*, London: Sage.

Leece, J. (2000) 'It's a matter of choice: making direct payments work in Staffordshire', *Practice*, **12**(4): 37–48.

Leete, E. (1989) 'How I perceive and manage my illness', *Schizophrenia Bulletin*, **15**(2): 197–200.

Leff, J., Trieman, N. and Gooch, C. (1996) 'Teams Assessment of Psychiatric Services (TAPS) Project 33: prospective follow-up study of long-stay patients discharged from two psychiatric hospitals', *American Journal of Psychiatry*, **153**(10): 1318–24.

Leonard, P. (1997) *Postmodern Welfare: Reconstructing an Emancipatory Project*, London: Sage.

Lewis J. (2001) 'Older people and the health-social care boundary in the UK: half a century of hidden policy conflict', *Social Policy and Administration*, **35**(4): 343–59.

Lewis, J. and Glennerster, H. (1996) *Implementing the New Community Care*, Buckingham: Open University Press.

Lewis, L.A. (1984) 'The coming-out process for lesbians: integrating a stable identity', *Social Work*, **29**(5): 464–9.

Link, B.G. and Phelan, J.C. (2001) 'On the nature and consequences of stigma', *Annual Review of Sociology*, **27**: 363–85.

Link, B.G., Phelan, J.C., Bresnahan, M. et al. (1999) 'Public conceptions of mental illness: labels, causes, dangerousness and social distance', *American Journal of Public Health*, **89**: 1328–33.

Link, B.G., Struening, E.L., Rahav, M. et al. (1997) 'On stigma and its consequences: evidence from a longitudinal study of men with dual diagnoses of mental illness and substance abuse', *Journal of Health and Social Behavior*, **38**: 177–90.

Logan, J. (2001) 'Sexuality, child care and social work education', *Social Work Education*, **20**(5): 563–75.

Logan, J., Kershaw, S., Karban, K. et al. (1996) *Confronting Prejudice: Lesbian and Gay Issues in Social Work Education*, Aldershot: Arena.

Long, T. and Johnson, M. (2006) *Research Ethics in the Real World: Issues and Solutions for Health and Social Care Professionals*, Edinburgh: Churchill Livingstone.

Loosley, S., Drouillard, D., Ritchey, D. and Abercromby, D. (2006) *Groupwork with Children Exposed to Woman Abuse: A Concurrent Group for Children and their Mothers. Children's Program Manual*, London, Ontario: The Children's Aid Society of London and Middlesex.

Lorde, A. (1984) *Sister Outsider: Essays and Speeches*, Freedom, CA: Crossing Press.

Lorenz, W. (2004) 'Research and social work's ongoing search for identity', in R. Lovelock, K. Lyons and J. Powell (eds) *Reflecting on Social Work: Discipline and Profession*, Aldershot: Ashgate.

Loxley, A. (1997) *Collaboration in Health and Welfare*, London: Jessica Kingsley.

Lymbery, M. (2001) 'Social work at the crossroads', *British Journal of Social Work*, **31**(3): 369–84.

Lymbery, M. (2005) 'The partnership initiative in nursing and social services: practical collaboration in services for older people', *Research, Policy and Planning*, **23**(2): 87–97.

Lymbery, M. (2006) 'United we stand? Partnership working in health and social care and the role of social work in services for older people', *British Journal of Social Work*, 37(7): 1119–34.

Lymbery, M. (2007) 'Social work in its organisational context', in M. Lymbery and K. Postle (eds) *Social Work: A Companion for Learning*, London: Sage.

Lymbery, M. and Millward, A. (2000) 'The primary health care interface', in G. Bradley and J. Manthorpe (eds) *Working on the Fault Line: Social Work and Health Services*, Birmingham: Venture Press/Social Work Research Association.

Lyons, K. (1999) 'Social Work: What Kinds of Knowledge? The Place of Research in Social Work Education', paper for TSWR seminar, Belfast.

Lyons, K. (2004) 'Dame Eileen Younghusband', *Social Work and Society*, www.socwork.de.

McBeath, G. and Webb, S.A. (2002) 'Virtue, ethics and social work: being lucky, realistic, and not doing one's duty', *British Journal of Social Work*, **32**: 1015–36.

Macdonald, G. (1996) 'Ice therapy: why we need randomised controlled trials', in P. Alderson, S. Brill, I. Chalmers et al. (eds) *What Works? Effective Social Interventions in Child Welfare*, Barkingside: Barnardo's.

MacDonald, G. (1999) 'Social work and its evaluation: a methodological dilemma?' in F. Williams, J. Popay and A. Oakley (eds) *Welfare Research: A Critical Review*, London: UCL Press.

Macdonald, K.I. and Macdonald, G.M. (1999) 'Perceptions of risk', in P. Parsloe (ed.) *Risk Assessment in Social Care and Social Work*, London: Jessica Kingsley.

McGrail, S. (2003) 'It's raining plans', *Druglink*, **18**(4): 6–7.

McLaughlin, H. (2007) 'Ethical issues in the involvement of young service users in research', *Ethics and Social Welfare*, **1**(2): 176–93.

McMillan, S. (1989) 'Lesbians and gay men need services too', *Social Work Today*, 4 July: 31.

McSweeney, T., Stevens, A., Hunt, N. and Turnbull, P.J. (2006) 'Twisting arms or a helping hand? Assessing the impact of "coerced" and comparable "voluntary" drug treatment options', *British Journal of Criminology*, **46**(5): 1–21.

Mair, G. (2002) 'Arrest referral schemes: first port of call for drug users in the criminal justice system', *Criminal Justice Matters*, **47**: 16–17.

Malin, N., Manthorpe, J., Race, D. and Wilmot, S. (1999) *Community Care for Nurses and the Caring Professions*, Buckingham: Open University Press.

Mallon, G.P. (1999) *Let's Get This Straight: A Gay- and Lesbian-affirming Approach to Child Welfare*, New York: Columbia University Press.

Mallon, G.P. (ed.) (2008) *Social Work Practice with Lesbian, Gay, Bisexual, and Transgender People*, 2nd edn, Binghamton: Haworth Press.

Mallon, G.P. and Betts, B. (2005) *Recruiting, Assessing and Supporting Lesbian and Gay Carers and Adopters*, London: British Association for Adoption and Fostering.

Mama, A. (1996) *The Hidden Struggle: Statutory and Voluntary Sector Responses to Violence against Black Women in the Home*, London: Whiting & Birch.

Mandelstam, M. (2005) *Community Care Practice and the Law*, 3rd edn, London: Jessica Kingsley.

Manthorpe, J. (2003) 'Nearest and dearest? The neglect of lesbians in caring relationships', *British Journal of Social Work*, **33**: 753–68.

Manthorpe, J., Stevens, M., Rapaport, J. et al.

(2008) 'Safeguarding and system change: early perceptions of the implications for adult protection services of the English individual budget pilots: a qualitative study', *British Journal of Social Work*, Advance Access, doi:10.1093/bjsw/bcn028.

Marchant, R., Lefevre, M., Jones. M. and Luckock, B. (2007) 'Necessary Stuff': The Social Care Needs of Children with Complex Health Care Needs and their Families, London: SCIE.

Marfleet, P. (2006) *Refugees in a Global Era*, Basingstoke: Palgrave Macmillan.

Marks, L. (1991) *Home and Hospital Care: Redrawing the Boundaries*, London: King's Fund.

Marlow, C. (2001) *Research Methods for Generalist Social Work*, 3rd edn, Pacific Grove, CA: Brooks/Cole.

Martinson, R.L. (1974) 'What works? Questions and answers about prison reform', *The Public Interest*, **35**: 22–54.

Maslow, A.H. (1954) *Motivation and Personality*, New York: Harper.

Mason, J. (2006) 'The Climbié inquiry: context and critique', *Law and Society*, **33**(2): 221–43.

Masson, H. and Hackett, S. (2003) 'A decade on from the NCH report 1992: adolescent sexual aggression, policy and service delivery across the UK', *Journal of Sexual Aggression*, **9**(2): 1–22.

Mattinson, J. (1975) *The Reflection Process in Casework Supervision*, London: Institute of Marital Studies.

Mauthner, M., Birch, M., Jessop, J. and Miller, T. (eds) (2002) *Ethics in Qualitative Research*, London: Sage.

Mayer, J.E. and Timms, N. (1970) *The Client Speaks: Working Class Impressions of Casework*, London: Routledge & Kegan Paul.

Means R. and Smith R. (1998) *From Poor Law to Community Care*, 2nd edn, Bristol: Policy Press.

Measham, F. (2002) 'Doing gender – doing drugs: conceptualising the gendering of drugs cultures', *Contemporary Drug Problems*, **29**(2): 335–73.

Measham, F. (2004) 'The decline of ecstasy, the rise of "binge" drinking and the persistence of pleasure', *Probation Journal*, special edition: Rethinking drugs and crime, **51**(4): 309–26.

Measham, F., Parker, H. and Aldridge, J. (1998) *Starting, Switching, Slowing and Stopping: Report for the Drugs Prevention Initiative Integrated Programme*, Drugs Prevention Initiative Paper No. 21, London: Home Office.

Mezirow, J. (1991) *Transformative Dimensions of Adult Learning*, San Francisco: Jossey-Bass.

Middleton, J. (2007) *Beyond Authority: Leadership in a Changing World*, Basingstoke: Palgrave Macmillan.

Mies, M. (1993) 'Feminist research: science, violence and responsibility', in M. Mies and V. Shiva (eds) *Ecofeminism*, London: Zed Books.

Millie, A., Jacobsen, J., McDonald, E. and Hough, M. (2005) *Anti-social Behaviour Strategies: Finding a Balance*, Bristol: Policy Press.

Milligan, D. (1975) 'Homosexuality: sexual needs and social problems', in R. Bailey and M. Brake (eds) *Radical Social Work*, London: Edward Arnold.

Mills, S. (1997) *Discourse*, London: Routledge.

Milner, J. and O'Byrne. P. (2002) *Assessment in Social Work*, 2nd edn, Basingstoke: Palgrave – now Palgrave Macmillan.

Moffat, K. (1999) 'Surveillance in government of welfare recipients', in A.S. Chambon, A. Irving and L. Epstein (eds) *Reading Foucault for Social Work*, Chichester: Columbia University Press.

Molyneux, J. (2001) 'Interprofessional teamworking: What makes teams work well?', *Journal of Interprofessional Care*, **15**(1): 39–35.

Mooney, J. (2000) *Gender, Violence and the Social Order*, Basingstoke: Palgrave – now Palgrave Macmillan.

Moore, R., Gray, E., Roberts, C. et al. (2004) *ISSP: The Initial Report*, Oxford: Centre for Criminological Research, University of Oxford.

Moran, P., Jacobs, C., Bunn, A. and Bifulco, A. (2006) 'Multi-agency working: implications for an early intervention social work team', *Child and Family Social Work*, **11**: 1–9.

Morgan, G. (1986) *Images of Organization*, London: Sage.

Morley, R. and Mullender, A. (1994) *Preventing Domestic Violence to Women*, Police Research Group, Crime Prevention Unit Series, Paper 48, London: Home Office.

Morrow, D.F. and Messinger, L. (eds) (2006) *Sexual Orientation and Gender Expression in Social Work Practice: Working with Gay, Lesbian, Bisexual, and Transgender People*, New York: Columbia University Press.

Mullender, A. (2004) *Tackling Domestic Violence: Providing Support for Children Who Have Witnessed Domestic Violence*, Home Office Development and Practice Report, London: Home Office.

Mullender, A. and Burton, S. (2000) 'Dealing with perpetrators', in J. Taylor-Browne (ed.) *Reducing Domestic Violence: What Works?*, London: Home Office.

Mullender, A. and Hague, G. (2000) 'Women survivors' views on domestic violence services', in J. Taylor-Browne (ed.) *Reducing Domestic Violence: What Works?*, London: Home Office.

Mullender, A. and Humphreys, C. (2000) *Children and Domestic Violence*, Totnes: Dartington Social Research Unit.

Mullender, A., Hague, G., Imam, U. et al. (2002) *Children's Perspectives on Domestic Violence*, London: Sage.

Munford, R., Sanders, J., Veitch, B. and Conder, J. (2008) 'Ethics and research: searching for ethical practice in research', *Ethics and Social Welfare*, **2**(1): 5–19.

Munro, E. (2002) *Effective Child Protection*, London: Sage.

Mwenda, L. (2005) *Drug Offenders in England and Wales 2004*, Home Office Statistical Bulletin 23/05, London: Home Office.

Myers, S. (2001) 'The registration of children and young people under the Sex Offenders Act 1997: Time for a change?', *Youth Justice*, **1**(2): 40–8.

Myers, S. (2008) 'Revisiting Lancaster: more things that every social work student should know', *Social Work Education*, **27**(2): 203–11.

Myers, S. and Milner, J. (2007) *Sexual Issues in Social Work*, Bristol: Policy Press.

Mynott, E. (2002) 'Nationalism, racism and immigration control: from anti-racism to anti-capitalism', in S. Cohen, B. Humphries and E. Mynott (eds) *From Immigration Controls to Welfare Controls*, London: Routledge.

NAO (National Audit Office) (2004) *The Drug Treatment and Testing Order: Early Lessons*, London: TSO.

NCH (National Children's Homes) (1992) *Report of the Committee of Inquiry into Children and Young People Who Sexually Abuse Other Children*, London: NCH.

Neill, S. (2008) *Disruptive Pupil Behaviour: Its Causes and Effects*, Interim Report, National Union of Teachers/University of Warwick.

Nellis, M. (1995) 'Probation values for the 1990s', *The Howard Journal*, **34**(99): 19–44.

Newburn, T. (1999) 'Drug prevention and youth justice', *British Journal of Criminology*, **39**(4): 609–24.

Newman, B.S. (1989) 'Including curriculum content on lesbian and gay issues', *Journal of Social Work Education*, **25**: 202–11.

Newman, J. (1996) *Shaping Organisational Cultures in Local Government*, London: Pitman/Institute of Local Government Studies.

Newman, T., Roberts, H., and Oakley, A. (1996) 'Weighing up the evidence', *Guardian*, 10 January.

Nixon, P. (2008) *Relatively Speaking: Themes and Patterns in Family and Friends. Case Research and Implications for Policy and Practice*, Dartington: RiP.

Northouse, P.G. (2007) *Leadership: Theory and Practice*, Thousand Oaks, CA: Sage.

Nosowska, G. (2004) 'A delay they can ill afford: delays in obtaining attendance allowance for older terminally ill cancer patients and the role of health and social care professionals in reducing them', *Health and Social Care in the Community*, **12**(4): 283–7.

NSPCC (National Society for the Prevention of Cruelty to Children) (1997) 'NSPCC Concerned re Inclusion of Juvenile Offenders on Sex Offenders Register', press release, 24 October.

NTA (National Treatment Agency) (2005) *Retaining Clients in Drug Treatment*, London: NTA.

O'Brien, C.-A. (1999) 'Contested territory: sexualities and social work', in A.S. Chambon, A. Irving and L. Epstein (eds) *Reading Foucault for Social Work*, New York: Columbia University Press.

O'Keefe, M., Hills, A., Doyle, M. et al. (2007) *UK Study of Abuse and Neglect of Older People Prevalence Survey Report*, London: NatCen.

O'Neill, O. (2002) *A Question of Trust: The BBC Reith Lectures 2002*, Cambridge: Cambridge University Press.

O'Sullivan, T. (1999) *Decision Making in Social Work*, Basingstoke: Macmillan – now Palgrave Macmillan.

O'Sullivan, T. (2005) 'Some theoretical propositions on the nature of practice wisdom', *Journal of Social Work*, **5**(2): 221–42.

Oliver, P. (2003) *The Student's Guide to Research Ethics*, Maidenhead: Open University Press/ McGraw-Hill Education.

Orme, J. (1995) *Workloads: Measurement and Management*, Aldershot: Avebury/CEDR, University of Southampton.

Orme, J. and Glastonbury, B. (1994) *Care Management: Tasks and Workloads*, Basingstoke: Macmillan – now Palgrave Macmillan.

Owen, H. (1997) 'One of the hardest jobs in the world: attempting to manage risk in children's homes', in H. Kemshall and J. Pritchard (eds) *Good Practice in Risk Assessment and Risk Management 2: Protection, Rights and Responsibilities*, London: Jessica Kingsley.

Palfrey, C. and Harding, N. (1997) *Social Construction of Dementia: Confused Professionals?*, London: Jessica Kingsley.

Parker, H. (2001) 'Unenforceable? How young Britons obtain their drugs', in H. Parker, J. Aldridge and R. Egginton (eds) *UK Drugs Unlimited: New Research and Policy Lessons on Illicit Drug Use*, Basingstoke: Palgrave – now Palgrave Macmillan.

Parker, H., Aldridge, J. and Measham, F. (1998) *Illegal Leisure: The Normalization of Adolescent Recreational Drug Use*, London: Routledge.

Parker, H., Williams, L. and Aldridge, J. (2002) 'The normalisation of "sensible" recreational drug use: further evidence from the north west England longitudinal study', *Sociology*, **36**(4): 941–64.

Parton, N. (1991) *Governing the Family: Child Care, Child Protection and the State*, Basingstoke: Macmillan – now Palgrave Macmillan.

Parton, N. (1998) 'Risk, advanced liberalism and child welfare: the need to rediscover ambiguity and uncertainty', *British Journal of Social Work*, **28**(1): 5–27.

Parton, N. (1999) 'Reconfiguring child welfare practices: risk, advanced liberalism and the government of freedom', in A.S. Chambon, A. Irving and L. Epstein (eds) *Reading Foucault for Social Work*, Chichester: Colombia University Press.

Parton, N. (2000) 'Some thoughts on the relationship between theory and practice in and for social work', *British Journal of Social Work*, **30**(4): 449–63.

Parton, N. (2001) 'Risk and professional judgement', in L.-A. Cull and J. Roche (eds) *The Law and Social Work*, Basingstoke: Palgrave – now Palgrave Macmillan.

Parton, N. and O'Byrne, P. (2000) *Constructive Social Work: Towards a New Practice*, Basingstoke: Palgrave – now Palgrave Macmillan.

Parton, N., Thorpe, D. and Wattam, C. (1997) *Child Protection: Risk and the Moral Order*, Basingstoke: Macmillan – now Palgrave Macmillan.

Patton, M.Q. (1980) *Qualitative Evaluation Research*, Newbury Park, CA: Sage.

Pawson, R. and Tilley, N. (1997) *Realistic Evaluation*, London: Sage.

Paylor, I. (2008a) 'Degrees of substance', *Druglink*, **22**(7): 28.

Paylor, I. (2008b) 'Social work and drug use', in K. Wilson, G. Ruch, M. Lymbery et al. (eds) *Social Work: An Introduction to Contemporary Practice*, Harlow: Pearson Longman.

Paylor, I. (2009) '"Be healthy": tackling children's drug and alcohol issues', in K. Broadhurst, C. Grover, J. Jamieson and C. Mason (eds) *Safeguarding Children: Critical Perspectives*, Oxford: Blackwell.

Paylor, I. and Orgel, M. (2004) 'Sleepwalking through an epidemic: why social work should wake up to the threat of hepatitis C', *British Journal of Social Work*, **34**(6): 897–906.

Payne, M. (1998) 'Social work theories and reflective practice', in R. Adams, L. Dominelli and M. Payne (eds) *Social Work: Themes, Issues and Critical Debates*, 2nd edn, Basingstoke: Macmillan – now Palgrave Macmillan.

Payne, M. (2000) *Teamwork in Multiprofessional Care*, London: Routledge.

Payne, M. (2005) *The Origins of Social Work: Conti-*

nuity and Change, Basingstoke: Palgrave Macmillan.

Payne, M. (2006) *What is Professional Social Work?*, 2nd edn, Bristol: Policy Press.

Payne, M. (2007) 'Partnership working: the interdisciplinary agenda', in M. Lymbery and K. Postle (eds) *Social Work: A Companion for Learning*, London: Sage.

Payne, M. (2008) Staff support', in M. Lloyd-Williams (ed.) *Psycho-social Issues in Palliative Care*, Oxford: Oxford University Press.

Payne, M. (2009) *Social Care Practice in Context*, Basingstoke: Palgrave Macmillan.

Pearson, G. (1999) 'Drugs at the end of the century', *British Journal of Criminology*, **39**(4): 477–87.

Pearson, G. and Hobbs, D. (2001) *Middle Market Drug Distribution*, Home Office Research Study No. 227, London: Home Office Research, Development and Statistics Directorate.

Peay, J. (1996) *Inquiries after Homicide*, London: Duckworth.

Pence, E. (1987) *In Our Best Interest: A Process for Personal and Social Change*, Duluth, MN: Minnesota Program Development.

Penn, D.L., Komman, S., Mansfield, M. and Link, B.G. (1999) 'Dispelling the stigma of schizophrenia, II: the impact of information on dangerousness', *Schizophrenia Bulletin*, **25**(3): 437–46.

Phillips, C., Palfrey, C. and Thomas, P. (1994) *Evaluating Health and Social Care*, Basingstoke: Macmillan – now Palgrave Macmillan.

Phillipson, J. and Riley, M. (1991) Women for a Change, unpublished MPhil, Cranfield Institute.

Philp, M. (1979) 'Notes on the form of knowledge in social work', *Sociological Review*, **27**(1): 83–111.

Pincus, A. and Minahan, A. (1973) *Social Work Practice: Model and Method*, Itasca, IL: F.E. Peacock.

Pitts, J. (2003) 'Changing youth justice', *Youth Justice*, **3**(1): 3–18.

Polanyi, M. (1983) *The Tacit Dimension*, Magnolia, MA: Peter Smith.

Police Foundation (1999) *Drugs and the Law: Report of the Independent Inquiry into the Misuse of Drugs Act 1971*, the Runciman Report, London: Police Foundation.

Preston-Shoot, M. (2007) *Effective Groupwork*, 2nd edn, Basingstoke: Palgrave Macmillan.

Prins, H. (1988) 'Dangerous client: further observations on the limitations of mayhem', *British Journal of Social Work*, **18**: 593–609.

Prins, H. (1999) *Will They Do It Again? Risk Assessment and Management in Criminal Justice and Psychiatry*, London: Routledge.

Pritchard, J. (2000) *The Needs of Older Women*, Bristol: Policy Press.

Prochaska, J. and DiClemente, C. (1994) 'Cycle of change', in J. Prochaska, C. Diclemente and J. Norcross (eds) *Changing For Good*, New York: Avon Books.

Pugh, S. (2005) 'Assessing the cultural needs of older lesbians and gay men: implications for practice', *Practice*, **17**(3): 207–18.

QAA (Quality Assurance Agency) (2000) *Benchmark for Social Policy and Administration and Social Work*, Gloucester: QAA.

Quinton, D., Rushton, A., Dance, C. and Mayes, D. (1998) *Joining New Families: A Study of Adoption and Fostering in Middle Childhood*, Chichester: Wiley.

RADAR (Royal Association for Disability and Rehabilitation) (2007) *Doing Work Differently*, London: RADAR.

Rai, D.K. and Thiara, R.K. (1997) *Re-defining Spaces: The Needs of Black Women and Children in Refuge Support Services and Black Workers in Women's Aid*, Bristol: WAFE.

Read, J. and Harre, N. (2001) 'The role of biological and genetic causal beliefs in the stigmatisation of "mental patients"', *Journal of Mental Health*, **10**(2): 223–35.

Read, J. and Law, A. (1999) 'The relationships of causal beliefs and contact with users of mental health services to attitudes to the "mentally ill"', *International Journal of Social Psychiatry*, **45**(3): 216–29.

Read, J., Haslam, N., Sayce, L. and Davies, E. (2006) 'Prejudice and schizophrenia: a review of the "mental illness is an illness like any other" approach', *Acta Psychiatrica Scandinavica*, **114**: 303–18.

Reason, P. and Bradbury, H. (eds) (2005) *Handbook of Action Research*, London: Sage.

Refugee Council (2002) *The Nationality, Immigration and Asylum Act 2002: Changes to the Asylum System in the UK*, briefing paper, London: Refugee Council.

Refugee Council (2005) *Asylum Seekers with Special Needs*, www.refugeecouncil.org.uk/publications/researchreports.

Reinharz, S. (1992) *Feminist Methods in Social Research*, Oxford: Oxford University Press.

Reissman, C. (2002) 'Narrative analysis', in M. Huberman, and M. Miles (eds) *Qualitative Researcher's Companion*, Thousand Oaks, CA: Sage.

Reissman, C. (ed.) (1994) *Qualitative Studies in Social Work Research*, Thousand Oaks, CA: Sage.

Reissman, C. and Quinney, L. (2005) 'Narrative in social work: a critical review', *Qualitative Social Work*, **4**(3): 391–412.

Repper, J., Sayce, L., Strong, S. et al. (1997) *Tall*

Stories from the Back Yard: A Survey of 'Nimby' Opposition to Community Mental Health Facilities Experienced by Key Service Providers in England and Wales, London: Mind.

Repper, J.M. and Perkins, R.E. (2003) *Social Inclusion, Recovery and Mental Health Practice*, London: Ballière Tindall.

Rhead, A. (1994) 'Age of innocence', *Community Care*, **1029**: 18.

Rich, A. (1980) 'Compulsory heterosexuality and lesbian existence', *Signs*, **5**: 631–60.

Richards, M. and Payne, C. (1990) *Staff Supervision in Child Protection Work*, London: NISW.

Richmond, M. (1917) *Social Diagnosis*, New York: Russell Sage Foundation.

Rinaldi, M. and Hill, R. (2000) *Insufficient Concern*, London: Merton Mind.

Rinaldi, M., Perkins, R., Hardisty, J. and Souza, T. (2006) 'Not just stacking shelves', *Life in the Day*, **10**(1): 8–14.

Roberts, H. (ed.) (1981) *Doing Feminist Research*, London: Routledge & Kegan Paul.

Roberts, H. (ed.) (1995) *Doing Feminist Research*, 2nd edn, London: Routledge & Kegan Paul.

Robinson, G. (2003) 'Technicality and indeterminacy in probation practice: a case study', *British Journal of Social Work*, **33**(5): 593–610.

Robson, C. (2000) *Small-scale Evaluation: Principles and Practice*, London: Sage.

Roe, S. and Man, L. (2006) *Drug Misuse Declared: Findings from the 2005/06 British Crime Survey, England and Wales*, Home Office Statistical Bulletin 15/06, London: Home Office.

Rolfe, G., Freshwater, D. and Jasper, M. (2001) *Critical Reflection for Nursing and the Helping Professions: A User's Guide*, Basingstoke: Palgrave – now Palgrave Macmillan.

Romaine, M./BAAF (British Association for Adoption and Fostering) (2003) *Assessing Lesbian and Gay Foster Carers and Adopters*, London: BAAF.

Rose, N. (1998) 'Governing risky individuals: the role of psychiatry in new regimes of control', *Psychiatry, Psychology and Law*, **5**(2): 177–95.

Rossiter, A. (1996) 'Finding meanings for social work in transitional times: reflections on change', in N. Gould and I. Taylor (eds) *Reflective Learning for Social Work*, Aldershot: Avebury.

Rumgay, J. (2000) *The Addicted Offender: Developments in British Policy and Practice*, Basingstoke: Palgrave – now Palgrave Macmillan.

Rumgay, J. (2003) 'Partnerships in the probation service', in W. Hong Chui and M. Nellis (eds) *Moving Probation Forward*, Harlow: Pearson Longman.

Rumgay, J. and Cowan, S. (1998) 'Pitfalls and prospects in partnership: probation programmes for substance misusing offenders', *The Howard Journal*, **37**(2): 124–36.

Rummery, K. (2003) 'Disability, citizenship and community care: a case for welfare rights', *Health and Social Care in the Community*, **11**(2): 186–7.

Rutter, M. (2007) 'Sure Start local programmes: an outsider's perspective', in J. Belsky, J. Barnes and E. Melhuish (eds) *The National Evaluation of Sure Start: Does Area-based Early Intervention Work?*, Bristol: Policy Press.

Ryan, T. (1999) *Able and Willing*, London: Values Into Action.

Safer Society (2007) 'A new direction', **2**: 5–8.

Sales, R. and Hek, R. (2004) 'Dilemmas of care and control: the work of an asylum team in a London borough', in D. Hayes and B. Humphries (eds) *Social Work, Immigration and Asylum*, London: Jessica Kingsley.

Samele, C., Seymour, L., Morris, B. et al. (2006) *A Formal Investigation into Health Inequalities Experienced by People with Learning Disabilities and/or Mental Health Problems*, Area Studies Report, London: DRC.

Sanders, J. and Munford, R. (2005) 'Activity and reflection: research and change with diverse groups of young people', *Qualitative Social Work*, **4**(2): 197–209.

Sarason, S.B. and Lorentz, E.M. (1998) *Crossing Boundaries: Collaboration, Coordination, and the Redefinition of Resources*, San Francisco: Jossey-Bass.

Sargent, K. (1999) 'Assessing risks for children', in P. Parsloe (ed.) *Risk Assessment in Social Care and Social Work*, London: Jessica Kingsley.

Sarup, M. (1993) *An Introductory Guide to Post-structuralism and Postmodernism*, London: Harvester Wheatsheaf.

Sayce, L. (1995) 'Response to violence: a framework for fair treatment', in J. Crighton (ed.) *Psychiatric Patient Violence*, London: Duckworth.

Sayce, L. (1999) 'Parenting as a civil right: supporting users who choose to have children', in A. Weir and A. Douglas (eds) *Child Protection and Mental Health: Conflict of Interest?*, Oxford: Butterworth Heinemann.

Sayce, L. (2000) *From Psychiatric Patient to Citizen: Overcoming Discrimination and Social Exclusion*, Basingstoke: Macmillan – now Palgrave Macmillan.

Sayce, L. (2003) 'Beyond good intentions: making anti-discrimination strategies work', *Disability and Society*, **18**(5): 625–42.

Sayce, L. (2004) 'Tackling social exclusion across Europe', in M. Knapp, D. McDaid, E. Mossialos and G. Thornicroft (eds) *Mental Health Policy and Practice Across Europe*, Buckingham: Open University Press.

Sayce, L. (2008) 'Equality and rights: overcoming social exclusion and discrimination', in T. Stickley and T. Bassett (eds) *Learning about Mental Health Practice*, Chichester: Wiley.

Sayce, L. and Boardman, A.P. (2003) 'The Disability Discrimination Act 1995: implications for psychiatrists', *Advances in Psychiatric Treatment*, **9**: 397–404.

Sayce, L. and Curran, C. (2007) 'Tackling social exclusion across Europe', in M. Knapp, D. McDaid, E. Mossialos and G. Thornicroft (eds) *Mental Health Policy and Practice Across Europe*, London: Open University Press.

Schoenberg, R., Goldberg, R.S. and Shore, D.A. (eds) (1984) *Homosexuality and Social Work*, New York: Haworth Press.

Schön, D.A. (1971) *Beyond the Stable State*, London: Temple Smith.

Schön, D.A. (1983) *The Reflective Practitioner: How Professionals Think in Action*, New York: Basic Books.

Schön, D.A. (1987) *Educating the Reflective Practitioner*, San Francisco: Jossey-Bass.

Schön, D.A. (1991) *The Reflective Practitioner: How Practitioners Think in Action*, 2nd edn, Aldershot: Avebury.

SCIE (Social Care Institute for Excellence) (2003) *Practice Guide 1: Managing Practice*, London: SCIE, www.scie.org.uk/publications/practiceguides/bpg1/files/pg01.pdf.

SCIE (Social Care Institute for Excellence) (2005) *What is the Impact of Environmental Housing Conditions on the Health and Well-being of Children?*, SCIE Research Briefing 19, London: SCIE.

SCIE (Social Care Institute for Excellence) (2008) *Poverty, Parenting and Social Exclusion*, London: SCIE, www.scie.org.uk/publications/elearning/poverty/index.asp.

Scott, D. (1990) 'Practice wisdom: the disregarded source of practice research', *Social Work*, **35**(6): 564–68.

Scottish Executive (2002) *It's Everyone's Job to Make Sure I'm Alright*, Report of the Child Protection Audit and Review, Edinburgh: Scottish Executive.

Scottish Executive (2004) *Protecting Children and Young People: Framework for Standards*, Edinburgh: Scottish Executive.

Scottish Executive (2006) *MAPPA Guidance*, Edinburgh, Scottish Executive.

Seddon, D. (2006) *Immigration, Nationality and Refugee Law Handbook*, London: Joint Council for the Welfare of Immigrants.

Sewpaul, V. and Raniga, T. (2005) 'Producing

results', in R. Adams, L. Dominelli and M. Payne (eds) *Social Work Futures*, Basingstoke: Palgrave Macmillan.

SFR (Statistical First Release) (2008) *Pupil Absence in Schools in England 2006–7, including Pupil Characteristics*, SFR 05/2008, London: DCSF.

Shaw, I. (1999) 'Seeing the trees for the wood: the politics of evaluating in practice', in B. Broad (ed.) *The Politics of Social Research and Evaluation*, Birmingham: Venture Press.

Shaw, I. and Norton, M. (2007) *The Kinds and Quality of Social Work Research in UK Universities*, London: SCIE.

Shaw, I., Arksey, H. and Mullender, A. (2006) 'Recognizing social work', *British Journal of Social Work*, **36**(2): 227–46.

Sheldon, B. (2000) *Evidence-based Practice*, Lyme Regis: Russell House.

Sheldon, B. (2001) 'The validity of evidenced-based practice in social work: a reply to Stephen Webb', *British Journal of Social Work*, **31**(5): 801–9.

Sheldon, B. and Chivers, R. (2000) *Evidence-based Social Care*, Lyme Regis: Russell House.

Shepherd, G., Boardman, A.P. and Slade, M. (2008) *Making Recovery a Reality*, London: Sainsbury Centre for Mental Health.

Sheppard, M. (1995a) *Care Management and the New Social Work: A Critical Analysis*, London: Whiting & Birch.

Sheppard, M. (1995b) 'Social work, social science and practice wisdom', *British Journal of Social Work*, **25**(3): 265–93.

Sherman, E. and Reid, W.J. (eds) (1994) *Qualitative Research in Social Work*, New York: Columbia University Press.

Shiner, M. (2003) 'Out of harm's way? Illicit drug use, medicalization and the law', *British Journal of Criminology*, **43**(4): 772–96.

Silver, E. and Miller, L.L. (2002) 'A cautionary note on the use of actuarial tools in social control', *Crime and Delinquency*, **48**(1): 138–61.

Simey, M. (2000) 'How and where I found independence', in M. Simmons (ed.) *Getting a Life: Older People Talking*, London: Peter Owen/Help the Aged.

Sinclair, R., Garnett, L. and Berridge, D. (1995) *Social Work and Assessment with Adolescents*, London: National Children's Bureau.

Skeates, J. and Jabri, D. (eds) (1988) *Fostering and Adoption by Lesbians and Gay Men*, London: London Strategic Policy Unit.

Smith, C. (2001) 'Trust and confidence: possibilities for social work in high modernity', *British Journal of Social Work*, **31**(3): 287–305.

Smith, D. and Vanstone, M. (2002) 'Probation and

social justice', *British Journal of Social Work,* **32**: 815–30.

Smith, G.W. (1990) 'Political activist as ethnographer', *Social Problems,* **37**(4): 629–48.

Smith, L. (1999) *Decolonising Methodologies: Research and Indigenous People,* London: Zed Books.

Smith, R. (2004) 'A matter of trust: service users and researchers', *Qualitative Social Work,* **3**(3): 335–46.

Social Services Inspectorate Wales (1999) *In Safer Hands,* Cardiff: National Assembly for Wales/ Social Services Inspectorate.

Sondhi, A., O'Shea, J. and Williams, T. (2002) *Arrest Referral: Emerging Findings from the National Monitoring and Evaluation Programme,* DPAS Briefing Paper 18, London: Home Office.

Soothill, K. (1997) 'Rapists under 14 in the news', *Howard Journal of Criminal Justice,* **36**(4): 367–77.

Soper, K. (1993) 'Postmodernism, subjectivity and the question of value', in J. Squires (ed.) *Principled Positions,* London: Lawrence & Wishart.

Souhami, A. (2007) *Transforming Youth Justice: Occupational Identity and Cultural Change,* Cullompton: Willan Publishing.

Speer, S.A. and Potter, J. (2000) 'The management of heterosexist talk: conversational resources and prejudiced claims', *Discourse & Society,* **11**(4): 543–72.

Spencer, L., Ritchie, J., Lewis, J. and Dillon., L. (2003) *Quality in Qualitative Evaluation: A Framework for Assessing Research Evidence,* London: Cabinet Office, www.gsr.gov.uk/ downloads/evaluating_policy/a_quality_ framework.pdf.

Spivey, C.A. (2006) 'Adoption by same-sex couples: the relationship between adoption worker and social work student sex-role beliefs and attitudes', *Journal of GLBT Family Studies,* **2**(2): 29–56.

Spratt, T. (2001) 'The influence of child protection orientation on child welfare practice', *British Journal of Social Work,* **31**: 933–54.

Stalker, K. (2003) 'Managing risk and uncertainty in social work', *Journal of Social Work,* **3**(2): 211–33.

Stanley, K. (2001) *Cold Comfort: Young Separated Refugees in England,* London: Save the Children.

Stanley, L. and Wise, S. (1997) *Breaking Out: Feminist Consciousness and Feminist Research,* 2nd edn, London: Routledge & Kegan Paul.

Stanley, N. (2007) 'Exploring the relationship between children's and adult services', *Child Abuse Review,* **16**: 279–82.

Stanley, N., Manthorpe, J. and Penhale, B. (eds) (1999) *Institutional Abuse: Perspectives Across the Life Course,* London: Routledge.

Steedman, P.H. (1995) 'On the relations between seeing, interpreting and knowing', in F. Steier (ed.) *Research and Reflexivity,* London: Sage.

Stein, M. (1997) *What Works in Leaving Care,* Barkingside: Barnardo's.

Sudermann, M., Marshall, L. and Loosley, S. (2000) 'Evaluation of the London (Ontario) community group treatment program for children who have witnessed woman abuse', *Journal of Aggression, Maltreatment and Trauma,* **3**: 127–46.

Swift, P. (2007) 'Champions that can leap hurdles', *Community Care,* 6 September.

SWSI/MWC (Social Work Services Inspectorate/ Mental Welfare Commission) (2004) *Investigations into Scottish Borders Council and NHS Borders Services for People with Learning Disabilities,* Edinburgh: Scottish Executive.

Taylor, A. and Kroll, B. (2004) 'Working with parental misuse: dilemmas for practice', *British Journal of Social Work,* **33**(4): 115–32.

Taylor, B.J. (2006) 'Risk management paradigms in health and social services for professional decision making on the long-term care of older people', *British Journal of Social Work,* **36**(8): 1411–29.

Taylor, C. and White, S. (2006) 'Knowledge and reasoning in social work: educating for humane judgement', *British Journal of Social Work,* **36**: 937–54.

Taylor, P. and Gunn, J. (1999) 'Homicides by people with mental illness: myth and reality', *British Journal of Psychiatry,* **174**: 9–14.

Terry, J. (1999) *An American Obsession: Science, Medicine, and Homosexuality,* Chicago: University of Chicago Press.

Thane, P. (1996) *Foundations of the Welfare State,* London: Longman.

Thomas, C. (1999) *Female Forms: Experiencing and Understanding Disability,* Buckingham: Open University Press.

Thomas, T. (2003) 'The sex offender register: the registration of young people', *Childright,* **194**: 10–11.

Thomas, T. (2007) 'A year of tackling anti social behaviour: some reflections on realities and rhetoric', *Youth and Policy,* **94**: 5–18.

Thompson, K. (1998) *Moral Panics,* London: Routledge.

Thompson, N. (1993) *Anti-discriminatory Practice,* Basingstoke: Macmillan – now Palgrave Macmillan.

Thompson, N. (2006) *Anti-discriminatory Practice,* 4th edn, Basingstoke: Palgrave Macmillan.

Thornicroft, G. (2006) *Shunned: Discrimination against People with Mental Illness,* Oxford: Oxford University Press.

Thyer, B. and Kazi, M. (eds) (2004) *International Perspectives on Evidence-based Practice in Social Work*, Birmingham: BASW.

Tievsky, D.L. (1988) 'Homosexual clients and homophobic social workers', *Journal of Independent Social Work*, **2**: 51–62.

Timmins, N. (1996) *The Five Giants: A Biography of the Welfare State*, London: Fontana.

Timmins, N. (2006) *Designing the 'New' NHS: Ideas to Make a Supplier Market in Health Care Work*, London: King's Fund.

Tonry, M. (2004) *Punishment and Politics: Evidence and Emulation in the Making of English Crime Control Policy*, Cullompton: Willan Publishing.

Topss England (Training Organisation for the Personal Social Services) (2002) *The National Occupational Standards for Social Work*, Leeds: Topss England.

Torkington, C., Lymbery, M., Millward, A. et al. (2004) 'The impact of shared practice learning on the quality of assessment carried out by social work and district nurse students', *Learning in Health and Social Care*, **3**(1): 26–36.

Townsend, M. (2006) 'Teens and guns: the shocking truth', *Observer*, 3 September.

Trevillion, S. (2000) 'Social work research: what kinds of knowledge/knowledges? An introduction to the papers', *British Journal of Social Work*, **30**(4): 429–32.

Trevillion, S. (2008) 'Research, theory and practice: eternal triangle or uneasy bedfellows?', *Social Work Education*, **27**(4): 440–50.

Trinder, L. (1996) 'Social work research: the state of the art (or science)', *Child and Family Social Work*, **1**(4): 233–42.

Trinder, L. (2000) 'Evidence-based practice in social work and probation,' in L. Trinder and S. Reynolds (eds) *Evidence-based Practice: A Critical Appraisal*, Oxford: Blackwell Science.

Trotter, C. (1999) *Working with Involuntary Clients*, London: Sage.

Trotter, J., Kershaw, S. and Knott, C. (2008) 'Editorial: updating all our outfits', *Social Work Education*, **27**(2): 117–21.

Truman, C. (1999) 'User involvement in large-scale research: bridging the gap between service users and service providers?', in B. Broad (ed.) *The Politics of Social Work Research and Evaluation*, Birmingham: Venture Press.

Tulloch, J. and Lupton, D. (2003) *Risk and Everyday Life*, London: Sage.

Tunstill, J., Aldegate, J. and Hughes, M. (2007) *Improving Children's Services Networks: Lessons from Family Centres*, London: Jessica Kingsley.

Turnbull, P.J., McSweeney, T., Webster, R. et al. (2000) *Drug Treatment and Testing Orders: Final Evaluation Report*, Home Office Research Study 212, London: Home Office.

Turner, W.B. (2000) *A Genealogy of Queer Theory*, Philadelphia: Temple University Press.

Tutty, L., Bidgood, B. and Rothery, M. (1993) 'Support groups for battered women: research on their efficacy', *Journal of Family Violence*, **8**: 325–43.

UN (United Nations) (1989) *UN Convention on the Rights of the Child*, Geneva: UN.

UN (United Nations) (2002) *Concluding Observations of the UN Committee on the Rights of the Child, United Kingdom*, Geneva: Office of the UN Commissioner for Human Rights.

Ungar, S. (2001) 'Moral panic versus the risk society: the implication of the changing sites of social anxiety', *British Journal of Sociology*, **52**(2): 271–91.

Usher, P. (1997) 'Challenging the power of rationality', in G. McKenzie, J. Powell and R. Usher (eds) *Understanding Social Research: Perspectives on Methodology and Practice*, Brighton: Falmer Press.

Usher, R. and Edwards, R. (1994) *Postmodernism and Education*, London: Routledge.

Vaid, U. (1995) *Virtual Equality: The Mainstreaming of Gay and Lesbian Liberation*, New York: Anchor Books.

Van Bilsen, H.P. (1986) 'Heroin addiction: morals revisited', *Journal of Substance Abuse*, **3**(4): 279–84.

Van Brussel, G.H. (1998) 'Service: the Amsterdam model', in R. Robertson (ed.) *Management of Drug Users in the Community*, London: Arnold.

Vickery, A. (1977) *Caseload Management: A Guide for Supervisors of Social Work Staff*, London: NISW.

Vincent, J. (1999) *Politics, Power and Old Age*, Buckingham: Open University Press.

Walby, S. and Allen, J. (2004) *Domestic Violence, Sexual Assault and Stalking: Findings from the British Crime Survey*, Home Office Research Study 276, London: Home Office Research, Development and Statistics Directorate.

Wald, M.S. and Woolverton, M. (1990) 'Risk assessment: the emperor's new clothes?', *Child Welfare*, **69**(6): 483–511.

Walden, J. and Mountfield, H. (1999) *Blackstone's Guide to the Human Rights Act*, London: Blackstone.

Wallace, E. and Rees, S. (1988) 'The priority of client evaluations', in J. Lishman (ed.) *Evaluation: Research Highlights in Social Work 8*, 2nd edn, London: Jessica Kingsley.

Wallace, S. (2000) 'Responding to the Human Rights Act', *Probation Journal*, **47**(1): 53–6.

Walsh, M. (2000) *Nursing Frontiers: Accountability and the Boundaries of Care*, Oxford: Butterworth Heinemann.

Walters, I., Nutley, S., Percy-Smith, J. et al. (2004) *Improving the Use of Research in Social Care Practice*, London: SCIE.

Ward, L. and Wintour, P. (2006) 'State supernannies to help struggling parents', *Guardian*, 22 November.

Warner, R. (1985) *Recovery from Schizophrenia: Psychiatry and Political Economy*, London: Routledge.

Washington, S. (2003) 'Ruddock's secret report', *Business Review Weekly*, 9–15 October: 18.

Webb, S. (2001) 'Some considerations on the validity of evidence-based practice in social work', *British Journal of Social Work*, 31(1): 57–79.

Webb, S. (2006) *Social Work in a Risk Society*, Basingstoke: Palgrave Macmillan.

Weeks, J. (1985) *Sexuality and its Discontents: Meanings, Myths and Modern Sexualities*, London: Routledge & Kegan Paul.

Weeks, J. (2003) *Sexuality*, 2nd edn, London: Routledge.

Weinberg, G. (1972) *Society and the Healthy Homosexual*, Garden City, NY: Doubleday Anchor.

Weinstein, J., Whittington, C. and Leiba, T. (2003) *Collaboration in Social Work Practice*, London: Jessica Kingsley.

Wenger, E. (1998) *Communities of Practice: Learning, Meaning and Identity*, Cambridge: Cambridge University Press.

White, S. (2001) 'Auto-ethnography as reflexive inquiry: the research act as self-surveillance', in I. Shaw and N. Gould (eds) *Qualitative Research in Social Work*, London: Sage.

White, V. (1995) 'Commonality and diversity in feminist social work', *British Journal of Social Work*, 25(2): 143–56.

Whitmore, E. (2001) '"People listened to what we had to say": reflections on an emancipatory qualitative evaluation', in I. Shaw and N. Gould (eds) *Qualitative Research in Social Work*, London: Sage.

Whittaker, D.S. and Archer L.L. (1990) 'Using practice research for change', *Social Work and Social Sciences Review*, 2(1): 29–37.

Whittington, R. (2001) *What is Strategy – and Does it Matter?*, 2nd edn, London: Thomson.

WHO (World Health Organization) (1973) *Continuing Education for Physicians*, Technical Report Series No. 534, Geneva: WHO.

WHO (World Health Organization) (1979) *Primary Health Care in Europe*, Euro Report No. 14, Geneva: WHO.

WHO (World Health Organization) (1988) *Learning Together to Work Together for Health: The Team Approach*, Steering Group on Multiprofessional Education, Geneva: WHO.

Whyte, G. (1998) 'Recasting Janis's groupthink model: the key role of collective efficacy in decision fiascoes', *Organisational Behaviour and Human Decision Processes*, 73(2/3): 185–209.

Wilding, P. (1982) *Professional Power and Social Welfare*, London: Routledge & Kegan Paul.

Wilson, A. and Beresford, P. (2000) 'Anti-oppressive practice: emancipation or appropriation', *British Journal of Social Work*, 30(5): 553–73.

Winter, R. and Munn-Giddings, C. (eds) (2001) *A Handbook for Action Research in Health and Social Care*, London: Routledge.

Wise, I. (2003) 'The Children Act and young prisoners', *Howard League Magazine*, 21(2): 15.

Wisniewski, J.J. and Toomey, B.G. (1987) 'Are social workers homophobic?', *Social Work*, 32(5): 454–5.

Wolfensberger, W. (1994) 'A personal interpretation of the mental retardation scene in the light of the "signs of the times"', *Mental Retardation*, 32(1): 19–33.

Woodman, N., Tully, C. and Barranti, C. (1995) 'Research in lesbian communities: ethical dilemmas', *Journal of Gay and Lesbian Studies*, 3(1): 57–66.

Worth, A. (2001) 'Assessment of the needs of older people by district nurses and social workers: a changing culture', *Journal of Interprofessional Care*, 15(3): 257–66.

Wright, D.J. and Easthorne, V. (2003) 'Supporting adults with disabilities', *Nursing Standard*, 18(11): 37–42.

Young, A. ([1972]1992) 'Out of the closets, into the streets', in K. Jay and A. Young (eds) *Out of the Closets: Voices of Gay Liberation*, London: Gay Men's Press.

Younghusband, E. (1959) *Social Workers in Local Authority Health and Social Services*, London: Ministry of Health.

Younghusband, E. (1960) *Training for Social Work in Hong Kong*, Hong Kong: Government Printer.

Zarb, G. (1992) 'On the road to Damascus: first steps towards changing the relations of disability research production', *Disability, Handicap and Society*, 7(2): 125–39.

Author index

Subject index

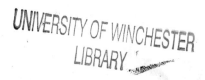